AF361399

Communication in Surgical Practice

Communication in Surgical Practice

Edited by
Sarah J. White and John A. Cartmill

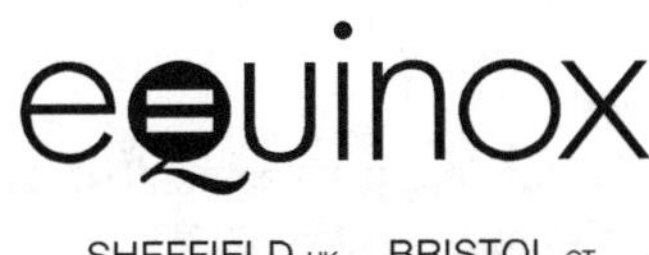

SHEFFIELD UK   BRISTOL CT

Published by Equinox Publishing Ltd.

UK: Office 415, The Workstation, 15 Paternoster Row, Sheffield, South Yorkshire S1 2BX
USA: ISD, 70 Enterprise Drive, Bristol, CT 06010

www.equinoxpub.com

First published 2016

British Library Cataloguing-in-Publication Data
A catalogue record for this book is available from the British Library.

ISBN-13 978 1 78179 050 2 (hardback)

Library of Congress Cataloging-in-Publication Data
Communication in surgical practice / edited by Sarah J. White and John A. Cartmill.
pages cm
  Includes bibliographical references and index.
  ISBN 978-1-78179-050-2 (hb)
1. Surgery. 2. Communication in medicine. I. White, Sarah J. II. Cartmill, John A.
  RD32.C688 2016
  617–dc23
                            2015031041

Typeset by S.J.I. Services, New Delhi
Printed and bound by Lightning Source Inc. (La Vergne, TN), Lightning Source UK Ltd. (Milton Keynes), Lightning Source AU Pty. (Scoresby, Victoria).

To our teachers:
Warwick, Ross, Judy and Alexandra (SW)
Amanda, Tim, Marilyn, Tom, Hannah and David (JC)

Contents

Section II: The Operating Theatre

Section III: The Aftermath

1 Exploring Communication in Surgical Practice

Sarah J. White and John A. Cartmill

Surgery is a remarkable human achievement; altruistic and uncompromising, it is a pragmatic, cooperative fusion of the best of humanity, culture and the sciences. Surgery owes much of its modern success to rigorous quantitative analysis and yet the humanity and communication that allow it to happen at all have largely been taken for granted; invisible, tacit or at least posing questions that are too difficult for those quantitative methods that surgeons prefer. So we are fortunate to have qualitative researchers take an expert, objective interest in what we do. Fortunate as surgeons because qualitative insights can allow us to do a better job (after all "quality" shares the same etymological root) and fortunate as a broader society because the extraordinary evolved behaviours and communicative phenomena of the operating room and surgery more generally might be made explicit and thus available to other fields.

This volume has been compiled for linguists and social scientists, surgeons and their patients, medical educators and policy-makers. The linguist can enjoy the secure footing of one of a number of trusted methodologies (conversation analysis, pragmatics, systemic functional linguistics) to explore the realm of surgery while the surgical reader will appreciate the insights of a multidimensional view of that which is so quotidian and familiar (the consultation, influence, consent, surgery itself, mishap) and yet made strange through the lens of qualitative research. The patient will find reassurance in the knowledge that we have the means of understanding how surgical care is achieved. Medical educators will appreciate the multiple approaches of this venture to make sense of the surgical world. Researchers will find areas of particular interest to pursue themselves and will no doubt find opportunities for original research in the less developed parts of this analysis.

Surgeons communicate profoundly with a variety of systems and people: patients, family, nurses and allied staff, each other. And for a variety of purposes – determining the problem, explaining the procedure and its alternatives and risks, facilitating decision-making, participating in and often leading a team, document-ing, handing over, managing mishap. Communication is co-constructed and surgi-cal communication constantly balances expertise and deep background knowledge with folklore and intuition, powerful primal emotion with nuanced mitigation and pragmatism. While systematic research has captured some of the dimensions of the surgical treatment journey, the complexity and layering of these most human of phenomena confound any single methodology.

The book is divided into three main sections: the consultation, the operating the-atre, and the aftermath, and applies a breadth of qualitative methodology to surgery. At heart, this is an analysis of the non-technical elements of surgical practice but it can also be considered a review or at least a sampler of qualitative research meth-ods. The purpose of this book is threefold – to improve our understanding of what occurs in communication in surgical practice, to provide an overview of current research, and to suggest future research and educational directions.

1.1   Approaches

The diversity of approaches reflects the complexity and importance of the topic. Analytic methods used in these chapters fall across a spectrum of methodologies including conversation analysis, discourse analysis, interaction analysis, systemic functional linguistics and pragmatics. Collectively these methodologies focus for the most part on authentic interactions captured as they happen with digital record-ings, which allows us access into the naturally-occurring interactional behaviours within surgical practice. It is not possible to record everything and the sensitive topic of disclosure, for example, is addressed through anecdote. Nor are the con-tributors all linguists. The chapter about communicating with tissue, while sur-gically authentic, is relatively naive linguistically and has been reframed for the linguist reader in the form of a dialogue. There may be frustrations for readers from a particular "school" at the perceived standards or annotation style or even subject matter of particular chapters and we hope that will serve as an incentive for their own research rather than an irritant.

1.2   Studies of Communication in Surgical Practice

1.2.1   The Consultation

While the more routine interaction (for patients) of visiting the general practitioner has been studied extensively, research into surgeon-patient communication is still poorly developed. The chapters in this section demonstrate that interactions between surgeons and patients differ from those in primary care and warrant independent study. These six chapters consider different aspects of the surgical consultation. The first (Chapter 2), by Sarah White, Maria Stubbe, Lindsay Macdonald, Anthony Dowell, Kevin Dew and Rod Gardner, highlights the unique interactional structure and epistemic environment of the referred (as opposed to the self-referred) consultation. This is followed by a chapter that considers consultation for non-native English speaking International Medical Graduates (IMGs) in Australia (Lynda Yates and Maria Dahm), examining how IMGs enact patient-centred care through their existing linguistic resources. Gavriel Ansara's review of psychological framing and influence by the surgeon effectively introduces the three following chapters on decision-making and treatment recommendation, including an examination of informed consent (Maria Dahm and Israel Berger) followed by a chapter from Maria Stubbe, Sarah White, Lindsay Macdonald, Anthony Dowell, Rod Gardner and Kevin Dew which addresses an implied default preference for surgery while Shannon Clark and Pamela Hudak consider treatment suggestions as part of a negotiation between surgeon and patient.

1.2.2   The Operating Theatre

The operating theatre is the inevitable focus of any thought or discussion about surgery. Highly developed, evolved, consequential and anticipatory, the theatre or operating room is literally a stage where people and technology, training and optimism converge. The operating theatre is such a multidimensional and layered complexity that no single methodology can do it justice. This section focuses inevitably on interaction: interaction between participants, interaction between layers of meaning and interaction between operators and tissue.

David Butt, Alison Moore and John Cartmill introduce the section with a perspective on the complexity of the operating theatre in the context of the health system as a whole. There follow three analyses of the interactions between members of the operating team, by Lorenza Mondada; Tehri Korkiakangas, Sharon-Marie Weldon, Jeff Bezemer and Roger Kneebone; and Alison Moore. Then Israel Berger and Sarah White present a chapter on the interaction between the operating team and the (awake) patient; and the section concludes with John Cartmill and David Butt's chapter seeking to describe the physical act of surgery as meaning-making and to discern the grammatical rules of surgery.

1.2.3   The Aftermath

Surgery does not occur in temporal isolation and nor does it always turn out as planned. Beyond the clinic and theatre, surgeons interact with patients, families and colleagues in order to continue patient care and to work within their broader professional practice in research and education. These areas of surgical practice have had the least analytic attention to date. Peter Roger, Maria Dahm, John Cartmill and Lynda Yates explore the inter-professional handover, and Stewart Dunn considers the challenges and rewards of the disclosure of mishap.

The collective knowledge represented in this book embodies a range of communicative activities that occur within and around surgical practice – from the consultation room, to the theatre, and beyond. This is put into context with a consideration of communication education and learning for surgeons and surgical trainees by Suzanne Kurtz in the final chapter.

Much of this book focuses on the everyday and the ordinary (at least from the surgical point of view) and there is much to learn from things going well. The individual projects presented here were realized after (appropriately) exhaustive ethics submissions, and that is how it should be. It is valuable to look closely at processes going well, but surgery does not always go well. Making sense of, explaining, and learning from unexpected, unfortunate and even catastrophic surgical outcomes remains an imperative. These events can be relatively infrequent, difficult to capture as they occur, and bewildering in retrospect. Surgery is a very human phenomenon and has been able to evolve and improve by reflecting on its performance. It is hoped that the methods and the level of analysis evident in this book might be brought to bear on such surgical mishaps "captured" for qualitative analysis.

This collection provides a view of many, but not all, of the communication activities within the practice of surgery. In each chapter the authors point to areas for further analytic inquiry and there are aspects of communication in surgical practice that this book does not touch on. In exploring consultations, for instance, we might analyse the different consultation types and their structures, such as post-operative visits, other types of follow-up, routine post-cancer check-ups – the list goes on. Additionally, we can compare the specialties and sub-specialties: does a consultation for breast surgery differ from neurosurgery, from orthopaedic surgery, from cosmetic surgery? We can ask other questions too: Does the structure of the clinic (with a nurse, with registrars, with students) change what is said and how it is said? How do different types of explanatory aids affect the progressivity of the consultation? Are there varied benefits in drawing pictures versus using models versus using digital presentations?

In the theatre, we might consider the critical interactions between surgeons and anaesthetists. When operating, we could take the analysis of teamwork further to look at the neuroscience of cooperation. Then after the operation we can again look at explanatory aids, and the operation record.

Further beyond the clinic and the theatre, we might consider other team environments, such as ward rounds, case conferences, journal clubs, research groups, or morbidity and mortality meetings, all of which can be recorded, observed and analysed. We can also continue to analyse how communication is taught and learned by surgeons and trainees within surgery. We might analyse supervision as well, since the apprenticeship model continues to be the primary approach to surgical training. All of these situations come with variables – native language, level of training, type of training, level of experience and specialty, to name a few. These variables create a wealth of research opportunity, of experiences that can benefit from in-depth analysis.

Surgery is a fine achievement but there is no reason to stop; it can be better. The focused attention of researchers and communication experts on a field so dependent on communication is an important step in the ongoing development and improvement of surgical practice and is welcomed by the surgical community.

Sarah J. White is a qualitative health researcher and linguist with a particular interest in using conversation analysis to understand communication in surgical practice. She is a Senior Lecturer at the Faculty of Medicine and Health Sciences at Macquarie University, Sydney. Sarah was awarded her PhD from the University of Otago, Wellington in 2011 and has professional and academic experience in clinical communication, quality and safety in healthcare, and medical education.

John A. Cartmill is a senior consultant surgeon at Nepean Public and Macquarie University Private Hospitals and a founding Professor in the Faculty of Medicine and Health Sciences at Macquarie University, Sydney. Professor Cartmill has played a leading role in developing the emerging area of postgraduate surgical education in Australia. A fortunate introduction to David Butt and Alison Moore has led to a fascination with the power of linguistics to unlock many of the (hitherto) intangibles of the specialty he enjoys so much.

SECTION I
THE CONSULTATION

2 The Referred Consultation

Sarah J. White, Maria Stubbe, Lindsay Macdonald,
Anthony C. Dowell, Kevin Dew and Rod Gardner

2.1 Introduction

Early research in doctor-patient communication describes a typical overall structure of the general practice consultation, with Byrne and Long who sought to "discover what patterns of behaviour doctors appeared to follow in their consulting rooms and the degree to which the patterns were repetitive among doctors" (1976: 20–1). Byrne and Long concluded that the logical sequence of activities they discovered demonstrated that it was possible to analyse doctor-patient consultations and "from that analysis derive information which should be beneficial to the process of doctor training" (1976: 190). Other descriptions of the overall structure of medical consultations have followed, including Cohen-Cole (1991), Helman (1981), Neighbour (1987), Pendleton and colleagues (1984), Stewart and colleagues (2003) and Stott and Davis (1979). Of particular note is the Calgary-Cambridge Model (Silverman, Kurtz and Draper 2013) that is now used around the world in medical education (cf. Chapter 16 in this volume). As the purpose of these models has generally been to inform communication education, they are generalizations of what occurs or what should occur in the consultation. Actual practice, however, differs from these models as the consultation is co-constructed turn-by-turn by the participants and is inevitably influenced by their individual goals, previous knowledge of each other, the presenting problem and other "contextual" factors. Robinson argues that in these models "no one has yet demonstrated the internal validity of the proposed project or its consequences for physicians' and patients' communication behaviour" (Robinson 2003: 32).

A recent systematic review (Levinson, Hudak and Tricco 2013) highlighted not only the paucity of research specific to surgeon-patient communication but also that while a range of areas of the surgical consultation have been explored, none has yet considered the overall structure and few have used an interaction-focused methodology such as conversation analysis. In this chapter we explore the differences between the primary care consultation and the referred surgical consultation. This follows from the hypothesis that visit types and settings other than acute general practice, which is the most described and analysed consultation type, are likely to have a different canonical structure and would likely be influenced by the goals of the visit. Through the analysis of differences and similarities in the overall structure of the surgeon-patient consultation as compared to primary care consultations, we propose that the interactional structure of referred surgeon-patient consultations is different from acute primary care interactions. We focus on the activities that are oriented to and performed by the participants at a local level, such as eliciting a problem and giving a diagnosis, as well as the overall structural organization of the consultation. We follow Robinson's (2003) "project" of activities and modify it to demonstrate the way in which the medical activities within the referred surgeon-patient consultation are structured in order to achieve certain goals.

2.2   Method and Data

Conversation analysis does not focus on the *why* of social action, but on the *what* and the *how* (Clayman and Gill 2004). It is directed at finding patterns in conversational structure and understanding and explaining their logic (ten Have 1999). Conversation analysis (CA) uses recorded, naturally occurring data that is transcribed in detail. The analysis begins with transcription, where repeated exposure to the data allows researchers to "notice" interesting features. This is followed by a more systematic analysis of the data, which is analysed with reference to the basic structures found in everyday, mundane conversation. It is increasingly being used to study medical interactions with the theory that: "It is by acting together that doctor and patient assemble each particular visit with its interactional textures, perceived features, and outcomes" (Heritage and Maynard 2006b: 19). Its inclusive, teamwork-based system of analysis is well-suited to the multidisciplinary field of clinical communication research and it has become an established methodology in the field (Heritage and Clayman 2010; Heritage and Maynard 2006a). Conversation analysis has been used to research clinical communication since the early 1980s (e.g., Peräkylä 1998) and has since developed into "an established presence in the field of medicine, where it is used to examine everything from genetic counselling to surgery" (Heritage and Clayman 2010: 1). Conversation analysis can be used to study doctor-patient interaction as the conversational tools and techniques used by participants are those that are used in everyday conversation, even though they may be restricted by the institutional normative orientations of the participants.

In this research we have used what is known about the generic orders of organization of conversation (Schegloff 2007) to analyse the turn-taking, sequence organization and turn design of 35 video-recorded consultations, all recorded in New

Zealand.[1] The data in this study come from two sources within the same larger corpus: the Interaction Study collected between 2003 and 2005, and the Surgeon Study collected in 2006 (White 2011). Ethics approval was granted by the Central Regional Ethics Committee in New Zealand.

Thirty-five video-recorded consultations between surgeons and patients were analysed using conversation analysis. Consultations were recorded over a number of clinics for both the Interaction Study and the Surgeon Study. Written consent was obtained from all participants (surgeons, trainee interns, nurses, patients, and family and/or friends of patients). Five surgical specialties were included in the research design: general (five surgeons), vascular (one), breast cancer (two), orthopaedic (one) and cardiothoracic (one). These specialties reflect the willingness of surgeons and their clinic staff to participate in the study. Ten surgeons participated, two of whom were female. Three surgeons (including a female surgeon) were registrars or trainee surgeons.[2] There were 35 patients in total, 15 male and 20 female. Twenty-one of these patients were seen in general surgery clinics, two in vascular, two in orthopaedic, three in cardiothoracic, and seven in the breast cancer clinic.

This chapter is drawn from the detailed analysis of each of the activities in these 35 consultations and is illustrated through the course of one consultation, so that the reader might see the progression of the consultation through the overall project of activities, how the institutional goals of the referred surgeon-patient consultation are achieved over the course of the whole interaction and how each activity creates a relevant local environment for the next activity.

2.3   Overall Project of Activities

The visits in this study were recorded in New Zealand, a country with a health system that requires referrals from other doctors, usually general practitioners, in order for patients to access secondary care services such as visiting a surgeon. Referrals

---

1   This research forms part of the work by the Applied Research on Communication in Health (ARCH) group based in the Department of Primary Health Care and General Practice at the University of Otago, Wellington. This multidisciplinary team and its research associates, who have varying backgrounds in primary health care, public health, sociolinguistics, psychology, sociology, ethnomethodology and conversation analysis, conduct research not only on surgeon-patient consultations, but on a variety of health professional communication events. The data collected by the team include ethnographic observations, demographic information, written materials and, most importantly, video recordings of actual communication events.

2   The term "surgeon" is used here to refer to both fully qualified surgeons and surgeons in training. In these consultations the surgeons in training were fulfilling the role of fully trained surgeons.

are formal letters either sent directly to the clinic or surgeon or given to the patient to give to the surgeon. The referral letters vary from minimal descriptions to long case histories and can include diagnostic test results. Despite these differences, they all provide the same function of allowing the patient access to the surgeon. This referral system, similar to that in Australia and the UK, is an important consideration when understanding these visits. As Robinson notes, "[i]f different types of medical business make relevant different interactional structures of social action, then it is imperative that researchers incorporate these distinctions into their analyses, theorizing, and recommendations for behavioural modification" (Robinson 2003: 52). As such, a distinction between visit types was made in the analysis, with only referred visits (also known as initial consultations) considered here.

For these visits, we found the following overall activity structure (Table 2.1). These activities display interdependence, with each activity dependent on the one that preceded it and creating a context for the next activity (White et al. 2013).

The analysis presented here provides an overview of how surgeons and patients orient to the normative structures of consultations in order to establish the patient's problem, reformulate that problem (based on information from the patient, the referral and the examination) and recommend next steps, such as treatment or further testing. While the analysis is based on 24 referred visits, one consultation is used to demonstrate the overall activity structure. This consultation was chosen as it provides a particularly clear example of the activities that occur in referred surgeon-patient consultations. It is a consultation between a general surgeon and a male patient in his early to mid twenties. Both are native English speakers. The patient has been referred to this surgeon from another surgeon who has already

Table 2.1: Activity structure of referred surgeon-patient consultations compared to acute primary care consultations

Referred surgeon-patient consultations (this chapter)		Acute primary care consultations (Robinson 2003)	
Activity 1:	Establishing mutual understanding of the referral and achieving alignment		
Activity 2:	Eliciting the patient's description (and perspective) of their problem	Activity 1:	Establishing a new medical problem as the reason for the encounter
Activity 3:	Gathering further information through verbal and/or physical examination	Activity 2:	Gathering additional information (history taking and/or physical examination)
Activity 4:	Reformulating the problem	Activity 3:	Diagnosis delivery
Activity 5:	Proposing next steps	Activity 4:	Treatment recommendation
Activity 6:	Closing the consultation		

diagnosed the problem (sigmoid volvulus) but is retiring, so is handing over his patients for operations.

2.4   Activities 1 and 2: Establishing mutual understanding of the referral and achieving alignment; Eliciting the patient's description (and perspective) of their problem

A referral letter is a type of clinical handover, involving the transfer of responsibility and accountability of patient care (Australian Commission on Safety and Quality in Health Care 2008). The referral recognition sequence (White et al. 2014), which reliably occurs at the start of referred visits, serves to *establish mutual understanding of the referral and achieve alignment*, not only between the surgeon and the patient, but also with the referring doctor. In this opening activity, the participants orient to the reason why the patient is there; that is, not their presenting problem, but that they were referred by another doctor to the surgeon. Mutual understanding at this level is essential for the progressivity of the consultation, as without it there would be no way forward as there would be no agreement as to the reason that the patient is there (that is, that they were referred). Alignment between the three parties regarding the reason for the visit is not as essential. Although the surgeon and patient must align before the consultation can proceed, a compromise can be made to achieve that alignment if the referral letter does not align with the patient's understanding of why they have been referred for the visit. A referral recognition sequence can be seen in Extract 1, which occurs at the very beginning of the consultation.

Extract 1: IS-SP03-02

```
1 SG:     (how's things.) >i got a letter from my colleague< mister samson.
2         (0.4) °and ah°
3 PT:     °ye[s,°
4 SG:        [(write to me) say you've been (0.8) having a bit of trouble
5         with: (0.7) volvulus. (0.5) or twisting of the bow:el.=
6 PT:     =yeah,=
7 SG:     =yep,=
8 PT:     =yeah.
9         (0.6)
10 SG:    if you c'd jus' tell me a little bit about >jus' tell me a little
11        bit about yourself.< (0.7) jason (to start). how old are you now?
12 PT:    i:'m twenty-six now.=
```

In Extract 1, the surgeon begins the consultation with a referral recognition sequence (lines 1–2, 4–5), after a greeting, to which the patient is not given an opportunity to respond. In this sequence, which is analysed further in Chapter 6 of this volume, the surgeon obtains agreement from the patient regarding the referral letter. As soon as the patient and surgeon agree on the nature of the presenting problem, mutual understanding is established. Because this mutual understanding is the same as that supposedly presented in the referral letter, as evidenced in the surgeon's turn (lines 1–2, 4–5), alignment between all three parties is also achieved. After the alignment is achieved, the surgeon then continues with asking the patient about his age and occupation, including some social conversation in that sequence (not shown).

Opening elicitors are those utterances delivered by surgeons in order to *elicit the patient's presenting problem*. As these typically occur near the beginning of the visit, patients orient to this sequential positioning and will respond to a variety of different opening elicitors (from *how are you* to *tell me about your knee*) as being in the service of eliciting their problem presentation. By attempting to elicit the patient's presenting problem, the surgeon is orienting to the relevance of the problem presentation not only in establishing the reason why the patient is at the clinic but also "in the service of at least the activity of diagnosis" (Robinson 2003: 38).

In this particular consultation, which is a first visit, the patient has already been diagnosed by another doctor (as evidenced in the referral recognition sequence). Thus, the goal of eliciting the patient's problem (Extract 2, lines 57–9) is likely to be in order to work towards confirming that diagnosis, while also building rapport and allowing the patient to tell their story and thus participate in this activity (which is a key point for patient agency in consultations [Heritage and Clayman 2010]). As it is this surgeon who will ultimately recommend treatment, ensuring that he agrees with the diagnosis that has already been made is an important consideration.

Extract 2: IS-SP03-02

```
57 SG:   okay, (.) .hhhhh (.) alright >so if you could jus' tell me a
58       little bit abou:t<(.) what's (.) what's it you've noticed with the
59       bow:els and so on.
60       (0.4)
61 PT:   si:nce (.) [i was (in ho-)]
62 SG:              [jus- th- the ] whole de- (kinda) the whole story even
63       going back to:=
64 PT:   =uh:m
65 SG:   childhood ado[lescence.
66 PT:                [>i know i know< it first happen:ed. (0.5) well
67       looking back i as- i assume this is what it was (0.2) when i was
68       in about standard four:?
69 SG:   °right°
```

In Extract 2, the patient does not present his problem right away, instead delaying his response which prompts the surgeon in line 62 to specify how much of the patient's problem should be presented. This relates to the interactional norm that requires speakers not to tell listeners that which they already know (Heritage 1984; Maynard 2003). That is, as the patient is cognizant that the surgeon has received a referral letter, he must therefore judge how much information he needs to give the surgeon. The surgeon then specifies his request (lines 62–3, 65), ask-ing the patient to retell his whole story, thereby addressing the patient's orien-tation to the interactional norm that would otherwise prevent him from doing so. After this clarification of the opening elicitor, the patient begins his problem presentation in Extract 3 (line 79).

Extract 3: IS-SP03-02

```
79 PT:   uh::m (.) yeah there w- it was sort of same thing i jus' (1.5)
80       pretty much my whole life i've remembered i've always had like i
81       aw-i always called the guts aches,
82       (0.2)
83 SG:   [yeah
84 PT:   [where i just=
85 SG:   [<right>
86 PT:   [=wouldn't be able to stand up straight an'=
87 SG:   =right
88       (0.4)
89 PT:   °an'° (.) but it it would never be too: bad.
90 SG:   [yeah
91 PT:   [i just sort ev have tuh
92       (1.2)
93 PT:   °um° (.) i w'dn't be able to do much for a whi:le but
94 SG:   y[eah
95 PT:    [it was never like intense pain or anything, it was ju[s'=
96 SG:                                                          [yeh
97 PT:   =really (0.2) uncomfortable.
98 SG:   yep
99       (0.5)
```

The patient begins by noting that he has experienced episodic symptoms his *whole life* (line 80). The patient then continues with a description of his symp-toms and historical experience of the illness, which continues in narrative form for another 63 lines. By presenting his problem, in the way requested by the surgeon, the patient and the surgeon are co-constructing the problem presentation. This demonstrates their orientation to the activity at hand, that is to *elicit the patient's description (and perspective) of their problem*, as well as to the overall project, as patients present their problems "*in the service of having them remedied*, and this remedy is implicated by their production" (Robinson 2003: 34, emphasis in original).

2.5   Activity 3: Gathering further information through verbal and/or physical examination

The transition from problem presentation to history taking is managed primarily through the doctor identifying the zone of transition in which he can ask the first history-taking question (Heritage and Clayman 2010). This zone is often identifi-able by the presentation of current symptoms, though the doctor may wait until the patient uses an exit device, stating in some way that they have finished their problem presentation (ibid.). In Extract 4, the surgeon begins history taking in line 163. Note that he does so, not after the presentation of a current symptom, but after the patient presents an occurrence of the problem, which is an episodic illness rather than an ongoing symptom, and then does not continue after line 161.

Extract 4: IS-SP03-02

```
147 PT: <an' the second ti:me was uh::m (0.7) °ah:: what was it° (0.8)
148     second start a- second university? >i [was um
149 SG:                                        [yes
150     (0.6)
151 PT: <twentyish?>=
152 SG: =right
153     (1.0)
154 PT: uh::m (1.3) tch (0.6) an' it was jus' one night i'd actually gone
155     to sleep an' then i woke up in the middle of the night (0.2) <an'
156     it was just unbelievable.>
157 SG: °yeh°
158 SG: [whe-
159 PT: [i was like=
160 PT: [rolling out of bed.]
161 SG: [(              ).] mm
162     (.)
163 SG: whereabouts do you feel the pain.
164     (0.5)
165 PT: ↑uh:m (0.8) aw jus' generally,=
166 SG: =jus' across the middle?
167 PT: yeh.
168 SG: yeh?
169 PT: basically=
170 SG: =[okay]
171 PT: =[i] (.) i c'dn't really (0.7) s- (0.2) c'ldn't say it with a
172     whole lot of [clarity=
173 SG:              [<right>
174 PT: =exact[ly where=
175 SG:       [e hhhhh
176 PT: =i felt it but at the=
177 SG: =[<right>]
178 PT: =[at the ] [time=
179 SG:           [.hhh
180 PT: =it w's?
181     (1.0)
182 SG: okay
183 PT: j'st (.) feels like a ma:ssive (0.9) i mean the THIRD one w's
184 SG: °yeah°
185     (0.5)
186 SG: yeah
187     (0.6)
188 SG: so (.) how many of these is that you've had [three?
189 PT:                                             [i'm pretty yeah=
190 SG: =[yeah
191 PT: =[that was the third one i had when i actually
192     (0.2)
193 PT: well the second one i did come to a an' e [and
194 SG:                                           [yeah
195     (.)
196 PT: on the way in on the drive in
197 SG: yep
```

```
198       (.)
199 PT:  it it [cleared itself¿
200 SG:        [(>it cleared itself so<)
```

Due to the episodic nature of the illness, the surgeon would be unable to rely on waiting for the patient to present a current symptom and instead must judge the zone of transition based on what could be considered the most recent episode. At first, it appears that the patient has indeed finished presenting his problem as he responds to the surgeon's questioning (starting at line 165). As he continues to answer the question at line 183, however, he cuts off the start of his utterance and returns to his problem presentation. The patient, nevertheless, does not describe the third episode until after the surgeon has confirmed the number of episodes, which allows the surgeon to best judge when to restart taking the patient's history. Here we can see how the surgeon and the patient "negotiate the boundaries of each of the main activity components" (Heritage and Maynard 2006b: 15), and by doing so demonstrate their orientation to the overall project.

History taking, or verbal examination, is characterized by question and answer sequences (cf. Heritage and Clayman 2010). This activity involves *gathering further information through verbal and/or physical examination*, which Robinson argues is oriented to by the participants "as being in the service of diagnosis" (Robinson 2003: 39). The activities of verbal and physical examination can be ordered either way and are more often than not intertwined. One or other can also be omitted, depending on the information needs of the surgeon. Through examination, the participants can be seen to be orienting to the necessity of further information for two distinct purposes: (1) to aid diagnosis, including the process of differential diagnosis; and (2) to assist the surgeon in assessing the patient's eligibility for treatment, particularly for surgery, as certain existing conditions may preclude the patient from being recommended for surgical treatment. Thus, examination is not only conducted in the service of diagnosis, but also in the service of treatment recommendation. In Extract 5, the surgeon recommences history taking in lines 201–2.

Extract 5: IS-SP03-02

```
201 SG:  .hhhhhh (0.6) what are yuh bowels like between attacks, are they
202      are they kind of
203       (.)
204 PT:  yeah: i wouldn't i wouldn't say they're classic.
205 SG:  n[o
206 PT:   [ah:: yih know like standard? (0.8) like >quite often< (0.2)
207      °uh° (0.5) sort of sittin' there for a while and not much is
208      goin' on but i jus' FELT like (um)
209       (0.6)
210 SG:  °right°
211       (0.9)
212 SG:  would you how often would you go to the toilet (during the day)
213      how many times a week (0.2) for example w'ld you
214       (1.1)
215 PT:  °(mm::)°
216       (2.7)
```

```
217 PT: °aw jeez i don't know?° (1.4) *uh::m* a- i- i- i try an' go once
218     a day but uh:m (2.4) yea:h it's NOT (1.0) yeah there's no real
219     (.) real pattern to it.=
220 SG: =right [okay¿
221 PT:        [°(>i'd say?<)°
222     (0.5)
223 SG: so yuh not a regular
224 PT: [nah: not=
225 SG: [a regu-
226 PT: =not really
```

The surgeon starts with a question (lines 201–2) that invites the patient to complete his sentence, ending his turn with the word *of*. The patient responds in line 204 with his assessment. The surgeon continues with this problem-specific history taking, asking about regularity (line 212) and then respecifying the question before the patient can respond (line 213), and summarizing the patient's response to confirm his understanding (line 223). This problem-specific question and answer sequence continues for another 16 lines (not all shown) before the surgeon and patient transition into comprehensive history taking, shown in Extract 6.

Extract 6: IS-SP03-02

```
242 SG: okay (.) .hhh anybody else in yuh family suffer from (.) similar
243     sort of problems?
244     (1.2)
245 PT: not that i've heard of,
246 SG: n[o
247 PT:  [uh::m
248     (1.1)
249 PT: °yeah°
250     (1.4)
251 SG: okay (.) .hhhh y- your general health otherwise.
252     (1.5)
253 SG: [>pretty good<?
254 PT: [y:eah:?
255     (0.2)
256 SG: [(pretty healthy)?
257 PT: [no complaints?
258     (.)
259 SG: [yeah?
260 PT: [yeah.
261 SG: yeh.
262     (1.2)
263 PT: i tend to always seem to be the last one to get get the flu. an'=
264 SG: =right
265 PT: an' NOT really as bad as (ev- any other) person.
266 SG: yep (.) okay?
267     (3.2)
268 SG: no serious illnesses or operations,
269 PT: °mm° ((shakes head))
270     (1.3)
271 SG: you on medications for anything?
272     (0.7)
273 PT: °nah°
274     (1.3)
275 SG: any allergies to medicines you've had previously¿
276     (0.5)
```

```
277 SG:  °no°
278       (2.6)
279 SG:  °kay°
280       (4.0)
281 SG:  okay huh:m?
282       (1.2)
```

In Extract 6, the surgeon begins the transition from problem-specific history taking to comprehensive history taking by using a bridging question in lines 242–3. This question can be categorized as both problem-specific, as it is in regard to the problem, and comprehensive, as it is not about the patient's own experience but rather his family history. In line 251, the surgeon continues with another comprehensive history-taking question, which is a non-specific enquiry after the patient's general health. The questions then become more specific as the surgeon not only establishes the status of the patient's health generally, but also gathers information that will allow him to assess the patient's suitability as a surgical candidate. The verbal examination then moves into the physical examination, as seen in Extract 7.

Extract 7: IS-SP03-02

```
321 SG:  =so yih know (0.6) a- th- at this stage we would t- if y'know
322       we're talking about surgery we would be talking about doing a
323       limited op operation to dea:l with the bit of bowel that's
324       causing the trouble,
325 PT:  yeah.=
326 SG:  =that's twisting it an' (i'll just strai-) take out that s- that
327       extra [length that's twisting?=
328 PT:        [>yeah sure<
          ((15 lines omitted))
344 SG:  =but at this stage (0.5) (y'know) in a young person like yourself
345       (w- would) i think one would deal with the (0.5) th- th- problems
346       that's really: °e- y- y-° [yih know=
347 PT:                            [*yeah*
348 SG:  =causing this twisting.
349       (0.2)
350 PT:  [(°mm°)
352       (0.8)
351 SG:  [an- then j'st (0.3) take it from there okay?
353 SG:  uh::m tch what i might do >is jus' pop you up on the couch jus'
354       have a little (look) at yuh tu:m:< ah: then we can jus' talk
355       throu:gh (1.0) y- the operation that's involved with taking out
356       this bit that's twisting.=and ah:
357 PT:  °mm°
358 SG:  how it's done, (0.9) <the um> the risks an' benefits and so
359       on.=okay?=so (1.8) we'll ask these folks here to (.) turn off
360       their recorder an' we'll .hh huh huhhuh .hh we'll examine you
361       okay?
362       (0.3)
363 SG:  alright?
364       (1.5)
365 SG:  now °mm ↑mm°
366       (0.7)
```

Here the surgeon indicates the probable treatment recommendation (lines 321–4, 326–7, 344–6, 348, 354–6, 358–9). Note that the surgeon has already been given a diagnosis by a more experienced surgical colleague through the referral. The surgeon begins by stating that surgery is only a possibility *at this stage*, using the word *if* in line 321. After positive uptake from the patient in lines 325 and 328, the surgeon then becomes more persuasive in his treatment talk, by arguing for surgery in lines 344–6 and 348, using the age of the patient to support his argument. All of this occurs prior to the physical examination, though after some diagnostic talk. The surgeon then requests the patient to move (lines 353–4). The examination begins around line 398 (Extract 8).

Extract 8: IS-SP03-02

```
398 SG: r:ight (jus' sit) (.) that's okay.
399     (0.7)
400 SG: jus' loosen you top (there)¿
401     (3.8)
402 SG: .hhh
403     (0.9)
404 SG: (°that's obviously t- (.) let's have a look.°)
405     (1.0)
406 SG: o:kay? just relax (    )?
407     (0.9)
408 SG: so have you had any other x rays of the bow:el apart from.
409     (0.9)
410 PT: the one when i w's
411 SG: you: had plain x rays, they put that tube up last time didn't
412     they,=
413 PT: =hyeah
414 SG: did that get rid of tha- did that relieve the pressure?
415 PT: oh h yeah [hhh
416 SG:          [yeah
417     (0.3)
418 PT: [instantaneously.
419 SG: [the whole (.) (the j'st all the gas 'n')
420     (.)
421 PT: [(oh my god it was)
422 SG: [( ) explosion.
423 PT: it [was fantastic apart from the whole uh:m=
424 SG:    [yeah
425 SG: =yeah the tube [thing
426 PT:               [(them having) to go up my=
427 PT: =[°bottom.°
428 SG: =[yeah ↓yeah yeah
429     (1.2)
430 SG: °okay°
431     (5.8)
432 SG: so when when you get these er g- y- d- did yuh stomach swell up?
433     is it really swollen?
434     (0.5)
435 PT: yeah (.) absolut- i mean normally i'm (sort of) quite fit and it
436     [sort of
437 SG: [well
438     (0.4)
439 SG: it j'st-
440     (0.3)
441 PT: yeah (.) just hh huh
442     (0.9)
443 PT: just a big mass.
444 SG: right,
```

```
445     (6.3)
446 SG: do you get rumblings with it or noises [or
447 PT:                                         [nah
448 SG: [yeah
449 PT: [ (mm)
450     (2.1)
451 SG: °mm°
452     (9.2)
```

In this consultation the video was switched off for the examination and the audio was captured on a separate audio recorder, thereby making it possible only to estimate the nonverbal actions of the participants. The surgeon gives the patient a number of instructions (lines 398, 400, 406) and then continues the verbal examination while conducting the physical examination, starting in line 408. This continues for another 44 lines.

Physical examinations can also include talk that is purely directive to aid the process of examination, as in Extract 9.

Extract 9: IS-SP03-02
```
455 SG: °↑jus- take a big breath for me?°
456     (1.1)
457 SG: °↓and right out.°
458     (0.7)
459 PT: hhh
460     (1.6)
461 SG: °↑and again?°
462     (0.5)
463 PT: .hhhh
464 SG: °an' right out.°
```

As can be seen here, the surgeon asks the patient to breathe in lines 455, 457, 461 and 464 (and this continues but is not shown). The relevant response is to perform the requested action, which the patient does (although we cannot see this, it is presumed as the consultation progresses smoothly and the action is sometimes audible, as in lines 459 and 463).

2.6   Activity 4: Reformulating the problem

As patients present their problems in the hope to have them remedied and doctors need to diagnose such problems in order to recommend a remedy, diagnosis not only builds on the problem presentation and examinations that have preceded it, but also projects a treatment recommendation (Robinson 2003). The activity of *reformulating the problem* is therefore key to the progressivity of the overall project of the consultation. It is important to note that in some surgeon-patient consultations, such as this one, a diagnosis may already exist prior to the visit. This may alter the sequential progression of the activities in the overall project as the diagnosis is not dependent on the previous activities. Thus, the processes of hearing the patient's story and gathering further information may also be in service of building rapport, confirming the diagnosis and developing treatment recommendations, as mentioned previously.

In this consultation, the surgeon reiterates the diagnosis (Extract 10, lines 283–4) that had previously been stated during the referral recognition sequence (see Extract 1).

Extract 10: IS-SP03-02

```
283 SG:  so (.) mister samson's explained to you you've got this (0.2)
284      you've got a very lo:ng bowel (and it) seems to [be twisting.
285 PT:                                                  [yeah:.
286      (0.5)
287 PT:  he said it was some (.) bottom (.) heh: (0.2) >he sort of kept
288      going like that,< there's like a bottom thing that
289      (0.8)
290 SG:  twis[ting
291 PT:      [*AH:: yeah? people giving me all sorts of hand signals.*
292 SG:  yeah hhheh °kay° it's basically like a .hhh the large bowel's
293      like a is a sort of like an inverted u shape tu:be. but (.) in
294      some people i- it it sort of looks (0.4) part of it's very
295      e:longated¿ (0.5) an' it's one quite a NARROW: (0.7) ( ) an' th-
296      an' that allows the whole thing to twist around=
297 PT:  =°yeah°=
298 SG:  =so it blocks off when it twists it, (0.4) the tube gets blocked
299      off at two points °(and they sort of gotten a)° closed system?
300      (0.9) ah:: an' that's obviously when yuh getting the pain an' so
301      on. (°kay°)
302      (.)
```

In this extract, which occurs prior to the examination, the surgeon uses the referring doctor (line 283) to support his diagnosis, which in turn will support and justify his treatment recommendation. The patient uses this opportunity to demonstrate his lack of understanding of the diagnosis (lines 287–8, 291). The surgeon responds to this by providing an explanation of the diagnosis that includes information about how the problem occurs (lines 292–320, not all shown). The surgeon has indicated what the likely treatment will be (see Extract 7).

Robinson notes (2003: 43), "[p]hysicians employ a variety of vocal practices that display their understandings that their treatment recommendation does not merely follow, but is an upshot or consequence of, their diagnoses. In these ways, physicians display that treatment recommendations relevantly and accountably follow diagnoses." Extract 11 occurs directly after the examination and prior to the treatment recommendation. This sequential position is important because this diagnosis, although it has already been stated previously, creates a local context for recommending treatment.

Extract 11: IS-SP03-02

```
529 SG:  now yuh x rays ar- i've got the report here (.) °which shows
530      (there was a obviously a sigmoid volvulus,°)
531      (1.4)
532 SG:  uh::m
```

```
533      (1.3)
534 SG:  okay
535      (2.3)
```

As with the reference to the referring doctor in Extract 10, the surgeon uses a report in lines 529–30 (from an investigation of the problem) along with medical terminology as evidence to strengthen his diagnosis and to support his treatment recommendation.

2.7   Activity 5: Proposing next steps

Another way surgeons orient to the overall project of the consultation is by initiating the activity of *proposing next steps* following the delivery of the diagnosis. The next relevant activity after diagnosis is treatment recommendation (Robinson 2003). In this way, both surgeons and patients orient to the overall project as moving towards remedying the presenting problem, which is done through an interrelated series of activities. In order to propose the next steps, even if these may involve further diagnostic testing or referring back to the doctor who referred the patient, the surgeon must first develop an understanding and formulate a diagnosis of the problem through the activities of *establishing mutual understanding of the referral and achieving alignment, eliciting the patient's description (and perspective) of their problem* and *gathering further information through verbal and/or physical examination*, and then must share that "diagnosis" with the patient through the activity of *reformulating the problem*. In Extract 12, the surgeon describes what is involved in the surgical treatment of this problem.

Extract 12: IS-SP03-02

```
550 SG:  .hhhh (0.4) a:lright okay (0.6) *so* (0.3) ((clears throat))
551      (0.3) so essentially what's involved (0.9) (°seems that°) if i
552      jus' sort ev (2.2) wh- with when you've got this condition with
553      this vo:lvulus th- the bowel's very (.) floppy and easily
554      accessible so we can do this through a fairly small ho:le. okay?
555 PT:  mm
556      (0.4)
557 SG:  right
558      (0.2)
559 SG:  we we could sort of do it pa:rtly through the keyhole technique
560      using a: (.) yih know jus- little (0.5) camera we put inside your
561      tu:m? (0.7) uh::m: (0.7) to be honest (0.3) ((coughs)) normally =
562      the bowel is so: floppy and so: mobile .hhh we can do it through
563      a tiny little hole anyway so (0.3) i think probably on balance we
564      can j'st we'll j'st do a little conventional (one) (0.6) jus' a
565      little cut down here on the left hand si:de.
566 PT:  mm
567      (0.3)
568 SG:  uh::m (1.7) i- it does remo:ve (0.2) so y- y- yih know we're
569      gonna take out (a a big) a lo:ng length of bowel that we're going
570      to take out an' then (0.5) straighten it out and then join the
571      two (0.4) en- ends together. (at [that)=
572 PT:                                  [yeah
```

As has been mentioned previously, this is not the first occasion where the surgeon has identified surgery as the possible treatment in the consultation (see Extract 7). On these previous occasions, the patient has not resisted the treatment recommendation, and thus the surgeon is at liberty to progress in the consultation by describing the treatment rather than needing to pursue agreement from the patient. Throughout the description the patient offers minimal feedback in lines 555 and 566 and at the end of the description provides the affirmative response of *yeah* (line 572).

One discussion that can occur during the treatment recommendation activity is that of informing the patient of the risks associated with the treatment. Extract 13 follows directly from 12, with the surgeon moving from describing the treatment, which had received positive uptake from the patient, to describing the risks associated with surgery.

Extract 13: IS-SP03-02

```
573 SG: =right so .hh it's it's a fAIrly straightforward operation?
574     (0.5) l:ike (0.4) like every operation ↓there are (sort of)
575     risks, (0.3) er which one has to take in= so the expected
576     outcome is that you be in hospital for ab- maybe abou- ter (0.5)
577     >i w'd think about< (0.3) four or five Day:s.
578     (0.3)
579 PT: yep=
580 SG: =ah: you be k- (0.2) you c'd go ho:me basically on a normal diet
581     with yih bowels working, (.) °okay° (0.4) °*alright,*° (0.7)
582     with- (.) with any:: (.) bowel surgery when we're sort of joi:n
583     two ends of the bowel together there's th- (0.3) (th-) the most
584     important thing risk of things that (uh) (.) could (.)
585     potentially go wrong is >that the< two ends don't heal, (0.3)
586     °kay° (0.3) °alright° (0.5) now that would happen in may:be:
587     (0.5) something in the order of one percent of people? (0.3)
588     >undergoing this surg-=(a) one in a hun[dred,<
589 PT:                                        [yeah,
590     (0.6)
591 SG: the bow:el WOULDn't hea:l (0.4) absolutely perfecly, an you get
592     what's called a leak, so there'd be some bowel contents w'd come
593     outsi:de, (0.6) er that's obviously a serious complication:. (.)
```

This shift, marked by the shift implicative *right* at line 573, begins with a noting of the occurrence of risks in line 574–5 followed by a contrasting statement regarding the normal, expected outcomes of the surgery. The surgeon then returns to the description of risks, starting at line 582. As this activity is primarily about informing the patient, there is minimal talk from the patient, although he does mark his attentiveness through the use of minimal feedback in lines 579 and 589. This risks informing activity continues for another 33 lines (not shown).

Patients also ask questions during the activity of treatment recommendation, as in Extract 14.

Extract 14: IS-SP03-02

```
628 PT:  someone told me like uh:: (0.3) >doctor samson told me< it was
629      like a MONTH OFF: is that?
630      (0.5)
631 SG:  yeh in terms of (0.4) ah recovry: uh:m (1.0) is very variable
632      from patient to patient? okay¿ so. (0.4) °it's ay° everybody
633      ah:f' an anaesthetic has what we call post operative fati:gue
634      syndrome where you feel j'st ti:red y'know it's not just (0.5)
635      not jus' the wound healing jus' generally in yourself, th' energy
636      levels (of) (.) are dow:n and they do: take a while tuh (0.3)
637      ↑tuh- (0.2) to pull back up¿
```

In Extract 14, the patient asks for information about how recovery from the surgery will affect his work life (lines 628–9). The surgeon then informs the patient of what is expected to occur after surgery (starting in line 631).

After describing the recommended treatment, the associated risks and answering the patient's question, all of which receive agreeing responses from the patient, the surgeon moves to close the activity of treatment recommendation by offering to organize the recommended treatment of surgery (Extract 15, lines 654–5).

Extract 15: IS-SP03-02

```
654 SG:  uh::m (.) so what i might do then is (.) is (0.4) or:ganise to:
655      (.) to do that. (.) uh::m,
656      (0.5)
657 PT:  it was actual- i've (.) i've got i'm working up until the: (.) i
658      think it's the fourth of july?
659      (0.4)
660 SG:  ri:ght.
661 PT:  (°*was on ↑the[re*°)
662 SG:              [fourth of july okay, (0.5) cos tyler said ju:ne
663      so¿
664 PT:  yeah
665      (0.2)
666 SG:  (>so we do it<) so ↑a:fter the fourth of july:.
         ((39 lines omitted))
705 SG:  so n- not before the fourth of july. okay? (0.4) >i mean< (1.0)
706      in terms ev (0.6) y'know i think if we uh still work fur *>mm
707      mm<* >sort ev< (0.5) >middle or end uh july:¿< (0.5) >would that
708      sound reas'nable?<
709      (0.3)
710 PT:  yeah
711 SG:  yep
712      (0.4)
713 SG:  okay.
714      (0.4)
```

This triggers a negotiation sequence between the surgeon and the patient, not as to the treatment type, but as to when it might occur because the patient hopes to fit in the surgery around his work schedule (lines 657–8). The participants reach an agreement and the sequence concludes at line 713. The surgeon returns again to the bureaucratic aspects of organizing surgery in lines 715–18 in Extract 16.

Extract 16: IS-SP03-02

```
715 SG: .hhh (0.5) *uh:m* (0.5) tch (0.7) °right° so a:ll i need to do
716     then j'st get the paperwork or:ganised and uh (0.9) we'll (.)
717     we'll try an' work tuh- towards those >sort ev< dates¿=i think
718     that's a reas- a sort of thing that needs to be done.
719         (0.9)
720 SG: yih know because it's it's GONNA happen again.
721         (0.4)
722 PT: [yeah: (>yeah that's right¿<)]
723 SG: [and   ah:   there's   NO  th]ere's no way or predicting when or where
724     or.=
725 PT: =yeah
726         (0.7)
727 SG: °yeah so it's it p- it (>certainly needs sorting.<) okay,°
728         (1.1)
```

2.8   Activity 6: Closing the consultation

Closing the consultation is an important activity as it demonstrates the participants'
orientation to the completion of the overall project (White 2012, 2015). In finishing
the activity of treatment recommendation, the relevant next activity is the closing,
as the presenting problem has in some way been remedied. In this consultation the
treatment recommendation phase has been completed with the necessary agreement
from the patient and so the surgeon moves to close the encounter. This final activity
is initiated in Extract 17, where in lines 729–30 the surgeon offers the patient the
opportunity to ask further questions regarding the agreed treatment (although it is
noteworthy that he does so using the negative polarity item *any*, which interactionally inhibits the patient from responding with a *yes* answer [Heritage et al. 2007]).
The patient delays his response, hesitates, pauses and then states that he does not
have any questions (line 732). Instead of closing the encounter, however, the surgeon restates the risks and then describes pain management directly following the
procedure.

Extract 17: IS-SP03-02

```
729 SG: >have you got any:< questions or concerns about (0.7) y' know
730     what we're proposing to do: or
731         (1.3)
732 PT: *uh::m* (2.8) not especially,=
733 SG: =yeh- you probably won't know until a:fter the operation [(what)=
734 PT:                                                           [yeah:
735 SG: =(want to ask)=
736 SG: =[b't
737 PT: =[oh yeah:
738 SG: imn uh- th- the in the most important thing is just th- the
739     sma:ll risk which (.) o- o- of an asmodic leak, (0.6) *ah::* the
740     OTHer complications w'd pre- be pretty uncommon,
741 PT: °yep°=
742 SG: =apart from wound infection=
743 PT: NN NN five days it's jus sort ev getting:
744         (0.3)
```

```
745 SG: yeah so a:fter what you'd ha:ve during y- ih- .hh (0.3)
746     >↑probably with an operation like that we just put some local
747     anaesthetic< (0.3) ( ) local anaesthetic round the wou:nd,
748 PT: uh okay,
749 SG: an' then give you little ↑pain pump like a mor:phine pump you c'd
750     you use yourself? you wouldn't need an epidural or anything like
751     that,
752 PT: °awh (sweet)°
```

The activity of closing is again made relevant in Extract 18, line 774, as the surgeon returns to the necessity of paperwork.

Extract 18: IS-SP03-02
```
774 SG: aw:lright so if that's: okay we'll (.) we'll get the paperwork
775     organised,
776     (0.3)
777 SG: o[kay?
778 PT:  [excellent.=
779 SG: =alrigh?
780     (0.4)
781 PT: and it'll jus be s- a letter get sent out to me.=
782 SG: =YEAH you'll you'll come in for what's called >pre assessment
783     anaesthetists jus'< like to have a look at you go over your
784     hear:t an' lu:ngs an' (0.3) just explain pain control an what
785     they're gunna do:. (0.6) ah: any blood tests they wanna do an'
786     then: uh:m (0.5) that happens about two weeks before the
787     operation¿ (0.3) er:: (1.0) yep?
788     (1.2)
789 PT: °excellent.°
790 SG: o:kay:?
791     (0.3)
792 PT: [>(yeah no problem at all?)<
793 SG: [alright? in terms ev uh:m:. (1.8) yep no that should be fi:ne
794     okay? (0.3) °very good?° okay? just hang on there we'll get the
795     paperwork all organised. alright-?
```

In this turn the surgeon also seeks further confirmation from the patient as to his agreement with the treatment recommendation, by stating that *if that's okay* then the bureaucratic procedures to book the surgery will be organized (line 774). This, however, is not responded to by the patient and the surgeon pursues agreement in line 777 using an upward intoned (or try-marked) *okay*. The patient then agrees using a very positive assessment, *excellent*. The closure of the consultation is then delayed again as the patient requests more information regarding the booking of the surgery (line 781). The surgeon not only answers the patient's enquiry but also explains other pre-operative procedures that will occur. Agreement is pursued (line 787) and received (line 789) and then repursued (line 790) and then re-received (line 792). Finally, the consultation closes as the surgeon asks the patient to wait as the paperwork is organized and then leaves the room.

2.9   Concluding Remarks

Through this analysis, we show that surgeon-patient consultations follow a similar overall structural organization to those described by Robinson (2003) and by others (Byrne and Long 1976; Cohen-Cole 1991; Helman 1981; Neighbour 1987; Pendleton et al. 1984; Silverman, Kurtz and Draper 2013; Stewart et al. 2003; Heron 1975). This is likely due to the logical progression of activities in problem solving (White et al. 2013). While there is similarity, there are also differences, particularly the key difference in Activity 1, which, by allowing for the establishment of a mutual understanding between the surgeon, the patient and the referring doctor of at least the existence of a referral and usually the reason for the visit, sets up not only a local context but also a course of action for the rest of the consultation (White et al. 2014).

Agency in each of the activities varies due to the interactional constraints directed by institutional identities and goals (Robinson 2003). Participants are oriented to the institutional goals that affect the relative passivity or interactional activity of the patient. Within this project of activities, there are points where the patient can more easily display greater agency, predictable by the purpose of the activity (ibid.). In the activity of history taking, for example, the surgeon is directing the course of action through a series of questions and answers, restricting the type of response the patient can give. However, as was seen in the consultation analysed above, the patient was able to answer outside of the constraints of the question in order to continue his problem presentation.

In the activity of diagnosis, the surgeon informs the patient of their problem and such descriptions do not necessarily require responses. In other activities, there is more scope for patient involvement. Due to the overall structure of the activities described, surgeons routinely allow patients points of interactional agency in the two activities that are most important for patient participation – defining the problem (through the referral recognition sequence and problem presentation) and deciding on treatment. These points of interactional agency are achieved through the requirement of the achievement of alignment in the referral recognition sequence, eliciting the patient's problem presentation and requiring the patient's agreement to the treatment recommendation.

The six activities of referred visits are interdependent and form an overall project designed to achieve the institutional goals of remedying the patient's presenting problem. As can be seen from the consultation analysed above, the various contingencies of the consultation (e.g., the referral may include symptoms, a tentative diagnosis or a confirmed diagnosis) can affect the ordering of these activities. However, as each activity is dependent on the occurrence of the activities that preceded it, the overall sequential organization of the project generally remains the same.

By demonstrating the distinctive features of referred surgeon-patient consultations, this research not only adds to the body of knowledge about clinical communication generally, but provides a basis on which later research that specifically focuses on surgical and other referred consultations can build. To further our understanding of surgeon-patient consultations, future research can refine the scope by focusing on particular specialties or on the level of training and experience when investigating the overall structure of the consultation. Future research might also investigate each of the activities within the consultation in greater depth and with a narrower scope than has been done previously (White 2011). Additionally, understanding the interactional structure that patients and surgeons routinely co-construct in clinic consultations supports the development of surgeon-specific education and training, as does much of the research in this volume (see Chapter 16).

This research brings to light considerations in the conceptualization of the role of the surgeon and the referred consultation in the broader patient journey and on the effectiveness of current practice (White et al. 2013). Explicitly establishing a mutual understanding of expectations of the consultation will assist in enhancing communication within the consultation, while engaging the surgical community in reflecting on these considerations is a key step forward in improving research and education specifically for communication in surgical practice.

Acknowledgements

We acknowledge the assistance from members of the Applied Research on Communication in Health (ARCH) group at the University of Otago, Wellington, New Zealand, for providing access to data archived in the ARCH Corpus of Health Interactions, and assisting with the recording and transcription of additional consultations. Any remaining errors or infelicities are solely our responsibility. Funding was provided through a University of Otago Postgraduate Scholarship and by the New Zealand Health Research Council and Marsden fund.

Contributions

SJW, MS, KD and RG designed the study. SJW and LM undertook the fieldwork and data collection. SJW had principal responsibility for data transcription and analysis, with SJW, MS, KD, RG, LM and AD all providing analytic input at various stages. SJW drafted the manuscript and all authors read and approved the final copy.

Transcription Notation

The transcription notations that are used in this research are taken from ten Have (1999: 213–14) and Gardner (2001: xi–xxi). These are based on the Jeffersonian transcription system (Jefferson 2004).

Sequencing

[	A single left bracket indicates overlap onset.
]	A single right bracket indicates the point at which an overlap terminates in relation to another utterance.
=	Equal signs, one at the end of one line and one at the beginning of the next, indicate no gap between the two turns. This is called latching.
>	A carat bracket is used within a speaker's utterance to indicate no gap between the speaker's turn constructional units.

Intervals

(0.0)	Numbers in parentheses indicate elapsed time in silence, in seconds and tenths of seconds. This works within a turn, within a turn constructional unit or between speakers. For example, (2.1) is a pause of two seconds and one tenth of a second.
(.)	A dot in parentheses indicates a tiny gap of less than 0.2 seconds within or between utterances.

Prosodic Features of Utterances

w<u>o</u>rd	Underscoring a word or part thereof indicates some form of stress.
::	Colons indicate prolongation of the immediately prior sound. Multiple colons indicate a more prolonged sound.
;	Semi-colon indicates a slight fall, continuative intonation contour.
–	A dash indicates a cut-off.
w-w-word	Stuttering is indicated by a repetition of the stuttered sound connected by hyphens.
*	An asterisk around an utterance or part thereof indicates creaky voice.
$	A dollar symbol around an utterance or part thereof indicates smiley voice.
.	A period indicates a stopping fall in intonation.
,	A comma indicates a slightly rising, continuing intonation.
?	A question mark indicates a rising intonation.
¿	A "Spanish question mark" indicates stronger rise than a comma but weaker than a question mark.
_	An underline symbol after the word indicates a level pitch contour.
x:x	An underlined colon within a syllable indicates that the intonation within the syllable falls then rises.

x<u>x</u>:	An underlined second letter within a syllable followed by a non-underlined colon indicates that the intonation within the syllable rises then falls.
	The absence of an utterance-final marker indicates some sort of "indeterminate" contour.
↑	An upward arrow indicates a marked shift into higher pitch in the utterance-part immediately following the arrow.
↓	A downward arrow indicates a marked shift into lower pitch in the utterance-part immediately following the arrow.
WORD	Upper case indicates especially loud sounds relative to the surrounding talk.
•word	Staccato talk is indicated by a bullet prior to the utterance-part
°word° °°word°°	Utterances or utterance-parts bracketed by degree signs are relatively quieter than the surrounding talk. Very quiet talk is indicated by two degree signs on each side.
<word>	Left/right carats bracketing an utterance or part thereof indicate slowing down as compared to the surrounding talk.
>word<	Right/left carats bracketing an utterance or part thereof indicate speeding up as compared to the surrounding talk.
.hhh	A dot-prefixed row of "h"s indicates an in breath.
hhh	Without the dot, the "h"s indicate an out breath.
w(h)ord	A parenthesized "h", or a row of "h"s within a word, indicates breathiness, such as can be heard in laughter and crying.

Transcriber's Doubts and Comments

()	The length of empty parentheses indicates the length of talk that the transcriber was unable to hear. Empty parentheses in the speaker designation column indicate inability to identify a speaker.
(word)	Especially dubious hearings or speaker identifications are indicated by parentheses around the utterance, utterance-part or speaker designation.
(())	Transcriber descriptions are indicated by double parentheses.

References

Australian Commission on Safety and Quality in Health Care. 2008. *Windows into Safety and Quality in Health Care 2008*. Sydney: ACSQHC.

Byrne, Patrick S., and Barrie E.L. Long. 1976. *Doctors Talking to Patients: A Study of the Verbal Behaviour of General Practitioners Consulting in Their Surgeries*, edited by Great Britain Dept. of Health and Social Security. London: HMSO.

Clayman, Steven E., and Virginia T. Gill. 2004. Conversation Analysis. In *Handbook of Data Analysis*, edited by Alan Byman and Melissa A. Hardy, 589–606. Beverly Hills, CA: Sage.

Cohen-Cole, Steven A. 1991. *The Medical Interview: The Three-Function Approach*. St. Louis, MO: Mosby-Year Book.

Gardner, Rod. 2001. *When Listeners Talk: Response Tokens and Listener Stance*. Amsterdam, PA: J. Benjamins Pub.

Helman, Cecil G. 1981. Disease versus Illness in General Practice. *Journal of the Royal College of General Practice* 31: 548–62.

Heritage, John. 1984. *Garfinkel and Ethnomethodology*. Cambridge: Polity Press.

Heritage, John, and Steven Clayman. 2010. *Talk in Action: Interactions, Identities, and Institutions. Language in Society* series, edited by P. Trudgill. West Sussex: Wiley-Blackwell.

Heritage, John, and Douglas W. Maynard. 2006a. *Communication in Medical Care: Interaction between Primary Care Physicians and Patients*. Cambridge: Cambridge University Press.

Heritage, John, and Douglas W. Maynard. 2006b. Introduction. In *Communication in Medical Care*, edited by John Heritage and Douglas W. Maynard, 1–21. Cambridge: Cambridge University Press.

Heritage, John, Jeffrey D. Robinson, Marc N. Elliott, Megan Beckett and Michael Wilkes. 2007. Reducing Patients' Unmet Concerns in Primary Care: The Difference One Word Can Make. *Journal of General Internal Medicine* 22(10): 1429.

Heron, John. 1975. A Six Category Intervention Analysis: Human Potential Research Project. Surrey: University of Surrey.

Jefferson, Gail. 2004. Glossary of Transcript Symbols. In *Conversation Analysis: Studies from the First Generation*, edited by Gene H. Lerner, 13–31. Amsterdam: Benjamins.

Levinson, Wendy, Pamela Hudak and Andrea C. Tricco. 2013. A Systematic Review of Surgeon–Patient Communication: Strengths and Opportunities for Improvement. *Patient Education and Counseling* 93(1): 3–17.

Maynard, Douglas W. 2003. *Bad News, Good News: Conversational Order in Everyday Talk and Clinical Settings*. Chicago: The University of Chicago Press.

Neighbour, Roger. 1987. *The Inner Consultation*. Lancaster: MTO Press.

Pendleton, David, Theo Schofield, Peter Tate and Peter Havelock. 1984. *The Consultation: An Approach to Learning and Teaching*. Oxford: Oxford University Press.

Peräkylä, Anssi. 1998. Authority and Accountability: The Delivery of Diagnosis in Primary Health Care. *Social Psychology Quarterly* 61: 301–20.

Robinson, Jeffrey D. 2003. An Interactional Structure of Medical Activities During Acute Visits and Its Implications for Patients' Participation. *Health Communication* 15(1): 27–59. doi: 10.1207/S15327027HC1501_2

Schegloff, Emanuel A. 2007. *Sequence Organization in Interaction: Volume 1*. New York: Cambridge University Press.

Silverman, Jonathan, Suzanne M. Kurtz and Juliet Draper. 2013. *Skills for Communicating with Patients*. 3rd ed. Oxford: Radcliffe Publishing.

Stewart, Moira, Judith Belle Brown, W. Wayne Weston, Ian R. McWhinney, Carol L. McWilliam and Thomas R. Freeman. 2003. *Patient-Centered Medicine: Transforming the Clinical Method*. 2nd ed. Oxford: Radcliffe Medical Press.

Stott, Nigel C.H., and Robert H. Davis. 1979. The Exceptional Potential in Each Primary Care Consultation. *Journal of the Royal College of General Practice* 29: 201–5.

ten Have, Paul. 1999. *Doing Conversation Analysis*. London: Sage.

White, Sarah J. 2011. A Structural Analysis of Surgeon-Patient Consultations in Clinic Settings in New Zealand. PhD dissertation, University of Otago.

White, Sarah J. 2012. Closing Surgeon-Patient Consultations. *International Review of Pragmatics* 4(1): 58–79. doi: 10.1163/187731012X632063

White, Sarah J. 2015. Closing Clinical Consultations. In *Handbuch Sprache in der Medizin [Handbook of Language in Medicine]*, edited by Albert Busch and Thomas Spranz-Fogasy. Berlin: De Gruyter.

White, Sarah J., Maria H. Stubbe, Kevin P. Dew, Lindsay M. Macdonald, Anthony C. Dowell and Rod Gardner. 2013. Understanding Communication between Surgeon and Patient in outpatient consultations. *ANZ Journal of Surgery* 83(5): 307–11. doi: 10.1111/ans.12126

White, Sarah J., Maria H. Stubbe, Lindsay M. Macdonald, Anthony C. Dowell, Kevin P. Dew, and Rod Gardner. 2014. Framing the Consultation: The Role of the Referral in Surgeon-Patient Consultations. *Health Communication* 29(1): 74–80. doi: 10.1080/10410236.2012.718252

Sarah J. White is a qualitative health researcher and linguist with a particular interest in using conversation analysis to understand communication in surgical practice. She is a Senior Lecturer at the Faculty of Medicine and Health Sciences at Macquarie University, Sydney. Sarah was awarded her PhD from the University of Otago, Wellington in 2011 and has professional and academic experience in clinical communication, quality and safety in healthcare, and medical education.

Maria Stubbe, PhD, is Research Director in the Department of Primary Health Care and General Practice and co-directs the Applied Research on Communication in Health (ARCH) group at the at the Wellington School of Medicine and Health Sciences, University of Otago. She has a background in interactional sociolinguistics and analysis of workplace/institutional discourse. Current research interests include shared decision-making in clinical encounters, communication in interpreter-mediated health encounters and patient experiences of health and illness.

Lindsay Macdonald, MA, is a Research Fellow in the Department of Primary Health Care and General Practice and co-directs the ARCH group, at the Wellington School of Medicine and Health Sciences, University of Otago. She is a registered nurse with a postgraduate degree in nursing and linguistics. Her research interests include aspects of health communication particularly in relation to managing long-term conditions, and how everyday communication can affect health outcomes.

Anthony C. Dowell, MBChB, is Professor of General Practice and Primary Health Care at the Wellington School of Medicine and Health Sciences, University of Otago, where he also co-directs the ARCH group. He is a General Practitioner at the Island Bay Medical Centre, Wellington, and a member of a WHO panel exploring classification issues in mental health for the ICD11 classification of disease. His current academic interests include research in mental healthcare, health services research, quality in healthcare and communication in healthcare consultation settings.

Kevin Dew, PhD, is Professor of Sociology at Victoria University of Wellington and before that was a senior lecturer in the Department of Public Health at the Wellington School of Medicine and Health Sciences. He is a founding member of the ARCH group. Current research activities include studies of interactions between health professionals and patients, cancer care decision-making in relation to health inequities, the social meanings of medications and the role of public health in contemporary society.

Rod Gardner, PhD, is Associate Professor in the School of Languages and Cultures at the University of Queensland in Brisbane. His academic and research interests include conversation analysis, second language interaction, indigenous Australian conversation and conversation analysis for classroom interaction and learning.

3 Doing Patient-Centred Consultations: Some Challenges for International Medical Graduates

Lynda Yates and Maria R. Dahm

3.1 Introduction

That surgeons also need to be skilful communicators is clearly reflected in the emphasis now given to leadership, teamwork and interpersonal communication in the core competencies for medical practitioners (Dedy et al. 2013; Royal College of Physicians and Surgeons of Canada 2005; RACS 2012), and in the focus on patient-centred approaches to care which treat the "whole person" and explore patients' perspectives to facilitate shared decision-making (Stewart et al. 2003). While surgeons from all backgrounds may benefit from training in patient-centred communication skills (Dedy et al. 2013), international medical graduates (IMGs), who have trained and practised in another language and culture, face particular challenges in adapting to a whole range of medical systems and approaches, and, crucially, to unfamiliar ways of communicating. These can be linguistic, that is, related to the language itself, but also cultural, that is, related to the way in which the cultural values of a community influence how members choose to speak to each other and the impact that different behaviours can have.

Internationally trained doctors are crucial to many first-world medical systems, including in Australia where they comprise about a quarter (25.4 per cent) of all practising doctors (Australian Institute of Health and Welfare 2011). In 2012, 1 in 13 surgeons practising in Australia had trained overseas (385 out of 4720),[1] and most (87.5 per cent) of those applying for skills assessment as surgical specialists originated from countries where English is the not the dominant language

---

1 The figure includes surgeons undertaking short-term specific training (215), practising as surgical specialists (118) and new RACS fellows (52).

(RACS 2013) and where approaches to medicine may also be markedly different. These surgeons may therefore need to become familiar with both patient-centred approaches to practice, and how to meet the communicative demands that they entail (Dahm 2011; Dahm and Yates 2013; Kaafarani 2009).

Traditional communications training, however, tends to provide advice that is quite general in nature, often without clear definitions of how and why communication issues occur. While general statements such as "Effective communication, ie, no poor phrasing, awkward statements, jargon" (Larkin et al. 2010: 288), or "Attentively listens to patients [and] sets an appropriate 'tone' for any communication with patients" (RACS 2012: 16) may be helpful in assisting native speakers of English who are already familiar with local communicative conventions, they fail to provide adequate concrete guidance for IMGs on exactly what it is that they are doing or not doing appropriately and, most importantly, it does not help them to understand why this is so (Dahm, Ogden et al. 2015). While native English speaking (NES) surgeons can draw on their implicit knowledge of how particular communicative effects can be achieved, non-native English speaking (NNES) doctors who have been raised and trained in a different language and communicative culture may not have either the linguistic forms or the cultural knowledge to do this on their own (Dahm 2011; Kaafarani 2009; Pilotto, Duncan and Anderson-Wurf 2007). Moreover, in Australia many IMGs work in remote areas where they have minimal opportunity to observe how other surgeons might communicate with patients. Appropriate communications training is therefore vital to help surgeons develop the communicative skills they need. Opportunities are, however, limited (McGrath et al. 2012) and where available, may lack the detail on the specific linguistic features that doctors use to engage patients within a patient-centred approach to medicine.

In this chapter we report on data from a series of studies designed to address these gaps. We first consider what is currently known about the features of communication that help to promote a patient-centred, empathetic environment in surgical communication. Drawing on analyses of complementary sets of authentic and elicited discourse data in surgical settings, we then highlight some of the specific challenges faced by NNES IMGs who are practising or preparing to practise in English. Finally, we consider how these challenges could be addressed in communications training and professional development for surgeons.

3.2   What Is Patient-Centred Care and How Do Doctors Do It?

Patient-centred care stresses the need to develop a close relationship with the patient while treating their disease (Epstein 2000; Stewart et al. 2003). To do this, a surgeon makes efforts to get to know the patient as a person, including their ideas and feelings about their illness, thus allowing the development of shared expectations for the surgical relationship (Stewart et al. 2003). Central to patient-centred care is the ability to communicate empathy in ways that are understood to be sincere and compassionate (Epstein 2000) and openness to the patient's perspective of approachability (Dahm and Yates 2013).

A common element in the many definitions of empathy is a mental state of compassion. However, the successful communication of that empathy relies on the use of specific communicative skills and behaviours (Suchman et al. 1997; O'Grady 2011). Empathy has consequently been defined as a two-step accomplishment: the ability (1) "to understand the patient's situation, perspective, and feelings" and (2) "to communicate that understanding to the patient" (Coulehan et al. 2001: 221). Similarly, while it is important as a first step for a surgeon to remain open to a patient's perspective, the ability to communicate that openness is also necessary. Surgeons therefore need to both understand and master the different ways in which they signal this approachability through the way they talk. Failure to do this runs the risk of signalling the opposite, that is, a lack of empathy and a reluctance to consider the views of the patient. Some of the subtle language features used to express empathy and approachability have been explored in recent studies summarized in Table 3.1 and discussed in more detail below.

Strategies that emphasize the interpersonal dimension of relationships help to establish a relaxed, patient-centred atmosphere in a consultation. These include the use of first name greetings, informal language, small talk and personal disclosure (Beach et al. 2004; Dahm, O'Grady et al. 2015; Dahm and Yates 2013; Hudak and Maynard 2011; Ragan 2000). Surgeons can make effective use of their "personal voice", that is, they can temporarily emphasize their personal experiences over their professional identity in order to promote solidarity and trust and gain greater insight into the patient's "life-world" (Cordella 2004; Mishler 1984; O'Grady et al. 2014; Roberts and Sarangi 1999). Thus patient-relevant self-disclosures can signal personal interest in the patient and offer reassurance which can help to build rapport and communicate empathy (Beach et al. 2004; Dahm, O'Grady et al. 2015; Stewart et al. 2003). Appropriate nonverbal behaviours such as maintaining eye contact, using an open body posture and mirroring patient movements have also been associated with perception of rapport and greater patient satisfaction (Hall, Harrigan and Rosenthal 1996; Harrigan, Oxman and Rosenthal 1985; Meadors and Murray 2014).

Crucial in communicating engagement and empathy are strategies that show the surgeon is actively listening and responding. Mirroring patient expressions and using minimal responses such as *hmm*, *uh-huh* or *yeah* (also referred to as back-channels or continuers) can signal interest in patients' narratives and encourage them to disclose their concerns, thereby laying the foundation for the expression of genuine empathy (e.g., Bensing 1991; Coulehan et al. 2001). Minimal responses that are followed by additions which reflect on or paraphrase the patient's point can help to show that the surgeon is really listening, and can also serve as a confirmation

Table 3.1: Discursive features that show empathy and approachability

Interpersonal strategies	– Greeting/introduction, forms of address (Dahm and Yates 2013; Moore, Yelland and Ng 2011; Wallace et al. 2009) – Small talk (Cordella 2004; Hudak and Maynard 2011; Ragan 2000) – Personal side sequence and self-disclosure (Beach et al. 2004; Dahm, O'Grady et al. 2015)
Nonverbal communication	– Bodily actions/position; eye contact (Coulehan et al. 2001; Hall, Harrigan and Rosenthal 1996; Harrigan, Oxman and Rosenthal 1985; Meadors and Murray 2014; O'Grady 2011)
Active listening	– Minimal responses (Bensing 1991; Cordella 2004; Coulehan et al. 2001; O'Grady 2011; Suchman et al. 1997) – Attentive silence (O'Grady 2011) – Mirroring (Cordella 2004)
Attentive responding	– Open (follow-up) questions (Suchman et al. 1997) – Paraphrasing and reflecting (Bensing 1991; Coulehan et al. 2001) – Requesting and accepting correction (Coulehan et al. 2001; Roberts et al. 2003)
Genuine statements	(Epstein 2000; Norfolk, Birdi and Walsh 2007; O'Grady 2011; Roberts et al. 2003)
Timing	(Coulehan et al. 2001; O'Grady 2011; Suchman et al. 1997)
Framing and signposting	(Coulehan et al. 2001; Roberts et al. 2003)
Tailored explanations	(Hadlow and Pitts 1991; Tannen and Wallat 1987; Street 2003)
Lexical choice	– Familiar words vs medical jargon (Dahm 2012a, b; O'Grady 2011; Roberts et al. 2003) – Informal language (Yates 2005)
Softening/tentative expression	(Adolphs, Atkins and Harvey 2007; Caffi 1999; Skelton and Hobbs 1999)

or request for clarification or additional information (Bensing 1991; Coulehan et al. 2001; Suchman et al. 1997). In this way, surgeons can express genuine empathy at an appropriate time and avoid the trap of offering premature reassurance in the form of unconvincing rehearsed empathetic statements (O'Grady 2011; Roberts et al. 2003).

Appropriate framing, that is, making explicit what is going on in various stages of the consultation using explanations and verbal "signposts" helps surgeons to involve patients as equal partners (Coulehan et al. 2001; Roberts et al. 2003; Tannen and Wallat 1987). Equally important is the clear explanation of conditions, procedures and management programmes in familiar lay language that the patient can understand. Failure to explain medical terminology can cause misunderstanding and cause anxiety, with negative impacts on patient satisfaction, compliance, participation and autonomy (Hadlow and Pitts 1991; Street 2003; Young, Humphreys and Norman 2008). In contrast, adopting or mirroring the patient's vocabulary, and tailoring explanations to address their concerns and level of understanding can help surgeons to display their engagement and reduce misunderstanding (Cordella 2004; Hadlow and Pitts 1991; Tannen and Wallat 1987). The use of non-technical, informal language can help to establish and maintain a patient-centred atmosphere in which patients feel more comfortable asking questions and playing an active role in decision-making (Dahm 2012a, b; Hall, Roter and Katz 1988). Similarly, the use of softening strategies to, for example, offer reassurance, soften the impact of unpalatable news and minimize (perceived) power distances can help to develop and maintain rapport (Adolphs, Atkins and Harvey 2007; Caffi 1999; Skelton and Hobbs 1999).

3.3   IMGs and Patient-Centred Care

While patient-centred approaches to medical care have been successful in improving outcomes for patients in other medical settings (Bauman, Fardy and Harris 2003; Stewart et al. 2003), they have not always been prioritized in surgical training, as indicated by two recent reviews (Dedy et al. 2013; Levinson, Hudak and Tricco 2013). Levinson and colleagues (2013), for example, found that while surgeons – both NES and NNES – generally explained procedures and conditions clearly to patients, they were less successful in enquiring about patients' feelings or showing that they were actively listening to what patients had to say and missed many arising empathic opportunities. This suggests a need for a greater focus on the practice of patient-centred communication in training and professional development among surgeons and trainees.

Both reviews (Dedy et al. 2013; Levinson, Hudak and Tricco 2013) suggest that interpersonal communication skills are "teachable" through role-plays, observations of authentic patient interactions, (peer) feedback on video-recorded interactions, or integration into the learning of new surgical procedures. As noted above, the need to address these aspects of communication is particularly acute for NNES international surgeons who may be uncertain about exactly what behaviours are culturally appropriate or how to express their intentions verbally and nonverbally (Pilotto, Duncan and Anderson-Wurf 2007). Research has highlighted particular areas of difficulty, including how to show active listening, how to pick up on patient cues, and knowing exactly how to respond sensitively to empathic opportunities when they are recognized (Fiscella and Frankel 2000; Pilotto, Duncan and Anderson-Wurf 2007; Dahm, Ogden et al. 2015). Limited proficiency in conversational as opposed to technical English may mean that some IMGs may only have a limited repertoire of empathic expressions on which to draw. They may therefore rely on formulaic phrases to communicate emotional support, a response that can be interpreted as detached or insincere and even "shut down" a genuinely interactive approach to exploring patients' feelings (Dahm 2011; O'Grady 2011).

Explicit feedback and training is therefore likely to be helpful for IMGs who may have had only limited opportunity to observe practising surgeons with exemplary communication skills (Gould 2010: 63), particularly since the aspects of interpersonal communicative behaviour that they need are often used unconsciously and are therefore difficult to identify (Yates 2010). Moreover, interpersonal communicative competence is not merely the ability to regurgitate at crucial points a range of set phrases that can be ticked off a list (see Larkin et al. 2010). Rather, the behaviours involved in engendering trust or communicating empathy must be understood as a complex set of interactive pragmatic skills of which native-speakers themselves may also not be wholly conscious (Dahm and Yates 2013; O'Grady 2011; Yates 2010). Therefore approaches to communications training for IMGs should be reflective and explicit about both the specific strategies and features that are used *and* why they are appropriate.

Reflective approaches to training generally make use of recordings or transcripts of authentic doctor-patient interactions and allow surgeons to make explicit their "tacit knowledge" about communication in order to adjust their own communication practices (Schön 1987; Skelton 2005). However, this approach assumes some shared understanding of those communication styles considered appropriate in a certain context. Where surgeons have been trained in a different communicative and medical culture, however, expectations and interactive practices may be different. Thus, while NNES IMGs will have the necessary tacit knowledge in their native language, there may well be gaps in their knowledge of exactly how empathy, attentiveness and approachability are signalled in English, and what might be appropriate in the Australian context. They may, for example, need additional assistance with the linguistic subtleties involved in exploring patient emotions and expressing empathy in an interactive and culturally appropriate manner. Yet very little is currently known about the specific linguistic features that facilitate empathy or approachability in medical interactions in English (Coulehan et al. 2001; Dahm and Yates 2013). Most previous research on IMGs' communicative competence has used elicited non-interactive data from interviews or focus groups with IMGs and their educators (e.g., McDonnell and Usherwood 2008; McGrath et al. 2012). We therefore lack an evidence base grounded in actual interactions between IMGs and patients on which we can draw for effective communications training.

To start addressing this gap, in this chapter we draw on a range of interactive data sets that include naturally-occurring surgeon-patient consultations and semi-authentic role-plays with both actual and standardized patients. We examine these data in order to:

(1) identify the discourse features used to successfully orient surgical consultations towards a patient-centred approach;

(2) investigate how effectively NNES IMGs use these features in surgical consultations; and

(3) consider the implications for a targeted approach to communications training for NNES IMG surgeons.

In the following section we outline in more detail the participants and methodology used to collect and analyse these data sets.

3.4   Methodology

3.4.1   Data Collection and Participants

In the analysis presented here we make use of audio recordings of authentic naturally occurring surgical consultations and video recordings of two types of elicited role-played interactions: simulated doctor-patient interactions conducted for training purposes, and mock Objective Structured Clinical Examinations (OSCEs). As naturally occurring data is difficult to collect and hard to control for extraneous variables (Bataller and Shively 2011), OSCEs and role-plays with standardized patients have been increasingly used to explore how IMGs interact with patients (e.g., Woodward-Kron, Stevens and Flynn 2011) as they afford a level of control and allow for comparison. Table 3.2 summarizes the three complementary data sets analysed here.

Table 3.2: Data sets

Data set	Type of recordings (n)	Doctors (n)	Type of interaction	Presenting complaints/Scenarios (n)
1	Audio (n=37)	NES (n=1)	Authentic	Various (n=37)
2	Video (n=2)	NNES (n=2)	Semi-authentic	(a) Prostatectomy & Kidney Stent (Consult 15) (n=1) (b) Bowel Cancer (Consult 16) (n=1)
3	Video (n=32)	NNES (n=32)	Elicited	(a) Lung Cancer (Station 12) (n=16) (b) Post-op Infection (Station 13) (n=16)

(1) NES surgeon in private practice

Thirty-seven consultations between a NES colorectal surgeon (pseudonym *James*) and consenting patients were audio-recorded in his private rooms between October 2011 and June 2012. These provide insight into the communication features used to promote a patient-centred environment in a naturally-occurring setting. The surgeon and his patients were volunteers. The latter were recruited by the researchers in his waiting room and could opt to be recorded with or without the researcher present.

(2) NNES IMGs and hospital patients

For training purposes, 16 NNES IMGs employed at registrar level at an Australian hospital were video-recorded interacting with 12 volunteer hospitalized patients or out-patients attending specialist clinics. The IMGs were instructed to take a history, conduct an examination and discuss management with the patient. Two of the recordings were directly related to surgical issues and these are included in the analysis here.

- Consult 15 (pseudonym *Thant*):
  Male patient after radical prostatectomy and kidney stent. Returned to hospital with abdominal pain/discomfort which resolved after removal of stent.
- Consult 16 (pseudonym *Ranjit*):
  Male cancer patient, bowel resection, new stoma bag. One week post-surgery.

(3) NNES IMGs and standardized patients

NNES IMGs were video-recorded interacting with standardized patients in role-play mock exams conducted during three bridging courses designed to prepare IMGs for the Australian Medical Council clinical exam. On each occasion, the IMGs completed 16 eight-minute OSCE stations covering a range of medical areas from psychology to surgery. Six of these were recorded for feedback purposes. The two that related to surgical issues are analysed here. Sixteen IMGs gave their consent for us to use their role-plays, giving a total of 32 performances in the following two role plays:

- Station 12: Lung Cancer
  Male patient with bronchogenic adenocarcinoma (T2N1MO), two months after tumour resection currently receiving chemotherapy and presenting with increasing breathlessness over the past two days.
- Station 13: Post-op Infection
  Female patient two days post cholecystectomy presenting with fever.

All studies were approved by the Human Ethics committee at the relevant university and hospital. Table 3.3 summarizes the background demographics of the IMG participants.

Table 3.3: IMG participant demographics

IMG participant demographics	Data set 2 (n=2)	Data set 3 (n=32)	
		S12 (n=16)	S13 (n=16)
Male, n (%)	2 (100)	12 (75)	10 (62.5)
Mean age (SD)	32 (2.8)	35.8 (5.9)	36.6 (5.8)
Mean years spent in Australia (SD)	2.5 (0.7)	3.9 (3.5)	3.0 (3.0)
Mean years practising in COO (SD)	3.5 (2.1)	5.9 (5.8)	9 (6.8)
Mean years practising in Australia (SD)	1.5 (0)	2.8 (3.6)	1.4 (1.7)
Region of origin, n (%)			
Northeast Asia		1 (6)	
Southern & Central Asia	1 (50)	7 (44)	5 (31)
Southeast Asia	1 (50)	10 (62.5)	3 (19)
North Africa & Middle East		2 (12.5)	6 (37.5)
Southern & Eastern Europe		1 (6)	
Sub-Saharan Africa		3 (19)	2 (12.5)

3.4.2 Analysis

The diverse and yet complementary nature of these data sets allowed a qualitative analysis focusing on pragmatic and discourse features. For this purpose, all recordings were transcribed, de-identified and assigned a unique code or pseudonym. Using an analytical framework drawn from the literature on the communication of empathy and approachability outlined above, we used a reiterative data-driven approach to explore how the doctors used various communicative features to put patients at ease and orient consultations towards a person-centred, rather than a medically-oriented, focus. Analytical techniques were drawn from discourse analysis, interactional sociolinguistics and inter-language pragmatics (Bardovi-Harlig and Hartford 2005; Roberts and Sarangi 2005; Harvey and Adolphs 2012; Jaspers 2012).

Initial analysis was conducted independently for each transcript, and the authors met to discuss preliminary findings. In this first iteration, we focused on the overall communication style and the achievement of empathy, approachability and patient-centredness in the consultations. The subsequent collaborative iterations were informed by the relevant literature on discourse features associated with communicative competence and empathic skills. Through reiterative analysis we became fully immersed in the data which allowed us to compare the use of linguistic features across all data sets. In the sections below, we use exemplary and unedited excerpts from the transcripts to illustrate and support our findings.

3.4.3   Findings and Discussion

Our analyses of these three data sets highlight a range of communicative behaviours associated with fostering a patient-centred approach and suggest a number of areas in which NNES surgeons might benefit from explicit training, in particular their use of approachability features and the ways in which they attended to and responded to empathic opportunities. While the NES surgeon demonstrated his attention to patients' feelings in a number of ways and used a variety of discourse features to increase his approachability and express empathy, many of the IMGs used a more limited range of strategies to do this. Some appeared to use certain features only superficially and to rely on formulaic expressions that, at times, had the tendency to project a demeanour that was uncaring, dismissive and authoritarian.

Below we illustrate how the NES surgeon and NNES IMGs made use of the discourse features outlined in Table 3.1 and discuss the implications for the surgeon-patient relationship.

3.5   Native English Speaking Surgeon (James)

James employed a variety of discourse features that communicated his empathy for and willingness to engage with his patients. These included small talk, conversational framing, banter and self-disclosure, the use of informal forms of address and language, signposting, softening techniques, active listening, open questions and various other techniques to make the most of the empathic opportunities that he saw. He used these throughout, adapting to each individual patient according to the demands of the situation, an approach that allowed him to set up the consultation as a conversation, establish and maintain rapport throughout, demonstrate his empathy and appear more approachable.

3.5.1   Small Talk

James routinely engaged in small talk with patients and any accompanying family members at the beginning of consultations, as in Excerpt 1. These sequences, often sprinkled with informal language (e.g., *bugger*) and humour (his failure to give himself a corner office), served to break the ice with new patients, ease tension and set up a more relaxed conversational and patient-centred atmosphere by helping to break down any perceived power distances between doctor and patient and their family members (Hudak and Maynard 2011; Ragan 2000).

Excerpt 1: 23_DG repeat male patient (51) with his wife. They are discussing how James chose his office.

```
Patient's wife: You must have the pick of the crop when you first got here.
Surgeon:        Well, I did but I thought, no, it's not quite the right way to
                do it.
Patient's wife: [Laughs].
Surgeon:        And, um...
Patient's wife: Already to go - they, they've all got a good view though.
Surgeon:        Yes. No, but today was the first time I've arrived and thought,
                bugger, I haven't got that corner office.
Patient's wife: [Laughs].
```

After a short small talk sequence, James usually progressed towards medical matters, all the while maintaining a conversational frame (Tannen and Wallat 1987) and involving the patient as an equal partner, as illustrated in Excerpt 2 below.

Excerpt 2: 16_SM new female patient (80) referred for a second opinion for a colonoscopy

```
Surgeon: Now, now, Dr [Berry]...
Patient: Yeah.
Surgeon: He's a nice fellow.
Patient: Yeah.
Surgeon: And he will have written a letter.
Patient: Yeah.
Surgeon: But I don't want to read it just yet. I'd like to hear from you what's,
         what's going on [unclear].
Patient: Well, this is a bit different. [Laughs]
Surgeon: What?
Patient: [laughing voice] Okay.
Surgeon: Well, no, I could read it.
Patient: [Laughs, high pitched, expresses high amusement]
Surgeon: But then I'd be...
Patient: Okay. Well... I'll tell
Surgeon: then I'd be going down his...his...
Patient: His path, okay.
Surgeon: ...not yours necessarily.
Patient: Okay.
```

James used an explicit discourse marker (*Now, now, Dr [Berry]*) to announce a shift from the preceding small talk to medical topics. Rather than relying on the information conveyed in the referral letter as is typical in such referral sequences (White et al. 2014), he elicited the patient's perspective through an open question (*I'd like to hear from you what's, what's going on*). The patient's comment and laughter (*Well, this is a bit different. [Laughs]*) suggests that this did not necessarily fit her preconceptions of how a consultation might proceed. James then made his motivation explicit (*Well, no, I could read it. But then I'd be...then I'd be going down his...his...*) to which the patient signalled her agreement by collaboratively completing the doctor's turn (*His path, okay*).

This strategy is a useful means of strengthening the patient-centred focus of the consultation and James used it regularly. It allowed him a perspective on the patients' feelings and the overall impact of the medical problem on their "lifeworld"

(Mishler 1984) that complemented the bio-medical focus of the referring letter. This opportunity for patients to divulge personal information allowed the establishment of a joint agenda for the consultation (see O'Grady et al. 2014; Stewart et al. 2003).

3.5.2   Banter and Self-Disclosure

The framing of the consultation as a conversation between equal parties also enabled both participants to freely introduce new topics, comment on earlier small talk, joke or banter throughout, as illustrated in Excerpt 3.

Excerpt 3: 18_SCN, new male patient (70s) referred for bleeding from bowel associated with constipation

```
Surgeon:  Alright.
Patient:  Pretty stressful year. We've just downsized, um...
Surgeon:  Okay.
Patient:  ...and, um, the building was late. And we rented for a while and all
          that sort of thing.
Surgeon:  You too.
Patient:  Yeah, ah...
Surgeon:  No, we are going through exactly, exactly the same thing.
Patient:  It's not, ah, it's not a great scenario, is it?
Surgeon:  No, I, I, I want to just sit here and tell you all my building problems.
Patient:  [Laughs]
```

James also used self-disclosing statements (*we are going through exactly, exactly the same thing*) to adopt a "personal voice" that would build solidarity, enhance rapport and increase his approachability (Beach et al. 2004; O'Grady et al. 2014).

3.5.3   Forms of Address, Signposts and Meta-Commentary

For new patients, James would usually enquire about their naming preferences, and in most of his consultations used informal forms of address (i.e., first names) often seamlessly blended with very casual empathic statements (*poor fella having to come and see me*).

Excerpt 4: 10_NN, new male patient (47) referred for colonoscopy, and hernia repair

```
Surgeon:  Okay, what should I call you?
Patient:  Herb.
Surgeon:  Herb. You poor fella having to come and see me, and I've got a letter
          there from Dr Smith...
Patient:  Yes.
Surgeon:  ...which I won't read just yet.
Patient:  Aha.
Surgeon:  I want to hear from you what's going on.
Patient:  Um.
Surgeon:  I'll, I'll take some notes on the computer.
```

The use of first names can convey feelings of closeness, familiarity and genuine concern (Moore, Yelland and Ng 2011; Wallace et al. 2009). The casual language James used in the self-deprecating expressions of empathy (*poor fella having to come and see me*) helped to alleviate anxiety and create rapport and trust (Chur-Hansen and Barrett 1996; Ragan 2000). The string of signposts made explicit his thought processes (*which I won't read just yet*) and anticipated actions (*I'll, I'll take some notes on the computer*), and fulfilled a range of functions such as signalling a shift in topic or transition to a different stage of the consultation (from history taking to examination and management), or outlining an agenda for the consultation (see Excerpt 5).

Excerpt 5: 10_NN

```
Surgeon:   ...and come a little... [Pause]. Okay. So we're going to talk about two
           things, then we'll do it very separately, so we'll have a colonoscopy
           talk...
Patient:   Aha.
Surgeon:   ...and then we'll have a hernia talk...
Patient:   Yes.
Surgeon:   ...and, you know, we'll probably, err, be able to fix them both at the
           same time like...
Patient:   Oh, excellent.
```

By making the next steps in the consultation transparent to the patient, and using the pronoun *we*, James reduced perceived power distances and allowed the consultation to become more collaborative (Robins et al. 2011; Silverman, Kurtz and Draper 2013). As in Excerpts 6 and 7, this kind of meta-commentary can help reduce anxiety (Robins et al. 2011). By explaining a line of thought, for instance, James reassured the patient who might have otherwise been concerned about the preceding silence (Excerpt 6).

Excerpt 6: 15_DC, repeat male patient (50s), post-op consultation following haemorrhoid artery ligation

```
Surgeon:   [3.0] And we took some biopsies from the stomach and from the...
Patient:   Alright.
Surgeon:   ...the bowel. I'm just sort of...
Patient:   Yeah.
Surgeon:   ...recreating this...
Patient:   Yeah.
Surgeon:   ...all in, in my mind.
```

Excerpt 7: 07_BH, repeat male patient (27), clearance for physical activity following fissure repair

```
Surgeon:   Can I have a little look at your tail? [...] I'm not going to put a fin-
           ger in your tail or anything like that. I just want to have a little...
Patient:   Yeah, no prob.
Surgeon:   ...just have a little gentle look and see if it's, see if it's healing.
```

By making transparent what he was planning (and not planning) to do during a rectal exam (Excerpt 7) James addressed in advance any fears the patient might have about examination (Silverman, Kurtz and Draper 2013). This demonstration of concern for the patient's anxiety illustrates his empathic communication skills (Coulehan et al. 2001).

3.5.4   Softening Strategies, Informal Language and Tailored Explanations

Also of note is his use of softening strategies (e.g., just, a little, or anything like that) and informal language (Excerpt 7: *a little look*; *tail* or Excerpt 8: *a little cushion; a little stitch*) as they reduce social distance, increase approachability and maintain a conversational climate which can strengthen rapport (Adolphs, Atkins and Harvey 2007; Caffi 1999; Yates 2005). The informal and euphemistic terms "tail" (Excerpt 7) and "cushion" (Excerpt 8) stand in marked contrast to the medical alternatives (rectum, anus, sphincter; haemorrhoid, piles). By explaining medical terms or employing familiar lay terms, James both specifically tailored information to his patients and guarded against the alienating effects of jargon. To the same end, he also often used drawings and/or everyday metaphors as in Excerpt 8 (*cushion almost filled with blood*) (Street 2003; Tannen and Wallat 1987).

Excerpt 8: 18_SCN, new male patient (70s) referred for bleeding from bowel associated with constipation

```
Surgeon:  [...] It, in fact, it sounds very like bleeding that's coming from
          what I'd call a haemorrhoid. And what I call a haemorrhoid's often
          different from what other people...
Patient:  Right.
Surgeon:  ...call a haemorrhoid. It's just...
Patient:  Yep.
Surgeon:  But a little, um, cushion almost filled with blood that can drip and
          squirt. And it's supplied by an artery. And in fact one modern way of
          fixing this is to put a little stitch through the artery.
```

3.5.5   Expressing Empathy: Minimal Responses and Open Questions

As described above, James routinely used the referral recognition sequence to invite patients to their share their own perspectives on their illness experience, used minimal responses (Excerpt 9, *yup, okay, yes*) to show that he was listening attentively and open questions to elicit more information (*Well, te-, tell me about that*).

3.5.6   Empathic Opportunities and Timing

James used what has been dubbed the "lasso effect" (Suchman et al. 1997), that is, the use of minimal responses to encourage the patient to keep talking in order to understand more about her experience. As illustrated in Excerpt 9, James let several (potential) empathic opportunities (e.g., *They thought it was a heart attack*) pass with only minimal reaction. This helped him to avoid the use of routine expressions and then give a more specifically tailored response to her experience and emotional state later (*Yeah, you must've had a really nasty fright*).

Excerpt 9: 04_KN, new female patient (61) with recurrent diverticulitis

```
Patient:   And I, and it's, I know that it manifests itself in, in a lot of dif-
           ferent ways, and quite scary ones [laughs] sometimes. Um...
Surgeon:   Well, te-, tell me about that.
Patient:   Well, I've had, you know, this is when it was first diagnosed, I was in
           casualty fo-, one time. They thought it was a heart attack, 'cause I
           had really severe pains up my arm and my neck...
Surgeon:   Yup.
Patient:   ...and across my chest. And that happened quite a lot. [...] And I tend
           to think when something like that happens, oh, it is, it is the GORD,
           or sometimes you, you wonder.
Surgeon:   Okay.
Patient:   And I've had [hesitates] - it doesn't - it really comes as what we
           would term heartburn, I guess
Surgeon:   Yes.
           [lines omitted]
Patient:   [...] lots of different symptoms - hard to explain - but I, usually I
           know when it, when it is. And I do normally get away with a lot. But,
           um...
Surgeon:   I'll write that down: I get away with a lot.
Patient:   [Laughs] I do, 'cause I know that some people, poor things, can't have
           anything.
           [lines omitted]
Patient:   I, I've completely changed what I - I haven't had any alcohol; I hav-
           en't had - I, I started drinking tea. I hate tea. But then I read you
           shouldn't have tea either, so I w-, I've been having half a cup of
           decaf every now and then.
Surgeon:   Oh, you poor thing.
           [lines omitted]
Patient:   ...and some Gaviscon as well. I'm sleeping sitting up. I'm doing -
           which is a nightmare in its-, well, it would be if you could get to
           sleep [laughs]. Um...
Surgeon:   Yeah, you must've had a really nasty fright.
```

He only interrupted her narrative to make a humorous aside (*I'll write that down*) in response to her admission *I get away with a lot.* This evoked laughter and reinforced the informal atmosphere (Ragan 2000).

3.5.7   Genuine Empathic Statements and Informal Language

Excerpt 9 also illustrates how James used informal language, and his "go-to" empathic statement (*poor thing/fella*, see also Excerpt 4), both of which served to reduce social distance. He used such strategies to great effect with patients from very different backgrounds. Excerpt 10 is taken from a consultation with a tall tattooed man who smelled strongly of alcohol. James was able align himself and demonstrate emotional reciprocity (Cordella 2004) with this repeat patient by using his more informal "personal voice" (Roberts and Sarangi 1999). As shown in the excerpt, James engaged with the patient's account of his ongoing pain following a hernia operation by shifting register and applying the informal metaphorical label "nightmare" to the patient, thus communicating his understanding of the patient's predicament.

Excerpt 10: 21_MD, repeat male patient (40s) with significant neuropathic pain

```
Patient:   It's always sore constantly down there...
Surgeon:   Yeah.
Patient:   ...always. And...
Surgeon:   Yeah.
Patient:   ...especially here. It's just - once - there, one spot there. Like it's
           real - oh, real sore all the time. Ah...
Surgeon:   What a nightmare you are.
Patient:   Yeah, it's all sore down here. And...
           [lines omitted]
Surgeon:   Did you? Just stopped them off your own bat?
Patient:   Yeah, well, I was sick of being drugged up all the time.
Surgeon:   Did you - were they spinning you out, were they?
Patient:   Yeah. Well, like...
           [Over speaking]
Patient:   ...I was getting - I'd have many of them I, I started like - I felt
           like I was always wasted like...
```

When discussing pain relief, James mirrored the patient's colloquial idiom "drugged up" with the similarly colloquial phrase "spinning out" and uses informal everyday language to reformulate the patient's statement (*I was sick of being drugged up all the time*) into an empathic tag question (*Did you – were they spinning you out, were they?*). By paraphrasing the patient in this way, James demonstrated his understanding and also invited further comment (Coulehan et al. 2001).

3.5.8   Cues, Paraphrasing and Reflecting

James was able to tailor the use of all these techniques to the individual needs of his patients, as illustrated in Excerpt 11 below.

Excerpt 11: 19_VI, new female NNES patient (57) seeking a second opinion following an inguinal hernia operation, accompanied by her niece

```
Surgeon:  Well, good afternoon.
Patient:  [very quietly] Good afternoon.
Surgeon:  You found us okay?
Niece:    Yeah, it was pretty good.
Surgeon:  Good.
Niece:    Yeah.
Patient:  [Even with me].
Niece:    I do. [Laughs].
Surgeon:  Okay. You look so nervous. Poor thing.
Niece:    Yeah, she's very nervous.
Surgeon:  Yeah.
Niece:    Well, she's been in a lot of pain for a long time, as well.
Surgeon:  Okay.
Niece:    I think she, I think she just wants answers now. [Laughs].
Surgeon:  Okay. What's been happening? What's been going on?
Patient:  It's my tummy. Always swelling, and always painful. I can't sit. I
          can't walk.
```

Although directly addressed in the greeting and follow-up question (*You found us okay?*), the patient's response was barely audible and then self-deprecating (*Even with me*). James interpreted her low voice and low self-esteem comment as a reflection of her anxiety and made this explicit (*You look so nervous*) before offering his empathy (*Poor thing*). The niece, speaking on behalf of the patient, agreed. James then reinforced his concern for the patient's feelings by inviting her to explain (*What's been happening? What's been going on?*)

This example nicely illustrates and summarizes the interactive and responsive nature of James's communicative competence and shows how strategies for showing empathy can be adapted and applied to individual patients through the use of different discourse features. He moved apparently effortlessly from recognizing a patient cue (O'Grady 2011) to displaying his understanding of her feelings through "paraphrase and reflection" (Bensing 1991; Coulehan et al. 2001) and the use of a direct empathic statement (O'Grady 2011), to following up with open questions (Roberts et al. 2003; Suchman et al. 1997).

While some IMGs in our data made use of similar strategies, there were differences in the extent to which they did this. In the following section we discuss some of those occasions where they missed opportunities or appeared to have difficulty communicating empathy and approachability, since these suggest some areas where explicit training may be useful.

3.6 International Medical Graduates

3.6.1 Greetings, Introductions and Nonverbal Communication

As noted above, for role-play Station 12 (S12) the IMGs were first required to discuss x-ray results with the examiner before taking a brief history and discussing management with a patient, thus five IMGs did not introduce themselves to the patient at all (neither first name, last name nor role) after talking with the examiner. For Station 13 (S13) they had to assess and manage a patient presenting with fever two days post cholecystectomy, and only two IMGs did not introduce themselves at all.

As discussed above, greetings and "How are you?" sequences are important in establishing a social rather than medically oriented atmosphere at the beginning of the consultation (Coupland, Robinson and Coupland 1994). While most IMGs used some sort of greeting and introduction, not all of these were successful in establishing rapport and reducing social distance. Excerpts 12 and 13 are taken from the same station (S13).

Excerpt 12: S13-IMG12

```
IMG12:     Hello I'm Dr [Last name]. How do you do?
Patient:   I'm, I'm okay...
IMG12:     I'm on the uh surgical...on call. Do you mind if I sit down next to you?
Patient:   Yeah.
IMG12:     I was actually rung by ward staff. [sits down] They wanted to uh me
           to come and have to come have a chat with you because um I understand
           you've been having some problems since your surgery.
```

Excerpt 13: S13-IMG23

```
IMG23:     Hello I'm Dr [Last name] how are you today?
Patient:   I'm not too good.
IMG23:     Mm-hm.
Patient:   A bit of pain in my gut area, and feeling a bit of hot and cold.
IMG23:     And uhm do you - How about your breathing? There's no problem with your
           breathing?
Patient:   No [no problem].
IMG23:     No difficulty, no chest pain?
Patient:   No.
```

IMG12 in Excerpt 12 took the time to introduce himself, greet the patient (*How do you do?*), ask permission to sit down and explain why he was there (*I was actually rung by ward staff*) using colloquial language (*have a chat with you*). Sitting down close to the patient's bed he also reduced the physical distance and equalized height differences. He thus used his initial 20 seconds to build a relaxed environment for the consultation. IMG23, in contrast, only briefly stated his name and role, offered only a short greeting (*how are you today?*) and after encouraging the patient to talk with a short backchannel (*mm-hm*) launched straight into the medical agenda with a series of closed questions. Moreover, he remained standing for the entire consultation. Like IMG23, half of the 16 IMGs (n=8) in S13 remained standing during the entire interaction, effectively towering over the patient rather than making use of the chair placed near the bed.

Other difficulties in nonverbal communication observed in some role-plays included the adoption of a "closed" posture, that is, standing or sitting with their arms crossed. While this may have been an unconscious reaction to the stress of being recorded, an unfortunate effect was to signal to patients a "lack of desire to interact" (Meadors and Murray 2014: 17). Other IMGs struggled to maintain eye contact with the patients, or at times offered explanations without looking in the direction of the patient (or examiner), another potential signal of disinterest (Harrigan, Oxman and Rosenthal 1985). A lack of eye contact also reduces the surgeon's means of checking for understanding and engaging the patient as an equal partner in shared decision-making. While such nonverbal aspects of communication are not specifically linguistic, their use varies across cultures, as does their relative importance in developing and maintaining rapport.

3.6.2 Forms of Address

The standardized patients in the mock exams were briefed to either state (S12) or withhold (S13) their name unless specifically asked at the beginning of their interaction. The patients in the simulated interactions did not receive any instruction in this regard (C15, C16).

Where patients or role-players did not give their name, only three of the 18 IMGs enquired about the patients' naming preferences, and only one of them addressed the patient by name more than once. In S12, all IMGs who received introductions used the patient's name at least once (usually to repeat and confirm it, or in a greeting), yet only five used it on any subsequent occasion (see Excerpt 14 below). As we saw in the data from James, however, the repeated use of first names can be very useful in putting a consultation on an interpersonal footing. IMG4 used this strategy very effectively:

Excerpt 14: S12-IMG4, examples of use of Geoff by IMG4 throughout the encounter

```
Patient:  Hello, I'm Geoff.
IMG4:     Geoff, nice to see you.
IMG4:     Sure, okay. Geoff I'd like to explain you what exactly we've found on
          - ah - your chest x-ray.
          There is some chance - there's unfortunately Geoff - ah - there is some
          chance - ah - there is some chance that the cancer [...]
          But Geoff there is something else - ah - they may need for you - [...]
          Geoffrey would you be happy with - ah - this mentioned plan [...]
          Geoffrey, any other questions?
```

Excerpt 14 illustrates nicely how IMG4 managed to repeatedly weave the patient's name into his signposts, explanations and while giving bad news. This allowed him to capture and hold the patient's attention at crucial points in the interaction and create a more personal environment (Moore, Yelland and Ng 2011; Wallace et al. 2009).

3.6.3 Interpersonal Strategies

While opportunities for small talk were somewhat constrained by the nature of the OSCE IMG-patient interactions, it was nevertheless quite noticeable that, in marked contrast to James, the IMGs made very little use of interpersonal strategies. There were no instances of self-disclosure and only rare occasions of banter or jokes (see, e.g., Excerpt 15), even in the two longer consultations with real patients where patient-initiated small talk was more prominent (data set 2).

As we see in Excerpt 15 (data set 2), for example, Ranjit's initial banter (*you're too young to be retired*) created affiliation through joint laughter, but the ensuing small talk surrounding the patient's work and social history was noticeably one-sided. While his backchannels (*yes, mm, okay*) encouraged the patient's narrative, Ranjit's only other contribution was an impersonal evaluative statement (*Okay, it's a good thing, then*) which effectively functioned to terminate that small talk sequence. He therefore missed the opportunity to foreground his personal voice and encourage a relaxed atmosphere.

Excerpt 15: C16 (Ranjit)

```
IMG:       You're retired, okay, so that you can take care of your sons now, but
           you don't look retired (...) you're too young to be retired.
           [Laughter]
           (...)
Patient:   They come along with a package that I couldn't refuse.
IMG:       Yes.
Patient:   And, um, that was 18 - but that was 12 months ago.
IMG:       Mm, okay.
Patient:   And, um
IMG:       [Sniffs]
Patient:   lucky I did take it because a place I went to here (...) a couple of
           months ago
IMG:       Mm-hm.
Patient:   to - they farewelled another - a - a - a - couple of my mates who worked
           in the same place.
IMG:       Mm-hm.
Patient:   And they didn't get half the packages I got and they've been there
           longer than me.
IMG:       Okay, it's a good thing, then.
Patient:   Mm.
           (...)
IMG:       Okay, so you don't have any other medical problems? Diabetes,
           hypertension...
```

IMGs who make less use of these strategies than their peers may be seen as less approachable. It is therefore important that they realize both the function interpersonal strategies play in consultations, and how to express them in an appropriately informal way (Dahm and Yates 2013).

3.6.4   Signposts and Softening

The majority of IMGs made good use of signposts and softening techniques to make their actions and reasoning more transparent to the patient. IMG12 in Excerpt 16, for instance, kept the patient informed about what he was planning (*I'd just like to outline what I'd like to do next*) and why (*And the reason I'm going to start you on is* [...]). He also mitigated his assessment of her current condition with a range of softeners (*I think* that you're *a bit* dehydrated, not too much but *a little bit*).

Excerpt 16: S13-IMG12

```
IMG12:    I'd just like to outline what I'd like to do next. So there will be
          several steps. One of the things that we'd like to do, you've already
          got one but I would like to start you on some fluids.
Patient:  Ok
IMG12:    And the reason I'm going to start you on is I think that looking at
          your physical findings, I think that you're a bit dehydrated, not too
          much but a little bit.
```

Other IMGs, however, were less successful. For example, in Excerpt 17, IMG17's signposting question *(Ah, can I ask you some more – more questions?)* framed the interaction as an interview and was followed by a series of bald questions.

Excerpt 17: S13-IMG17

```
IMG:      Okay. And now you're having some pain and fever. Ah, can I ask you some
          more - more questions?
Patient:  Yeah.
IMG:      Ah, do you smoke?
```

3.6.5   Explanations and Medical Language

It was noticeable that the IMGs frequently failed to tailor their explanations to their patients' level of understanding and tended to use medical terminology without either checking their understanding or providing adequate lay explanations.

Excerpt 18: C15 (Thant)

```
IMG:      And so do you have any hypertension?
          (...)
Patient:  Oh
IMG:      Hypertension?
Patient:  Well that's what we've got to try and find out at the moment.
IMG:      Alright.
Wife:     No, hypertension, high blood pressure.
```

We see in Excerpt 18 that the "real" patient, who was also suffering anxiety following a radical prostatectomy and kidney stent removal, was confused by the unexplained use of the medical term *hypertension*, but Thant failed to pick this up and it was left to the patient's wife to clear up the confusion.

Although their technical vocabulary is often excellent, colloquial language could be a particular challenge for IMGs who may not have had as much experience of informal English as they have had with medical English. This meant that they were not always able to supply appropriate lay explanations even when they noticed that patients could not understand certain medical terms.

Excerpt 19: S13-IMG15

```
IMG:      Er, the most common cause after surgery on Day 1 and Day 2 is atelec-
          tasis, which means, um, the lungs, um, there's something going on in
          your lungs.
```

While IMG15 in Excerpt 19 attempted to provide a lay explanation for a medical term, it was vague and inadequate (*there's something going on in your lungs*), and the false start and hesitations (*which means, um, the lungs, um*) could be interpreted as signalling a lack of medical expertise or a deliberate withholding of information rather than as a reflection of difficulties with language (Dahm 2012a). Lay explanations alone, however, do not guarantee a person-oriented consultation frame, as shown in Excerpt 20.

Excerpt 20: S13-IMG23

```
IMG:      [...] and as I've said earlier one of the causes also of fever is
          lung - problems in the lung like atelectasis, because initially uhm uh
          some patients on the first few hours may present difficulty breathing or
          fever and chest tightness and on x-ray they may have atelectasis, and
          then - are you familiar with atelectasis?
Patient:  No.
IMG:      Collapse of the lung. One part of the lung is collapsed.
Patient:  [overspeaking] [yeah, oh yeah?]
IMG:      It can manifest as fever and aside from difficulty in breathing, and
          also one of the causes also of fever is embolic episodes where uh a
          clot is lodged on one of mm uhm your bronchials or one of the parts of
          your lungs,[...]
```

While IMG23 checked for her patient's understanding (*are you familiar with atelectasis*) and provided a lay description (*One part of the lung is collapsed*), she did not, however, recognize the patient's verbal clue (*oh yeah?*) or realize the anxiety her explanation caused, but continued with a terminology-dense account which may have not only increased anxiety but also have had a distancing effect. Clearly, attention to the necessity of providing accessible explanations and the language to do this would be a useful addition to communications training for these doctors.

3.6.6 Exploring Patient Emotion and Expressing Empathy

While most IMGs used nonverbal signals such as nodding and verbal backchannels during patient narratives, their listening strategies were often only superficial and their responses sometimes inappropriate. As we see for example in Excerpt 21 (data set 3), IMG6 used backchannels (*mm-hm*) and mirroring (*very breathless*) to encourage the patient to speak, but the questions that followed the minimal responses (*right; okay*) failed to display an interest in his illness experience. On multiple occasions, she failed to acknowledge the patient's main concerns, explore his feelings or pick up on the empathic opportunities presented. Rather, she adopted an interrogatory stance and used series of closed questions to pursue a biomedical agenda (*Right. Have you got any cough?*). Even after he reiterated his concern about his delayed convalescence, she did not engage with or show concern for his anxieties (*Okay. You don't have any other – ah – ah – conditions like asthma or – ah...*). Moreover, her stream of questions effectively limited his ability to participate as an equal and thus limited opportunities for shared decision-making.

Excerpt 21: S12-IMG6

```
Patient:   Well a - after the operation and I had some - ah - chemotherapy
IMG6:      mm-huh
Patient:   - um - it seemed to be going all right but in the last couple of days
IMG6:      mm-huh
Patient:   I get - um - um - very breathless...
IMG6:      Very breathless.
Patient:   ...you know. I really have a lot of trouble getting my breath
IMG6:      Mmhm
Patient:   and I'm - I'm also getting really tired as well.
IMG6:      Right. Have you got any cough?
Patient:   No.
IMG6:      Fever?
Patient:   No.
IMG6:      Any chest pain on that side?
Patient:   No.
IMG6:      That side?
Patient:   No.
IMG6:      No.
Patient:   No.
IMG6:      Okay. I just - just only breathlessness.
Patient:   Yes, really hard to get my breath sometimes -
IMG6:      Mh-hum
Patient:   um - and - um - that - that makes tired as well
IMG6:      Mh-hum
Patient:   so you know I thought I was getting better really.
IMG6:      Okay. You don't have any other - ah - ah - conditions like asthma or
           - ah...
```

Some IMGs, like Thant (Excerpt 22), were more successful. He picked up on the implication of psychological difficulty in the patient's response that he was fine physically (*I'd say I'm all right, yeah, physically and that yeah*) and followed up with a series of questions (e.g., *So you said physically so*).

Excerpt 22: C15 (Thant)

```
Patient:   I'd say I'm all right, yeah, physically and that yeah. A few aches and
           pains ()
IMG:       So you said physically so
Patient:   I'm not sure quite sure what's going on with this thing. But I've been
           talking to a psych (...) the last couple of days
IMG:       Ah ha. So may I listen to what happened please?
Patient:   Uh, I've just had a talk with him that's all
           [...]
IMG:       So what did you feel? (...) Why why do you have to see psychologist?
Patient:   Uh, I just didn't feel (...) with this thing what's going on. What was
           (...) whether that's psychologically that's what the pain is or (...)
           so we're going to try to sort it out.
IMG:       Mm. So are you feeling (...) upset, depressed
Patient:   Better now yeah
IMG:       Better now. So you - you said better now means previously it was worse?
Patient:   Yeah, well the last couple of days I've been - and today I've been
           feeling really well.
IMG:       All right. Do you have any (...) ((hand gestures)) idea about (...)
           ((hand gestures)) I mean termination of your life or I mean
Patient:   No.
IMG:       No. So you don't have you didn't have (...) suicidal ideation?
Patient:   No I just didn't want to keep going, yeah.
```

Unfortunately, however, Thant's use of increasingly technical language as he struggled to find familiar words to name the patient's feelings, culminating in his question about "suicidal ideation", potentially distanced the patient and detracted from his approachability as a medial practitioner (Coulehan et al. 2001; O'Grady 2011; Roberts et al. 2003).

3.6.7   Tokenistic Reassurance and Empathy

Either as a result of not recognizing the opportunity or perhaps through difficulty in finding the appropriate expression, IMGs often missed opportunities to respond empathically by paraphrasing and reflecting. They tended to show empathy through direct reassurance, often in the form of empathic statements that run the risk of being perceived as tokenistic. For example, IMG10 (Excerpt 23), noticed his patient's feelings, but responded using only routine phrases (*I'm sorry; I understand it's a very difficult situation*) and medical reasoning, and did not explore the emotions underlying the patient's worried question (*More blood tests?*).

Excerpt 23: S12-IMG10

```
IMG:       Ah, we would like to do some [simple] blood tests.
Patient:   More blood tests?
IMG:       Yeah, I'm sorry.
Patient:   That's okay. If we have to...
IMG:       I understand it's a very difficult situation.
Patient:   Thank you. Yes, um, it is.
IMG:       Ah, because we also need to exclude the infection.
```

As discussed above, empathy is an interactive accomplishment dependent on responding to the individual patient, so that IMGs, who rely on ready-made phrases, can often be perceived as uncaring and unengaged. Direct reassurance statements may therefore do little to reassure patients and can even have the opposite effect (Epstein 2000; Roberts et al. 2003).

Excerpt 24 illustrates how the challenge of giving explanations may lead IMGs to give up and resort to direct reassurance. IMG20 specifically elicited any concerns the patient might have (*Do you have any other concern?*) and provided reassurance in the form of normalization (*it is a common infection for the woman*), but resorted to a direct reassurance statement (*Okay don't worry about that.*) when she experienced difficulty explaining the underlying reason.

Excerpt 24: S13-IMG20

```
IMG:      Okay. Do you have any other concern?
Patient:  Um is it serious and...
IMG:      Yeah it is a common infection for the woman because of - you are, you
          are - it should go away after completing the antibiotic. Okay don't
          worry about that.[...]
```

These findings suggest that communications training, on interactive approaches to the expression of empathy that are tailored to the individual patient, as well as on how to achieve this using informal English, would be useful for these IMGs.

3.7   Implications for IMG Surgical Communication Training

A focus on the kinds of features analysed in this chapter is important if non-native English speaker surgeons and native English speaker medical educators are to gain a more conscious understanding of the kinds of behaviours that contribute to successful patient-centred consultations. Like many NES medical novices, the IMG data discussed above include behaviours that Roberts and colleagues (2003: 195) describe as "retractive": a communication style characterized by a failure to listen actively, show genuine empathy or provide accessible explanations. However, the challenges faced by IMGs are compounded by their lack of experience of local, patient-centred approaches to medicine and the communicative and linguistic conventions expected in a community. Although often very competetent in technical English, they have not always had the training or the experiences that can provide the cultural understanding and spoken informal English skills that they will need in interactive, patient-centred contexts. They may be unfamiliar with the socio-cultural conventions of doctor-patient communication in Australia (or the U.S. or wherever they are now practising), and lack an awareness of the subtle linguistic features that facilitate culturally appropriate consultations in that community (Dahm 2011; Dahm and Yates 2013; McDonnell and Usherwood 2008;

McGrath et al. 2012). This is not simply a matter of learning more grammar or vocabulary, but also of gaining the relevant socio-cultural knowledge and learning how to apply and interpret subtle communicative features in ways appropriate to the communicative and medical culture (Dahm, Ogden et al. 2015).

Thus, for example, they may not use certain discourse features because they lack the socio-cultural knowledge that it is appropriate for a surgeon to acknowledge and explore patients' feelings within a patient-centred approach to care. They might also have a limited understanding of linguistic functions associated with certain discourse features, both in interpreting them when they are used by others, and in using them themselves. They may therefore have difficulty noticing the subtle patient cues implicit in loaded vocabulary items, for example, and recognizing these as possible signs of emotional distress. They might also use specific discourse features like "mmh" or "yeah" routinely without understanding the need to respond to and engage with the patient more actively (Roberts et al. 2003). Even highly proficient IMGs who are aware of the discourse features discussed above might not use them as frequently as native speakers because they are unclear as to their function and importance in their new context of practice. As argued above, and evident in the way James conducts his consultations, surgeons need not only to understand that it is important in patient-centred care to communicate empathy and approachability, but also to have the necessary communicative skills and use them interactively and sensitively in response to patient cues. That is, effective communication involves both the socio-cultural knowledge and the communicative skills to project approachability and empathy in a way that does not rely on the simple regurgitation of platitudinous rote-learned phrases.

The challenges faced by the IMGs in this study suggest some aspects of communication skills that could be usefully addressed in targeted communications training. Specifically, our findings suggest that IMGs may need explicit help to develop their interactive skills in empathy and approachability, and perhaps also to understand their importance in the communicative repertoire of the surgeon. Based on our findings, we suggest that surgical communications training for IMGs should target the ability to:

(1) develop an awareness and understanding of the local social and medical communicative conventions (i.e., what might be socially expected of them in their role as surgeons) and

(2) develop an understanding of the discourse features used in the local social and medical communicative context (i.e., how to use culturally appropriate language in their role as surgeons).

Our findings further suggest the importance of explicit attention to linguistic and communicative features used to do the following:

Show empathy through:

- Noticing and reacting to empathic opportunities
- Active, empathic responses to show that they are listening
- Paraphrasing and reflecting
- Providing explanations tailored to a patient's understanding and emotional state

Display their approachability through:

- Strategies that reduce social distance and put patients at ease
- Informal, conversational language
  - Greetings
  - Naming practices
  - Interpersonal strategies
  - Signposts and softening
- A willingness to deviate from the medical agenda

Realistic simulations using standardized patients can provide effective training for surgical trainees and can be supplemented by innovative teaching methods that combine the study of authentic doctor-patient interactions with interactive simulations. Videos or transcripts of authentic and semi-authentic interactions (as Excerpts 1–11 and 12–24 above), can illustrate how patient-centred communication discourse features can be more or less successfully applied in surgical contexts. Through guided analysis of such discourse data, IMGs can be encouraged to identify relevant recurrent linguistic features, discuss how and why these might be used, and reflect on how this consultation approach might differ from their own cultural expectations (Dahm and Yates 2013; O'Grady 2011; Newton 2004).

Overall, approaches that prioritize reflective practice (Candlin and Roger 2013; Spiro 1992) offer a more useful and sustainable alternative to the teaching of discrete skills as a checklist of behaviours or "a box of tricks" (Skelton 2005: 43). In this way, IMGs can benefit from a safe environment in which they can learn about the relevant socio-cultural conventions and associated language features, reflect on and experiment with such features, and thus develop the long-term strategies they will need in actual patient interactions (Dahm and Yates 2013; Epstein, Siegel and Silberman 2008; O'Grady 2011).

3.8   Concluding Remarks and Future Directions

The present study has focused only on one, albeit important, aspect of surgical communication: surgeon-patient consultations. However, IMG surgeons will face many communicative situations that will require them to understand both the socio-cultural conventions that underlie community expectations of appropriate interaction in general, and those that underlie medical communication in particular. They also need to know how to make use of the conversational resources of English to do this interactively, in ways that respond sensitively to different interlocutors and situations. In catering for their communicative needs, therefore, we need to specifically address the issue of cross-cultural variation in medical approaches, and the fact that this might not be immediately apparent to surgeons whose training and experience have been in a different culture and language. IMGs might not be fully aware of the expectations that their Australian patients or colleagues hold of them, nor be completely familiar with the range of specific discourse features that they can use to achieve particular effects in interaction. They therefore have particular educational needs that are best met through innovative reflective practice approaches that draw on authentic interactions and simulations. Reflections should explicitly address cultural and linguistic differences so that IMGs can be guided to see how key components of patient-centred communicative approaches are accomplished through talk. Our study makes a contribution to the evidence-base that is sorely needed to inform the development of communications training appropriate to this aim, that is, training that can provide IMG surgeons with an understanding of the nature of patient-centred communication *and* illustrate the linguistic resources they have at their disposal in English to make it work.

Transcription Notation

(. . .)	Silence shorter than two seconds.
(( ))	Nonverbal action.
–	Sudden cut off (hesitation, false starts).
[. . .]	Part of transcript omitted.
[3.0]	Silence to the nearest tenth of a second.
[text]	Doubt about accuracy of transcribed text.
. . .	Continuity of talk after listener backchannel or brief pause of less than 0.5 seconds.

References

Adolphs, Svenja, Sarah Atkins and Kevin Harvey. 2007. Caught between Professional Requirements and Interpersonal Needs: Vague Language in Healthcare Contexts. In *Vague Language Explored*, edited by Joan Cutting, 3–20. New York: Palgrave Macmillan.

Australian Institute of Health and Welfare. 2011. Medical Labour Force 2009: Detailed Tables. Table 9: Employed medical practitioners, by country of first qualification (a), states and territories. http://www.aihw.gov.au/workforce-data/

Bardovi-Harlig, Kathleen, and Beverly Hartford. 2005. *Interlanguage Pragmatics: Exploring Institutional Talk*. Mahwah, NJ: L. Erlbaum.

Bataller, Rebeca, and Rachel Shively. 2011. Role-Plays and Naturalistic Data in Pragmatics Research: Service Encounters during Study Abroad. *Journal of Linguistics and Language Learning* 2(1): 15–50.

Bauman, Adrian E., H. John Fardy and Peter G, Harris. 2003. Getting It Right: Why Bother with Patient-Centred Care? *Medical Journal of Australia* 179(5): 253–6.

Beach, Mary Catherine, Debra Roter, Susan Larson, Daniel E. Ford, Wendy Levinson and Richard Frankel. 2004. What Do Physicians Tell Patients about Themselves? A Qualitative Analysis of Physician Self-Disclosure. *Journal of General Internal Medicine* 19(9): 911–16. doi: 10.1111/j.1525-1497.2004.30604.x

Bensing, Jozien. M. 1991. Doctor-Patient Communication and the Quality of Care. *Social Science and Medicine* 32(11): 1301–10. doi: 10.1016/0277-9536(91)90047-g

Caffi, Claudia. 1999. On Mitigation. *Journal of Pragmatics* 31(7): 881–909.

Candlin, Sally, and Peter Roger. 2013. *Communication and Professional Relationships in Healthcare Practice*. Sheffield, UK: Equinox Publishing Ltd.

Chur-Hansen, Anna, and Robert John Barrett. 1996. Teaching Colloquial Australian English to Medical Students from Non-English Speaking Backgrounds. *Medical Education* 30(6): 412.

Cordella, Marisa. 2004. *The Dynamic Consultation: A Discourse-Analytical Study of Doctor-Patient Communication in Chilean Spanish*. Amsterdam: John Benjamins.

Coulehan, John L., Frederic W. Platt, Barry Egener, Richard Frankel, Chen-Tan Lin, Beth Lown and William H. Salazar. 2001. "Let Me See if I Have This Right...": Words That Help Build Empathy. *Annals of Internal Medicine* 135(3): 221–7.

Coupland, Justine, Jeffrey Robinson and Nikolas Coupland. 1994. Frame Negotiation in Doctor-Elderly Patient Consultations. *Discourse and Society* 5(1): 89–124.

Dahm, Maria R. 2011. Patient Centred Care: Are International Medical Graduates "Expert Novices"? *Australian Family Physician* 40(11): 895–900.

Dahm, Maria. 2012a. Coming to Terms with Medical Terms: Exploring Insights from Native and Non-Native English Speakers in Patient-Physician Communication. *Hermes – Journal of Language and Communication in Business* 49: 79–98.

Dahm, Maria R. 2012b. Tales of Time, Terms, and Patient Information-Seeking Behavior: An Exploratory Qualitative Study. *Health Communication* 27(7): 682–9. doi: 10.1080/10410236.2011.629411

Dahm, Maria R., Catherine O'Grady, Lynda Yates and Peter Roger. 2015. Into the Spotlight: Exploring the Use of the Dictaphone during Surgical Consultations. *Health Communication* 30(5): 513–20. doi: 10.1080/10410236.2014.894603

Dahm, Maria R., Kathryn Ogden, Lynda Yates, Kim Rooney and Brooke Sheldon. 2015. Enhancing International Medical Graduates' Communication: The Contribution of Applied Linguistics. *Medical Education* 49(8): 828–37. doi:10.1111/medu.12776

Dahm, Maria R., and Lynda Yates. 2013. English for the Workplace: Doing Patient-Centred Care in Medical Communication. *TESL Canada Journal* 30 (Special issue 7): 21–44.

Dedy, Nicolas J., Esther M. Bonrath, Boris Zevin and Teodor P. Grantcharov. 2013. Teaching Nontechnical Skills in Surgical Residency: A Systematic Review of Current Approaches and Outcomes. *Surgery* 154(5): 1000–8. doi: 10.1016/j.surg.2013.04.034

Epstein, Ronald M. 2000. The Science of Patient-Centered Care. *Journal of Family Practice* 49(9): 805.

Epstein, Ronald M., Daniel J. Siegel and Jordan Silberman. 2008. Self-Monitoring in Clinical Practice: A Challenge for Medical Educators. *Journal of Continuing Education in the Health Professions* 28(1): 5–13. doi: 10.1002/chp.149

Fiscella, Kevin, and Richard Frankel. 2000. Overcoming Cultural Barriers: International Medical Graduates in the United States. *JAMA* 283(13): 1751.

Gould, Jon C. 2010. Communications Skills for Surgeons. *Journal of Surgical Research* 160(1): 63.

Hadlow, Jan, and Marian Pitts. 1991. The Understanding of Common Health Terms by Doctors, Nurses and Patients. *Social Science and Medicine* 32(2): 193–6. doi: 10.1016/0277-9536(91)90059-1

Hall, Judith A., Jinni A. Harrigan and Robert Rosenthal. 1996. Nonverbal Behavior in Clinician-Patient Interaction. *Applied and Preventive Psychology* 4(1): 21–37.

Hall, Judith A., Debra L. Roter and Nancy R. Katz. 1988. Meta-Analysis of Correlates of Provider Behavior in Medical Encounters. *Medical Care* 26(7): 657–75.

Harrigan, Jinni A., Thomas E. Oxman and Robert Rosenthal. 1985. Rapport Expressed through Nonverbal Behavior. *Journal of Nonverbal Behavior* 9(2): 95–110. doi: 10.1007/bf00987141

Harvey, Kevin, and Svenja Adolphs. 2012. Discourse and Healthcare. In *The Routledge Handbook of Discourse Analysis*, edited by James Paul Gee and Michael Handford. New York: Routledge.

Hudak, Pamela L., and Douglas W. Maynard. 2011. An Interactional Approach to Conceptualising Small Talk in Medical Interactions. *Sociology of Health and Illness* 33(4): 634–53. doi: 10.1111/j.1467-9566.2011.01343.x

Jaspers, Jurgen. 2012. Interactional Sociolinguistics and Discourse Analysis. In *The Routledge Handbook of Discourse Analysis*, edited by James Paul Gee and Michael Handford. New York: Routledge.

Kaafarani, Haytham M.A. 2009. International Medical Graduates in Surgery: Facing Challenges and Breaking Stereotypes. *American Journal of Surgery* 198(1): 153–4. doi: 10.1016/j.amjsurg.2008.08.004

Larkin, Anne C., Mitchell A. Cahan, Giles Whalen, Demetrius Litwin, David Hatem, Susan Starr, Heather-Lyn Haley, Mark Quirk and Kate Sullivan. 2010. Human Emotion and Response in Surgery (HEARS): A Simulation-Based Curriculum for Communication Skills, Systems-Based Practice, and Professionalism in Surgical Residency Training. *Journal of the American College of Surgeons* 211(2): 285–92. doi: 10.1016/j.jamcollsurg.2010.04.004

Levinson, Wendy, Pamela Hudak and Andrea C. Tricco. 2013. A Systematic Review of Surgeon-Patient Communication: Strengths and Opportunities for Improvement. *Patient Education and Counseling* 93(1): 3–17. doi: 10.1016/j.pec.2013.03.023

McDonnell, Louise, and Tim Usherwood. 2008. International Medical Graduates: Challenges Faced in the Australian Training Program. *Australian Family Physician* 37(6): 481–4.

McGrath, Pamela, David Henderson, John Tamargo and Hamish A. Holewa. 2012. Doctor-Patient Communication Issues for International Medical Graduates: Research Findings from Australia. *Education for Health* 25(1): 48–54.

Meadors, Joshua D., and Carolyn B. Murray. 2014. Measuring Nonverbal Bias through Body Language Responses to Stereotypes. *Journal of Nonverbal Behavior*: 1–21. doi: 10.1007/s10919-013-0172-y

Mishler, Elliot George. 1984. *The Discourse of Medicine: Dialectics of Medical Interviews.* Norwood: Ablex Publishing Corporation.

Moore, Romayne, Michael Yelland, and Shu-Kay Ng. 2011. Moving with the Times: Familiarity versus Formality in Australian General Practice. *Australian Family Physician* 40(12): 1004–7.

Newton, Jonathan. 2004. Face-Threatening Talk on the Factory Floor: Using Authentic Workplace Interactions in Language Teaching. *Prospect: An Australian Journal of TESOL* 19(1): 47–64.

Norfolk, Tim, Kamal Birdi and Deirdre Walsh. 2007. The Role of Empathy in Establishing Rapport in the Consultation: A New Model. *Medical Education* 41(7): 690–7. doi: 10.1111/j.1365-2923.2007.02789.x

O'Grady, Catherine. 2011. Teaching the Communication of Empathy in Patient-Centred Medicine. In *English Language and the Medical Profession: Instructing and Assessing the Communication Skills of International Physicians*, edited by Barbara J. Hoekje and Sara M. Tipton, 43–72. Bingley: Emerald.

O'Grady, Catherine, Maria R. Dahm, Peter Roger and Lynda Yates. 2014. Trust, Talk and the Dictaphone: Tracing the Discursive Accomplishment of Trust in a Surgical Consultation. *Discourse and Society* 25(1): 65–83. doi: 10.1177/0957926513496354

Pilotto, Louis S., Geraldine F. Duncan and Jane Anderson-Wurf. 2007. Issues for Clinicians Training International Medical Graduates: A Systematic Review. *Medical Journal of Australia* 187(4): 225–8.

RACS. 2012. Becoming a Competent and Proficient Surgeon: Training Standards for the Nine RACS Competencies. Royal Australasian College of Surgeons of Australia and New Zealand. http://www.surgeons.org/media/18726523/mnl_2012-02-24_training_standards_final_1.pdf

RACS. 2013. 2012 Annual Activities Report. Royal Australasian College of Surgeons. http://www.surgeons.org/government/workforce-and-activities-reports/

Ragan, Sandra L. 2000. Sociable Talk in Women's Health Care Contexts: Two Forms of Non-Medical Talk. In *Small Talk*, edited by Justine Coupland. Harlow; New York: Longman.

Roberts, Celia, Annie Gillett, Val Wass, Roger Jones and Srikant Sarangi. 2003. A Discourse Analysis Study of "Good" and "Poor" Communication in an OSCE: A Proposed New Framework for Teaching Students. *Medical Education* 37(3): 192–201. doi: 10.1046/j.1365-2923.2003.01443.x

Roberts, Celia, and Srikant Sarangi. 1999. Hybridity in Gatekeeping Discourse: Issues of Practical Relevance for the Researcher. In *Talk, Work and Institutional Order: Discourse in Medical, Mediation and Management Settings*, edited by Srikant Sarangi and Celia Roberts, 473–503. Berlin: Mouton de Gruyter.

Roberts, Celia, and Srikant Sarangi. 2005. Theme-Oriented Discourse Analysis of Medical Encounters. *Medical Education* 39(6): 632.

Robins, Lynne, Douglas Brock, Saskia Witteborn, Lanae Miner, Larry Mauksch and Kelly Edwards. 2011. Identifying Transparency in Physician Communication. *Patient Education and Counseling* 83(1): 73–9. doi: 10.1016/j.pec.2010.05.004

Royal College of Physicians and Surgeons of Canada. 2005. CanMEDS Framework. http://www.royalcollege.ca/portal/page/portal/rc/common/documents/canmeds/framework/the_7_canmeds_roles_e.pdf

Schön, Donald A. 1987. *Educating the Reflective Practitioner*. 1st ed. San Francisco: Jossey-Bass.

Silverman, Jonathan, Suzanne M. Kurtz and Juliet Draper. 2013. *Skills for Communicating with Patients*. 3rd ed. Oxford: Radcliffe Publishing.

Skelton, John R. 2005. Everything You Were Afraid to Ask about Communication Skills. *The British Journal of General Practice: The Journal of the Royal College of General Practitioners* 55(510): 40–6.

Skelton, John R., and F.D. Richard Hobbs. 1999. Descriptive Study of Cooperative Language in Primary Care Consultations by Male and Female Doctors. *BMJ: British Medical Journal* 318(7183): 576–9.

Spiro, Howard. 1992. What Is Empathy and Can It Be Taught? *Annals of Internal Medicine* 116(10): 843–6. doi: 10.7326/0003-4819-116-10-843

Stewart, Moira, Judith Belle Brown, W. Wayne Weston, Ian R. McWhinney, Carol L. McWilliam and Thomas R. Freeman. 2003. *Patient-Centered Medicine: Transforming the Clinical Method*. 2nd ed. Oxford: Radcliffe Medical Press.

Street, Richard L. 2003. Communication in Medical Encounters: An Ecological Perspective. In *Handbook of Health Communication*, edited by Teresa L. Thompson, Alicia Dorsey and Katherine Miller, 63–89. Mahwah, NJ; London: L. Erlbaum Associates.

Suchman, Anthony L., Kathryn Markakis, Howard B. Beckman and Richard Frankel. 1997. A Model of Empathic Communication in the Medical Interview. *Journal of the American Medical Association* 277(8): 678–82.

Tannen, Deborah, and Cynthia Wallat. 1987. Interactive Frames and Knowledge Schemas in Interaction: Examples from a Medical Examination/Interview. *Social Psychology Quarterly* 50(2): 205–16.

Wallace, Lorraine S., David C. Cassada, William F. Ergen and Mitchell H. Goldman. 2009. Setting the Stage: Surgery Patients' Expectations for Greetings during Routine Office Visits. *Journal of Surgical Research* 157(1): 91–5.

White, Sarah J., Maria H. Stubbe, Lindsay M. Macdonald, Anthony C. Dowell, Kevin P. Dew and Rod Gardner. 2014. Framing the Consultation: The Role of the Referral in Surgeon-Patient Consultations. *Health Communication* 29(1): 74–80. doi: 10.1080/10410236.2012.718252

Woodward-Kron, Robyn, Mary Stevens and Eleanor Flynn. 2011. The Medical Educator, the Discourse Analyst, and the Phonetician: A Collaborative Feedback Methodology for Clinical Communication. *Academic Medicine* 86(5): 565–70. doi: 10.1097/ACM.0b013e318212feaf

Yates, Lynda. 2005. Negotiating an Institutional Identity: Individual Differences in NS and NNS Teacher Directives. In Bardovi-Harlig and Hartford (see above), 67–98.

Yates, Lynda. 2010. Pragmatic Challenges for Second Language Learners. In *Pragmatics across Languages and Cultures*, edited by Anna Trosborg, 287–308. Berlin; New York: Le Gruyter Mouton.

Young, Meredith E., Karin R. Humphreys and Geoffrey R. Norman. 2008. The Role of Medical Language in Changing Public Perceptions of Illness. *PLoS ONE* 3(12). doi: 10.1371/journal.pone.0003875

Lynda Yates, PhD, is currently Professor of Linguistics and Associate Dean International in the Faculty of Human Sciences at Macquarie University, Sydney. Her professional experience teaching adult TESOL and consulting to industry has fuelled an interest in research that can feed into the practical concerns of adult language learners and their teachers, and in particular the pronunciation and pragmatic needs of immigrants and transnational professionals. She has a strong commitment to the translation of research findings into professional practice.

Maria R. Dahm completed an Early Career Research Fellowship in Linguistics at Macquarie University, Sydney, and is currently working with the Australian Institute of Health Innovation at Macquarie where she combines her passion for patient-centred health research with her expertise in qualitative and mixed methods research. Her PhD (completed in 2012) examined the impact of medical terminology on English-medium consultations involving non-native speakers. Her research interests include communication and culture in intercultural health and other workplace contexts, health informatics and English for Specific Purposes.

4 Psychological Effects in Surgical Decision-Making: Evidence, Ethics and Outcomes

Y. Gavriel Ansara

4.1 Introduction

In recent years, there has been extensive debate in medicine regarding the extent to which individuals should be involved in decision-making about their own medical care and the role that medical professionals should play in decision-making processes. Currently, the preferred approach in many healthcare settings is *shared decision-making*. This model not only involves the consideration of patients' wishes (as in *patient-centred* healthcare), but also the active involvement of patients in directing and influencing decision-making processes to the extent that they wish to be involved. Thus in order to facilitate effective shared decision-making, health professionals need to be aware of how their presentation of information can affect patients' decisions as well as how they themselves have been affected by information presentation. This chapter will discuss the evidence regarding specific cognitive effects that can influence decision-making, including framing effects, amount of information provided, information source and indirect influences from popular culture, exploring both patients' and surgeons' decision-making.

We like to think that our decisions are rational choices, based on our careful consideration of available evidence. However, our decisions can be altered solely by changes to the way information is presented. This phenomenon is called a *framing effect*, a term for cognitive effects that occur when variations in the description and presentation of information influence people's preferences and/or decisions. Although these kinds of cognitive effects are often described as cognitive "biases", the term "bias" may be somewhat misleading, in that it can only be understood in reference to an assumed "neutral" standpoint. Despite widespread claims of "neutrality" within medical practice, human endeavours are, by their very nature, not ideologically neutral or "bias-free". Increasing recognition of this concern has led some scientists to strive instead for greater reflectivity and greater awareness of how personal, professional and communal values can influence ostensibly scientific judgements.

In the decades since Tversky and Kahneman's (1981) laboratory findings about the "risky-choice" gain-loss framing effect, psychological researchers of decision science have continued to identify and explore cognitive effects that influence choices. *Loss aversion* (Kahneman and Tversky 1984) refers to the finding that people can be more likely to prefer decisions that avoid losses than those that acquire gains. In one example of loss aversion, a study of 79 women university students found that those who received a pamphlet on breast self-examination focused on negative consequences (i.e., a loss-frame) had more positive attitudes toward breast self-examination, were more likely to intend to conduct breast self-examination and were more likely to carry out their intentions to conduct breast self-examination than participants who received a gain-frame or no-arguments pamphlet (Meyerowitz and Chaiken 1987). In this study, participants' desire to avoid loss appeared to provide an effective incentive to perform breast self-examination.

The cognitive effects of loss aversion and personal evaluations of risk perception can be invoked by subtle aspects of medical communication. These subtle communication strategies can have significant impact on patients' decisions. Some of the many aspects that can affect surgical decisions include whether risk is communicated as time intervals or only per total population (for small populations, Weinstein, Kolb and Goldstein 1996), whether risk/benefit is presented in relative or absolute terms (Malenka et al. 1993), whether risks are presented as gains (e.g., 90 per cent chance of survival) or losses (e.g., 10 per cent chance of death) (Gillotti, Thompson and McNeilis 2002), and how graphs are formatted (Ancker et al. 2006; Schapira, Nattinger and McHorney 2001).

Patients without medical training often use heuristics (cognitive short-cuts that are developed through experience) to help with decision-making and judgement about medical treatments. As a result, they may have very different perceptions of complication rates than surgeons (Lloyd 2001; Lloyd et al. 2001; Papagrigoriadis and Heyman 2003), whose professional judgements are typically informed by formal training, clinical algorithms and prior professional experience. Bogardus and colleagues (1999) discuss the potential uses of *anchoring bias*, the cognitive effect that occurs when patients base their decisions on a familiar reference point or on the first information they receive (their "anchor"). They discuss how anchoring bias can be used to help patients make more informed decisions and suggest providing patients with quantitative comparisons to more familiar occurrences such as automobile-related deaths or being injured in sport. They argue that by placing medical risks alongside non-medical risks, we help patients to form more accurate perspectives on the likelihood of a given risk. They also suggest letting patients choose their preferred format for communication about risk. This strategy may make it easier for clinicians to vary their communication style with each patient, rather than having to guess based on social cues and their prior familiarity with the patient.

Another cognitive effect is *ambiguity aversion*, the preference for known outcomes over unknown outcomes, as distinct from loss aversion (Fox and Tversky 1995). For example, Han et al. (2006) examined ambiguity aversion using data from the Health Information National Trends Survey (HINTS), a United States national survey, using data from 3375 participants aged 40 and over with no prior history of cancer. They found that 79 per cent reported high perceived ambiguity about cancer recommendations, but 70 per cent of all respondents still reported high belief in cancer preventability overall. The higher participants' perceived ambiguity ratings, the less they believed it was possible to prevent cancer overall. Although an awareness of uncertainty and ambiguity may decrease some patients' belief in the effectiveness of cancer prevention activities and their resultant engagement in such activities, different patients respond in different ways. Politi and colleagues (2011) found that patients to whom scientific uncertainty was communicated during cancer-related decision-making were more dissatisfied overall with their decisions. This dissatisfaction can have a direct impact on the patient-surgeon relationship and can reduce patient satisfaction with surgical outcomes. However, they also found that the communication of uncertainty had less of an association with patient satisfaction for patients who were involved in decision-making about their care.

Uncertainty may invoke patients' existing prejudices. Patients may treat uncertain information differently depending on demographic characteristics of the source. For example, a study by Cousin, Schmid Mast and Jaunin-Stalder (2013) found that the relation between uncertainty communicated by physicians and patient satisfaction varied by physician and patient gender. These findings documented a statistically significant effect of uncertainty on patient satisfaction only in the case of women physicians and men patients, but not with patients and physicians who were both women, both men, or with a man physician and a woman patient. The finding that men patients had lower patient satisfaction when women doctors communicated uncertainty than when men doctors communicated uncertainty is one of many examples of how sexism and other ideological influences can affect patients' evaluative cognitions of their medical care and the decisions they make based on these cognitions. The cognitive perception of the prototypical surgeon as a man positions surgeons who are women as a marked category and may promote disproportionate criticism of these surgeons (see Hegarty et al. 2013).

One difficulty in studying ambiguity or uncertainty is the lack of standardization in how authors have defined these constructs. Politi and colleagues (2007) identified many different kinds of ambiguity for people making medical decisions and documented that researchers defined and measured uncertainty in very different ways. Most studies have only addressed uncertainty about the probable outcomes, while ignoring how the presentation of uncertainty, personal characteristics and individual values could influence people's understanding of and reactions to uncertainty. For example, Schapira, Nattinger and McHorney (2001) found variable responses to uncertainty in risk estimates presented to patients, with some patients accepting scientific uncertainty and others losing trust in information for which risk estimates were presented as uncertain. Further research on the impact of ambiguity and uncertainty on medical decision-making can use clear operational definitions and measures to improve understanding of these phenomena.

Patients' risk assessments can be related to perceived ambiguity; patient choices may not reflect their preferences in obvious or simple ways. Amsterlaw and colleagues (2006) asked patients to make decisions based on a simple table that summarized two surgical options. The options differed only in death rate (20 per cent vs 16 per cent) and complication rate (1 per cent for each vs 0 per cent). They found that although 51 per cent of participants specified that they would prefer to live with complications rather than die, this stated preference was not reflected in their surgical decisions. Although psychologists have devised complex theoretical models for understanding decision-making processes, evidence from ecologically valid contexts continues to defy the tidy universalist assumptions of these models. The finding of Amsterlaw and colleagues reflects the "real world" logistics of decision-making, in that we not only wish to avoid undesirable outcomes but also must weigh risks in terms of probability rather than certainties when determining our own limits for acceptable risk.

4.2   Psychological Effects in Patients' Surgical and Other Medical Decisions

Experimental evidence has confirmed that multiple types of framing effects can influence patients' decisions in diverse fields of medicine, including but not limited to surgical specialties that range from general to cardiothoracic to gynaecological, obstetric and urological. Tversky and Kahneman's (1992) *cumulative prospect theory* proposed that people often make decisions in which low probability events are given greater weight than more frequent and typical events, a finding supported by their empirical research. Thus decision-making appears in many cases to be influenced by overt and subtle aspects of communication rather than based solely on rational choice as some psychological models for decision-making and planned human behaviour have claimed. The influence exerted by these overt and subtle aspects of communication can have especially important consequences for patient care, where decisions affect people's daily lives and physical outcomes.

In addition to cognitive effects based on the framing of information, the environment and the relational climate can affect decision-making. Fowler and colleagues (2012) analysed survey responses of fee-for-service Medicare-recipient patients who had interventions for prostate cancer or elective coronary artery stenting. These two procedures were selected as useful contexts for studying decision science, because of the limited-to-no difference in improved life expectancy of the prostate surgery or coronary artery intervention over conservative management, the potential consequences to quality of life and the non-immediacy of the need for clinical action. Fowler and colleagues explored the extent to which patients reported having received information about available options, having pros and cons discussed with them, and having their preferences reflected in treatment decisions. They found significant differences between the two procedures: prostate surgical candidates were more likely to report having been offered other treatment options, having been told about the benefits and drawbacks of the more intrusive intervention and having been asked for their preferences, than elective coronary artery stenting candidates. Patients who were aware of alternatives to surgery and more involved in the decision-making process were less likely to choose to undergo surgery.

The surgical decisions that patients make ultimately depend not only on their awareness of available options, but also on their personal values and their perception of how each option is likely to affect key aspects of life that matter to them. For example, although mastectomy and lumpectomy with radiotherapy have similar long-term survival prognosis, Veronesi and colleagues (2002) found that women with breast cancer who were concerned about the effects of radiation were more likely to choose mastectomy over lumpectomy with radiotherapy, whereas women who were more concerned about their spouse's view of their body were more likely to choose lumpectomy with radiotherapy. In addition to concerns about surgical outcomes, it appears that the decision-making model itself can also influence patients' choices. Hawley and colleagues (2009) found that breast cancer patients were more likely to choose mastectomy over lumpectomy with radiotherapy when decisions occurred within a patient-centred rather than surgeon-centred approach.

The aforementioned findings (by Fowler et al., Veronesi et al. and Hawley et al.) illustrate the importance of communicating available options to patients, discussing benefits and drawbacks of these options, and making sure patients' wishes are incorporated into surgical decision-making. As mentioned above, Politi and colleagues (2011) documented the dissatisfaction that cancer patients expressed when physicians communicated uncertainty. However, there was an interaction between patient decision involvement and communication of uncertainty in relation to decision satisfaction. Thus although communicating scientific uncertainty can lead to lower patient satisfaction with cancer treatment decisions, involving patients in the decision-making process can also increase satisfaction in the face of uncertainty.

While I was writing this chapter, numerous friends and colleagues from around the world expressed their interest in learning more about cognitive effects in surgical decision-making. Many voluntarily shared their own experiences as patients, physicians and surgeons. I have included some of these narratives in this chapter, where doing so seemed particularly useful to illustrate my point. All narratives have been de-identified through the use of compositing technique and pseudonyms, except for one surgeon who gave written consent to be mentioned by name. To illustrate how lack of information about treatment options can affect patient decision-making and outcome satisfaction, consider these experiences shared by "Andrew" and "Rita".

> I found out that I had an early stage prostate cancer when various tests confirmed that there was a nodule on my prostate. Aside from this symptom, I had no other way to tell something was wrong. My GP sent me to a urologist, who told me that I needed surgery. I was scared of having an operation, but the urologist told me that I would live longer if I had my prostate surgically removed. She showed me some graphs from studies of prostate cancer, but I was not convinced. I got a second opinion from a radiation oncologist, to explore non-surgical options. In the end, though, I decided to go ahead with surgery because the cancer was still in the early stages, I was fairly young and physically fit, and surgery could possibly cure my cancer completely. Since having surgery, I have not had any further problems with cancer. Having the surgery was scary and difficult, but I am much better off.
> – "Andrew", 68

Andrew's case illustrates how patient satisfaction can be influenced by a patient's sense that the options have been explored adequately prior to decision-making. In the case of non-aggressive prostate cancer, surgery is not universally considered the preferred, first-line treatment (Cookson et al. 2007).

In Rita's case, her enduring perception of the surgeon's overconfidence and failure to adequately discuss risk compounded her negative surgical experience:

> I had cataract surgery but still had blurry vision after my ophthalmologist removed the eye patch. He did some more tests and found that the lens was not at the right power for my vision. The ophthalmologist told me he would need to do another surgery to replace the lens. He assured me that this would solve the problem completely. I was desperate to regain my eyesight, so I said yes. The corrective procedure seemed to go fine, but when I went back the next day, all I could see were shadows and was now permanently blind. I discovered after the fact that I should never have been advised to have cataract surgery. Not only had my ophthalmologist made a mistake the first time that he calculated the intraocular lens power, but he also recommended unnecessary eye surgery for what had previously been tolerable and fairly minor blurry vision. Because of his bad advice, I am now permanently blind.
> – "Rita", 52

Andrew and Rita's experiences highlight the high stakes that can be involved in patients' surgical decision-making processes, the results of which can range from having a life free from cancer and with clear vision to incontinence, death or blindness. The stakes are also high for surgeons, whose influence on a patient's decision to accept or reject a particular surgery could lead to outcomes that range from lifelong appreciation and professional acclaim to loss of licensure or premature retirement. Given the profound consequences of surgical decision-making in both chronic and acute medical situations and the pivotal role that surgeons can play in influencing patients' surgical decisions, it seems surprising that most surgeons receive little to no formal training focused on how to communicate with patients about surgical procedures during the decision-making process.

It appears that the process of gaining consent (usually in the form of a written signature) is often confused with decision-making. In addition to questions about the extent to which surgeons and potential surgical candidates should be involved in decision-making about patients' care, medical communication used to ensure patients' "informed consent" is often conducted by professionals who will not themselves be involved in performing the surgical procedure. This can lead to inadequate disclosure of essential information such as the risks and benefits of the proposed surgical technique and of potential alternative techniques, the likely surgical outcomes, the extent to which possible complications can be remedied and the logistics of post-operative follow-up. Take the following experience shared by emergency medicine specialist "Dr Rashad", who described the ethical dilemma she encountered when being asked to obtain consent from patients for surgery during her medical residency:

> I am not a surgeon, but I was required to complete an orthopaedic rotation in order to complete my emergency medicine residency. At the beginning of my rotation, the orthopaedic senior resident would assign certain tasks that I knew to be outside my scope, such as consenting patients for surgery. It is essentially impossible for me to consent a patient for a procedure that I do not and will not do: I don't know the statistics to offer a patient or the realistic, possible outcomes. As such, I was not able to offer an honest risk/benefit/alternative analysis to a patient.
>
> After the first two episodes of sending me to "consent" a patient they stopped sending me: I would name the procedure to the patient and state that the purpose of the procedure was to try to fix their problem (e.g.: fractured femur). I would state that the basic risks to surgery are bleeding, infection and death, but if the patient wanted more information than that, I would be happy to call the operating surgeon, as I am not qualified to answer such reasonable questions. Naturally, the patients wanted more information, and it wasn't an unreasonable request on their part. I think the orthopaedic surgeons felt that the surgeries were routine, basic and low-risk, and as such, I should be able to consent them. These surgeries are routine to the surgeon, not necessarily to the person whose life will be changed, for better or worse, by the procedure. They are not routine to me; I've never scrubbed into an orthopaedic surgery. Still, I never truly felt pressured to lie to patients, as I knew my department would support ethical behaviour. And it was the right thing to do for my patients.
> – "Dr Rashad"

4.3   Role-Framing

Even the role descriptions of people who engage with medical services are cognitive frames that influence people's perceptions of their agency and function in decision-making processes. Medical sociologist Ewen Speed (2006) has explored how concepts such as "patient", "consumer" and "survivor" frame the discourses of people who use mental health services and can simultaneously influence and reflect how they interact with health systems and professionals. Patient discourses emphasize pathology and tend to objectify the person, treating them more as problems to be fixed than as individuals equipped with responsibility and agency (e.g., "they started me on medication"). Consumer discourses accept a pathologizing approach to the presenting issues, but problematize the passive relationship between patient and system that characterizes patient discourses. Consumer discourses typically promote a negotiated relationship between the service user and health services (e.g., "I did not like the medication, but instead asked to discuss alternative treatment options"). In contrast to patient and consumer discourses, survivor discourses emphasize the relation between the person and their wider environment and cast the person as the author of their own story (e.g., "To understand me, you have to understand the society I'm living in. The problem isn't solely inside my head, so medication might not fix it."). Survivor discourses often involve redefining the problem as interactional and variable, rather than as an intra-psychic property of an individual. In so doing, survivor discourses often highlight systemic service barriers, challenge the objectification and pathologizing of people with presenting issues in medical contexts, and expose the limitations of patient and consumer discourses.

Medical historian and critical disability studies scholar Geoffrey Reaume (2002) has documented how shifts in psychiatric approaches to people who have received psychiatric diagnoses have coincided with corresponding changes of framing, from positioning them first as "lunatics", then as "patients" and subsequently as "people". Although "patient" is likely to be one of the most familiar and ubiquitous concepts applied to people who engage the services of medical professionals, it is worth considering the assumptions contained in this construct. For example, some "patients" are also medical professionals, and most medical professionals will seek healthcare at multiple points across the lifespan. Although I use the "patient" discourse throughout this chapter, I do so reluctantly, due to practical considerations such as ensuring its broad intelligibility and familiarity among medical professionals. It is well worth considering the practical limitations of utilizing the "patient" ideology when communicating with people about important surgical decisions that may require them to engage in critical evaluation and agentic action beyond the typical "patient" role.

4.4 Influence of Celebrities, Mass Media and Television

Broad, high-penetrance cultural influences such as naming practices extend beyond simple communication to affect how we treat people, which decisions we make about them, and how they view themselves. Other cultural influences can also affect the decisions people make about themselves and their awareness of normative community responses to medical dilemmas. Many of the values people hold are shaped and perpetuated by their family culture and the intersecting cultural narratives shared in their communities of influence. The medical experiences recounted by celebrities, mass media and loved ones can determine how we perceive treatment options and the extent to which we consider ourselves susceptible to illnesses or complications.

Consider the narratives made familiar by mass media: the young patient stricken with a tumour that could kill her, her parents faced with the decision to approve surgery with a high death rate; the pregnant mother of three children who must choose between the risk of surgery that could kill her but save her baby or the procedure that could save her so that she can be alive for her other children, but risk the death of the foetus. Television medical dramas conjure these images in the minds of the public and train us to view medical decision-making in the broad brush strokes of black and white, and life and death. These shows train viewers to view surgeons as miracle-workers whose uncanny and even infallible judgements never cease to impress. Yet surgical decisions often involve far more subtle and nuanced questions. Often, the question is not "life or death", but instead a more existential question, "What kind of life is worth living to *you*?" or "How will these options affect my life goals?" (see, for example, Brody 1993). A nephrologist who heard about my chapter conveyed his concern that public attention to dramatic, "life-and-death" situations in television medical dramas can lead patients to overlook the importance of making careful surgical choices when dealing with routine and chronic medical situations, noting that some routine decisions would preclude future treatment options.

Decision science has produced compelling evidence that our judgements are shaped and influenced by cognitive effects and not determined solely by factual evaluation of probable outcomes. Our cognitive decision-making processes are also affected by external influences outside of laboratory conditions, such as television and other forms of mass media. The actions of celebrities and television characters create societal norms that can influence our behaviour. For non-surgeons, most knowledge about surgical decision-making that does not come from direct personal experience is likely to come from mass media, such as television, films and headline news. These scenarios are often sensationalist and extreme.

In addition to these television scenarios, we also have influences from celebrities. Two examples of celebrity influence are responses to actor and humanitarian

Angelina Jolie Pitt's double mastectomy and reactions to journalist Julie Chen's blepharoplasty. After testing positive for a mutation of the BRCA1 gene that is associated with breast cancer, Angelina Jolie Pitt announced her decision to undergo preventive double mastectomy. A resultant phenomenon known as "the Angelina Jolie effect" has occurred worldwide. For example, the United Kingdom has seen a sustained 2–2.5-fold increase in referrals for genetic testing for BRCA1/2 since Jolie Pitt announced the results of her test and her subsequent risk-reducing mastectomy (Evans et al. 2014).

Although greater awareness of a disease can lead to increased screening rates, as in the case of Angelina Jolie Pitt's disclosure of her surgery, the success of her breast reconstruction could lead to unrealistic expectations of breast reconstruction for other women. This problem of unrealistic expectations has been studied extensively in reference to depictions of cardiopulmonary resuscitation (CPR) on television. Studies have shown that television depictions of CPR can lead the public to hold unrealistic beliefs about survival and consequences, with the survival rates predicted by participants far exceeding the most optimistic survival rates reported in the medical literature (Diem, Lantos and Tulsky 1996; Donohoe, Haefeli and Moore 2006; Jones, Brewer and Garrison 2000). It is crucial to note that the procedure does not need to be depicted many times to distort viewers' perceptions; even a few dramatic depictions can affect participants' ratings regarding the likelihood of a successful outcome (Van den Bulck and Damiaans 2004). These findings document that outcomes portrayed on television can lead people to think that the successful CPR performed on a television character reflects a typical outcome in actual medical situations. We may assume that art imitates life when it comes to surgical heroism in life-threatening situations, but the evidence suggests that we are tragically and regrettably misinformed.

Journalist Julie Chen is credited widely with being a trendsetter in Asian women's beauty norms. Her decision to have blepharoplasty (cosmetic surgery to alter eyelid appearance) reflects the simultaneous normalization of stereotypically Anglo-American facial features and pathologizing of facial features typically associated with other ethnicities. As noted by Ginwala (2014: 13), "the language surrounding double eyelid surgery contributes largely to the issue of normalizing Anglo-European features. Advertising the procedure as 'removing excess skin' implies a flaw; excess that doesn't belong. It's as if by some design mishap, Chinese women are born with extra skin that must be corrected surgically." Julie Chen's professional success following blepharoplasty and media reports about the success of her surgery illustrate how ethnocentric prejudices about ideal appearance can alter perceptions of an Asian woman's face, with her natural features being labelled as "flawed" with "extra skin", whereas her surgically altered face is depicted as "beautiful" and "normal". The emphasis on surgical reinforcement of ethnocentric norms has the alarming result of downplaying the cosmetic and physical risks involved in facial surgery during the decision-making process.

4.5   Complexity of Decision-Making for Oneself

As may be apparent from the earlier examples in this chapter, decision-making does not necessarily follow an obviously systematic process, and information may come from multiple sources within and beyond the context of medical encounters (Steginga et al. 2002). Although many influences can affect decision-making across the population at large, no sole influence can accurately predict a given person's decision. In previous sections, I have addressed how communication in consultations and in broader societal contexts can affect surgical decisions. Individual, cultural and generational differences can also influence such decisions. People's reasons for deciding whether or not to have surgery can vary widely based on demographic characteristics (Rivera et al. 2000). Some studies suggest that older adults may be less averse to ambiguity (e.g., Sproten et al. 2010). Culture can affect not only which decisions are made, but also how decisions are made and the extent to which family members are involved in decision-making processes (e.g., Maly et al. 2006; Galavotti and Richter 2000; Ang et al. 2002). Some studies have found differences in the proportion of eligible women and men who receive particular surgeries independent of clinical factors, but the reasons for these reported gender differences in surgical treatment decisions are unclear (e.g., Poisson et al. 2010; cf. Tobin et al. 1987). Hyde (2005), in a review of 46 meta-analyses, found that there is a tendency to assume gender differences even where the sizes of the reported effects are minuscule and where the findings appear to document unexpected gender similarities. Thus people may be likely to assume that such divergence is due to inherent differences between women and men rather than variations in clinicians' judgements about and communications with patients of different genders.

Patients who have a high level of health literacy and who understand the risks and benefits of treatment are not necessarily immune from *affective forecasting errors*, a term that describes patients' mis-prediction of how they will be affected by post-intervention impairment, disability labels or complications. These errors may sometimes be mistaken for fatalism or depression. People who have previously been considered "healthy" are more likely to make affective forecasting errors and often have difficulty imagining that they will develop new coping mechanisms or physical adaptations. In contrast, people who have experienced similar complications may have a more accurate estimation of their ability to cope with such challenges (Halpern and Arnold 2008). Emotional distress can block patients' memories about good times and cloud their ideas about the future (Eich and Forgas 2003; Philippot and Schaefer 2001). Patients who are emotionally distressed may also distance themselves from the situation (Burgess et al. 2006). Thus it may be important for a surgeon to respond appropriately to the emotional distress that a patient or loved one is experiencing, prior to addressing possible cognitive effects and proceeding with the decision-making process. However, to further illustrate the complexity of coexisting cognitive effects, distress may sometimes lead to more accurate perceptions of time in a phenomenon known as *depressive realism* (Kornbrot, Msetfi and Grimwood 2013). Whereas some patients may find their perceptions impaired by distress, others who experience some level of depression may demonstrate more realistic perceptions of post-operative recovery duration.

Sleep deprivation can negatively impact aspects of cognition related to decision-making skills (Killgore et al. 2006), particularly for decisions that involve unexpected situations, creative thinking, concentration and effective communication (e.g., Anderson and Platten 2011; Harrison and Horne 1999; Lim and Dinges 2010; Martella et al. 2011). One strategy to improve the quality of patient decision-making is to time conversations about surgical decision-making in a way that ensures that patients and family members are adequately rested and have optimal stress levels; this advice may be far easier to give than it is to enact in time-critical situations. Medical professionals can also be aware that their own sleep deprivation can affect their responses to patients during crucial interactions and can increase their vulnerability to the adverse emotional consequences that can result from these encounters (Zohar et al. 2005).

Acute and chronic pain can also affect patients' cognitive decision-making skills. Apkarian et al. (2004) documented specific cognitive deficits in emotional decision-making among patients living with chronic back pain and patients living with chronic complex regional pain syndrome, although people living with chronic pain in this particular study did not differ from others in short-term memory, attention and intellectual ability. In their review of clinical and preclinical studies of how pain affects cognition, Moriarty et al. (2011) discussed both the direct and indirect cognitive effects of chronic pain, including deficits in attention, learning, working memory, information processing speed, perceptual learning ability, perceptual-motor coordination and executive functions such as initiating and planning actions, evaluating potential consequences of actions, organization, goal-directed behaviour, emotional decision-making and emotion regulation.

Given that people living with chronic pain often experience resulting fatigue, sleep disturbances, emotional distress and the need for analgesic medication that can affect cognition, it can be difficult to identify which underlying factors are responsible for the association between chronic pain and cognition. In a longitudinal case-control study, Seminowicz et al. (2011) found that patients with chronic low back pain who received effective spine surgery or facet joint injection treatment had increased cortical thickness in a previously thinner area, reduced pain, reduced physical impairment and improved performance on an attention-demanding cognitive task at six months after intervention. These findings suggest that adequate treatment for chronic pain can lead to functional and structural reversal of neurological and cognitive impairments and can facilitate subsequent restoration of impaired brain functions. However, these findings also highlight the importance of identifying and treating pain early to avoid such deficits.

Medical professionals often underestimate the magnitude of physical pain among patients and their consequent need for pain medications (Solomon 2001). The perceptual gap between patients and medical professionals can be particularly acute with patients from societally marginalized populations and those whose cultural norms for pain communication may differ from those of the medical professional, even when medical interpreters are used (e.g., Schouten and Schinkel 2014). Medical professionals' dismissal of children's self-reported pain often results in the traumatic experience of inadequate analgesic medication (e.g., Dong et al. 2012). Being alert to the wide variation in pain expression and communication – including signs of pain in cultures where the explicit communication of pain is taboo or stigmatized – can minimize the detrimental effects of pain on patient decision-making.

4.6   Influence of Cognitive Effects on Medical Professionals' Decisions

A broad range of factors can affect medical professionals' decisions and recommendations. Despite extensive training, medical professionals are not immune to cognitive effects in clinical decision-making. In their review of literature on doctors' decision-making biases, Bornstein and Emler (2001) identified a variety of cognitive effects or "biases" that can affect doctors' processes of information gathering, interpretation of evidence, diagnostic reasoning and treatment decisions. These include diagnostic effects such as:

(1) confirmation bias, the tendency to search for and privilege evidence that supports what one already believes;
(2) representativeness bias, the tendency to give undue weight to evidence that appears typically representative of a particular diagnosis or to assume that results from a small sample accurately reflect the general population;
(3) availability bias, the tendency to estimate the likelihood of an event based on how readily one can remember similar past events in one's own experience;
(4) hindsight bias, the tendency to retroactively alter one's evaluation of the likelihood and predictability of a clinical outcome or diagnosis, without a factual basis; and
(5) regret bias, the tendency to overestimate a negative clinical outcome or diagnosis due to anticipated regret in the event that a negative consequence would be missed.

Bornstein and Emler also found treatment biases such as:

(1) regret bias, as above, the tendency to overestimate a negative clinical outcome;

(2) outcome biases, the tendency to feel more responsible for negative outcomes that result from action than for those that result from inaction, an effect that may lead doctors to feel more hesitant to take action than to refrain from action and may lead them to take credit for positive outcomes more often than negative outcomes;

(3) framing effects described above; and

(4) number of alternatives, the uncertainty produced by seemingly similar options that can lead doctors to avoid starting a new treatment.

As mentioned earlier in this chapter, when discussing cognitive "biases", it is important to note that it is not possible to have a "neutral" or "unbiased" position, because people bring a variety of beliefs, emotions, past experiences and social influences to each situation. Instead of striving for an unobtainable clinical objectivity, it may be more practically useful for surgeons to reflect on how their personal motivations and beliefs may influence their views and to engage in critical thinking about their professional practices. Such reflexive habits will also challenge surgeons to learn more about patients' own motivations and beliefs, a process that can aid in understanding the need for treatment recommendations and decision-making processes to be tailored for a particular patient's beliefs, preferences and values. The multidisciplinary meeting can help to broaden medical professionals' perspectives, counteract systematic bias and validate treatment suggestions.

Disciplinary limitations can affect medical professionals' clinical perceptions and judgements. LeBlanc, Brooks and Norman (2002) tested medical students and experts by showing them head-to-shoulder photographs of patients that displayed obvious features of the presenting medical problems, with a majority of images taken from medical textbooks. The extent to which seemingly obvious features were identified was strongly influenced by context. LeBlanc and colleagues found that both participant groups identified more of the obvious features when the accepted diagnosis was suggested to them and that both groups experienced about 20 per cent increased diagnostic accuracy when key features that were clearly visible in the photographs were verbally described for them. For example, tan skin was misinterpreted as jaundice despite evidence of white sclerae (rather than the yellow sclerae typically associated with jaundice), and a round face was misinterpreted as facial oedema. Implicit suggestions such as having read a journal article on a particular topic recently could lead to not only more accurate positive identifications but also to more false positives; in these cases, normal human variations were misidentified as indications of pathology.

Even one's medical specialty can be a major factor in perceptions about which anatomical variations are natural, attractive or require surgery. Reitsma and colleagues (2011) showed 164 women and men who were gynaecologists, general practitioners and plastic surgeons four images of vulvae with labia minora of different sizes. Two had been surgically reduced, and two were natural. Participants rated each image on naturalness, attractiveness, their personal preference and society's ideal. The gynaecologists and plastic surgeons were asked whether they would perform a reduction on each image for physical complaints only, cosmetic complaints only, or both. The plastic surgeons were more likely than the GPs and gynaecologists to view the natural vulva with the largest labia minora as unnatural, distasteful and eligible for surgical reduction. Plastic surgeons were also more willing than gynaecologists to perform labia minora reduction for women, regardless of the specific labia minora size or whether the woman had a physical complaint. Men physicians were more likely to prefer surgical reductions than women physicians. Across all physician groups, an overwhelming majority believed that the very small labia minora characteristic of a post-surgical appearance represented society's ideal. This study illustrates how specialty-dependent aesthetics and personal preferences and values can influence a physician's surgical recommendations.

4.7 Surgeons' Decision-Making

Conscientious surgeons may underestimate the extent to which potential surgical candidates, their loved ones, and colleagues in multidisciplinary teams are influenced by the information they have received. Although all sources of information can influence those involved in surgical decision-making, the subtle linguistic framing in verbal and textual communications and the extra-linguistic framing in schematic diagrams and other visual aids can be particularly persuasive. The finding that people can be influenced to shift their preferences and even to change their decisions to give or withdraw consent based on how information is presented raises a number of ethical, legal and clinical concerns about how surgeons present information.

An awareness of framing effects and other cognitive influences in the psychology of surgical decision-making can improve surgical practice and clinical outcomes. Surgeons who wish to integrate an awareness of these effects into their professional interactions can consider carefully how they communicate surgical risks and benefits. General surgical resident "Dr Maliki" explained how she applies the science and art of framing effects to her communications with prospective surgical patients:

> Patients often want to know health professionals' opinions on what they should do or what the professional would do if they were in the patient's shoes. This can be a tricky situation, because patients are exercising their autonomy by seeking competent advice (whether from friends, the internet, or health professionals), yet we don't want patients to make decisions just because they want to do what we would do. There may be a few options that offer different risks and benefits.
>
> In this situation, I try to frame information in terms of the patient's own goals, priorities, and concerns and how the most common or major risks and benefits of each option would likely affect them. I try to present a balanced picture based on these

aspects of the patient's life. Most of the time, it is impossible to cover every possible risk and benefit, so we try to cover those that are common as well as the risks that can be devastating.

Dr Maliki stressed the importance of considering a patient's own values and priorities, when discussing surgical options:

Depending on what the patient seems to be looking for, I would then make a recommendation based on weighing my perception of their goals, priorities and concerns against the common or major risks and benefits to them. If a patient is likely to get great benefit from a treatment with few risks, then I stress this ratio, and the same if a treatment is likely to be high risk with little benefit. The difference is that I will probably not mention a high risk–low benefit treatment unless the patient is running out of options or has specific goals that make other treatments even less beneficial. Ultimately, my presentation of information depends on how well I understand the patient's goals and priorities – both in life and in their healthcare.

Plastic and reconstructive urological surgeon Dr Curtis Crane[1] shares Dr Maliki's belief that patients' own goals should guide how surgeons frame the information they provide for patients who are considering surgery:

I look at my role as a healthcare provider as a counsellor or as teacher. I try to, number one, figure out what my patient's surgical goals are and then, number two, make their surgical goals as safe as possible to obtain. So if I find that a patient is deviating from a safe path to an unsafe path and undertaking undue risk, then I proceed based on a series of assumptions: mainly that the patient is following a logical approach to their healthcare and also wants to mitigate as much risk as possible. With that assumption in mind, I describe in great detail my concerns with the risks and then immediately give a safer alternative to accepting those risks, which might be staging a surgery across two or three operations, having surgery at another time, or having a different surgery altogether.

After I sense that the patient has a very clear understanding, I let them make their own decision. Very rarely, there are cases where I feel like a patient is accepting too much risk for their desired goal. If that's the case, then I have to evaluate the patient's position and mental status. Number one, is the goal just so important to them that they will accept any risk to get to it – sometimes that is logical for that patient. In that case, I just make sure everything is spelled out in informed consent, because the ultimate goal is the patient's happiness. If, on the other hand, I think the patient is behaving irrationally or not understanding what I'm trying to explain, then I try to incorporate the assistance of other healthcare providers, or perhaps even a psych consult, to make sure that the patient is logical, rational, and has decision-making capacity to pursue risky surgery. That's the kind of decision-tree I use.

---

1   Dr Crane is the only surgeon with whom I spoke who gave me permission to use his name instead of a pseudonym, when quoting him for this chapter.

Dr Crane explained how he approaches sensitive discussions about surgical risks and benefits with patients who are considering gender affirmation surgery. As with many other surgical specialties, surgical decision-making in this context can involve the consideration of multiple options beyond whether or not to undergo surgery:

My practice usually involves patients making decisions between surgeries or combinations of surgeries rather than between having or not having a surgery at all. A common decision my patients make is whether to pursue urethral lengthening as part of their metoidioplasty or phalloplasty. In a patient who wants to stand to urinate, but they're extremely overweight and have a paucity of labial tissue, making it difficult to reconstruct a urethra, and I think the chances of being able to stand to urinate are pretty small, I say, "I'm concerned that you don't have enough local tissue. You also have an excess of subcutaneous fat, limiting the projection of your phallus, so I think there's a low chance for hygienic urethral lengthening, meaning you're not showering the front of your clothes with urine every time you urinate. I can save you 10–20 per cent of risk and around $10,000 (patients often understand money), if we just don't pursue urethral lengthening. I can make you a very nice phallus, but you would sit to urinate."

I don't want to completely destroy patients' dreams, so I usually follow with, "If standing to urinate is absolutely critical to your happiness, then we can pursue this – but these are the risks, and these are my concerns." If you're the kind of person who says, "Well I've been sitting all my life. That's a lot of money and a lot of risk for something that more than likely I will not be happy with and will not achieve my goals," then let's save you some time, some money and some risk, and the large majority of times in those situations, I have a patient who says "saving $10,000 sounds pretty good, and not having the risk of urethral fistula and stricture would certainly be nice", and then at that point, they often say "okay let's not do the urethral lengthening".

"Dr Hathaway", a general surgeon, described some of the strategies he uses to communicate the gravity of the situation and the options available to patients with serious illnesses:

I believe presentation is very important. When I have to deliver sombre news or discuss life and death situations with a patient and their family, I make sure to dress more formally – those are the days when I wear a jacket and tie. I want every aspect of my appearance, from my clothing to my body language, to show I take seriously the gravity of the situation... I also pay attention to the positioning of my body in terms of whether I am at the patient's eye level, the position of my hands, and the angle at which the chairs in my consulting room are positioned. I will also sometimes draw pictures for patients, based on their personal interests and area of knowledge. If I'm dealing with an athlete, I will try to discuss the situation using analogies related to their sport or activity.

Using these techniques, Dr Hathaway accomplishes the dual aims of presenting himself as a credible professional and demonstrating his accessibility and attentiveness to patients. His awareness of how physical alignment can affect patient perception is also likely to improve the communication quality and patient satisfaction.

4.8   Surgical Decision Aids/Strategies/Tools

In addition to these strategies used by the individual surgeons above, an increasing number of medical settings now employ surgical decision aids and tools in routine practice. Some tools for health professionals such as Adjuvant Online and Recurrence Online are designed to improve clinical decision-making skills, whereas others assist surgeons in determining how to best advise and treat individual patients. Adjuvant Online compiles statistical models from research findings to calculate the probability of disease-free survival, recurrence, death from cancer and death from other causes for various treatments using characteristics about the patient's cancer. Many decision aids are designed to assist patients in discussing and deciding on treatments with their doctors; these aids may be marketed directly to patients or used by clinicians during their interactions with patients.

Thinking strategically about framing effects can enhance surgical practice, improve surgical outcomes, and assist surgeons, patients and their loved ones in making evidence-based decisions. In addition to decision aids designed for patients, creative decision aids are available for surgeons and surgical trainees. The Surgical Improvement of Clinical Knowledge Ops game (Tsui, Lau and Shieh 2014), known by the acronym SICKO, is a game that uses virtual patients to simulate the surgical decision-making process for surgeons and surgical trainees. SICKO facilitates the evaluation of surgical trainee skills and can improve surgical training quality.

At the Boston-based Massachusetts General Hospital (MGH) (Bresnick 2014), the queriable patient interface dossier (QPID) (Campbell et al. 2012; Harvey, Krishnaraj and Alkasab 2014) functions as a predictive analytic system that can determine a patient's surgical risk and provide a corresponding red, yellow or green indicator. The QPID was first developed in 2007 by MGH-based radiologist Michael Zalis and software architect Mitch Harris, whose initial aim was to develop a method of extracting useful patient data from electronic health records. The QPID rapidly became a clinical decision-making aid based on machine learning. Machine learning is a field that involves the use of algorithms to learn from data and build models that can be applied to make predictions or inform decisions. According to MGH representatives, the American College of Surgery has discussed the possibility of routine application of the QPID across the U.S. However, standard use of the QPID would require electronic versions of paper charts and linkage of patient data from all medical providers involved in healthcare. At present, these limitations mean that predictive analytic tools can be most effective when combined with other elements of clinical decision-making. Clinical decision-making is not merely a technical process grounded in science, but also an art that requires consideration of interpretive, intuitive and experiential factors.

4.9 Guidelines for Optimal Surgical Decision-Making Outcomes

If the myriad psychological influences discussed in this chapter seem complex, consider that I have provided only brief coverage of some among many such effects and that the effects compound one another in complex ways that require further exploration in future research. Despite the complexity of variables and processes involved in surgical decision-making, it is possible to apply evidence-based communication strategies to assist people who are considering surgical procedures. For example, surgeons should be aware that patients might not be making decisions based on precise numbers (e.g., risk). Reyna (2008) found that patients retain information better when it is communicated in terms of the "gist" (i.e., the overall sense or big picture message, such as "this is a very low risk") rather than as a precise number ("the risk is .05 per cent"). It may also be helpful to note that reasoning functions independent of memory. Gist is more than a vague representation of risk; it incorporates insight from past experiences with new knowledge. Patients do not need to understand all of the specific risks to make decisions, if they have a sense of the gist. Being able to recall facts may not necessarily translate into better patient decision-making.

Siegel (2010) developed recommendations for clear communication of risk. These recommendations include the avoidance of solely verbal descriptions of risk, particularly the use of vague words such as "rare" or "common". Although the European Commission (Berry et al. 2003) recommended using "common" to describe risks of up to 10 per cent, participants interpreted "common" to refer to risks of 45 per cent on average. The EC also recommended using "rare" to refer to risks of .01–.1 per cent and "very rare" for risks of up to .01 per cent, but participants understood these to mean 8 and 4 per cent, respectively, on average. Siegel (2010) concluded that patients may be less likely to accept treatments based on these interpretations of risk. Berry and colleagues (2003) advised the use of multiple formats to communicate risk, including pictures when possible. When making comparisons, they suggested that medical professionals use a common denominator to avoid patients having to do their own calculations; use absolute numbers instead of relative numbers; when describing risk of less than 1 per cent use frequencies (e.g., 1 in every 1000); and individualize estimates rather than providing generic information.

The science of social influence is similar to the study of framing effects, in that the presentation of a request affects whether it will be accepted. Redelmeier and Cialdini (2002) discussed how social influence functions in medical practice. The aim of raising surgeons' awareness about social influence is not intended to negate patient autonomy, but rather to ensure surgeons understand how social influence can function to inhibit patient autonomy in subtle and unintended ways during medical interactions. This understanding can assist surgeons who wish to reinforce patient preferences and to prevent these preferences from being derailed by others. Redelmeier and Cialdini (2002) list seven principles of influence that can provide a useful framework for understanding not only patients' choices but also the subtle and unacknowledged ways in which medical professionals can influence patients' choices:

- reciprocation: e.g., initiating a surgical conversation by contributing something to the patient such as praise for previous decisions;
- concession: e.g., offering a more palatable (to the patient) option that may be less preferred by the surgeon;
- consistency: e.g., praising the patient for continuing on a multi-staged surgery;
- endorsement: e.g., telling a patient about other patients' successful surgical outcomes to establish a new social comparison group;
- liking: e.g., responding in a pleasant and supportive way to a patient who is facing negativity;
- authority: e.g., giving surgical advice and answering questions directly and not through intermediaries; and
- scarcity: e.g., identifying unique benefits of the treatment option.

Each of these strategies can make the proposed treatment option appear more attractive to patients, even when surgical treatment may not be the most appropriate method of achieving patients' desired outcomes. Surgeons and other health professionals can use these strategies to evaluate the ethical dimensions of their own use of influence with patients or to assist patients in making a firm and lasting decision about their preferred option. Surgeons can also take steps to avoid these forms of influence when attempting to present options that prioritize patients' own worldviews and preferences. Being aware of variability in how patients perceive and respond to surgeon factors can also be helpful, as discussed earlier regarding sexist reactions to women professionals.

Alignment with some aspects of patients' preferred communication style can also improve patient satisfaction. Cousin and colleagues (2012) found that a high caring communication style by a virtual physician was associated with greater patient satisfaction regardless of participants' preferences, whereas patient satisfaction with the level of sharing varied by individual preference for low versus high sharing. Although some patients will not wish to direct their own case, there may be similar aspects of communication and decision-making styles for which patient preferences can vary. Patient satisfaction can be improved by actively discussing patients' communication preferences and by attempting orientational alignment with patients' preferred levels of authority and agency. Whereas some patients will prefer to be provided with all possible information, others may experience high sharing as overwhelming or as information overload. Some patients will prefer to be directed by their surgeon, some will prefer to direct the surgeon, some will prefer to collaborate and others will prefer to involve additional people such as designated family and spiritual authorities in their decision-making processes. Understanding the worldview, values and preferences of patients can provide clinically useful guidance on whether a proposed surgical intervention is likely to result in patient satisfaction and on which of the available surgical options is most likely to result in an optimal outcome in terms of how each patient defines quality of life.

When multidisciplinary teams are used in a way that genuinely facilitates diverse perspectives and not merely as tokenistic exercises to re-create interdisciplinary hierarchies of influence, these teams can augment the available information with which patients and surgeons make their decisions. Attention to subtle aspects of ideology and values communicated in visual aids can also contribute to more carefully informed choices. Providing individuals with practical descriptions of the "best outcome", "worst outcome" and "most likely outcome" for a proposed surgical intervention can help people to imagine their reactions more accurately than general and impersonal discussions of population statistics. The urgency with which some surgical decisions must be made will limit opportunity to discuss patient preferences; this time limitation provides another rationale for engaging in such conversations at the earliest opportunity, before the onset of a medical crisis that may necessitate immediate action.

Acknowledgements

I am grateful to all of the people who gave permission for their narratives to appear in this chapter; to Israel Berger for editorial feedback on earlier drafts; and to Peter Hegarty and Freyja Quick for catalysing my interest in decision science.

References

Amsterlaw, Jennifer, Brian J. Zikmund-Fisher, Angela Fagerlin and Peter A. Ubel. 2006. Can Avoidance of Complications Lead to Biased Healthcare Decisions? *Judgment and Decision Making* 1(1): 64–75.

Ancker, Jessica S., Yalini Senathirajah, Rita Kukafka and Justin B. Starren. 2006. Design Features of Graphs in Health Risk Communication: A Systematic Review. *Journal of the American Medical Informatics Association* 13(6): 608–18.

Anderson, Clare, and Charlotte R. Platten. 2011. Sleep Deprivation Lowers Inhibition and Enhances Impulsivity to Negative Stimuli. *Behavioural Brain Research* 217(2): 463–6.

Ang, Dennis C., Said A. Ibrahim, Chris J. Burant, Laura A. Siminoff and C. Kent Kwoh. 2002. Ethnic Differences in the Perception of Prayer and Consideration of Joint Arthroplasty. *Medical Care* 40(6): 471–6.

Apkarian, A. Vania, Yamaya Sosa, Beth R. Krauss, P. Sebastian Thomas, Bruce E. Fredrickson, Robert E. Levy, R. Norman Harden and Dante R. Chialvo. 2004. Chronic Pain Patients are Impaired on an Emotional Decision-Making Task. *Pain* 108(1): 129–36.

Berry, Dianne C., D.K. Raynor, Peter Knapp and Elisabetta Bersellini. 2003. Patients' Understanding of Risk Associated with Medication Use: Impact of European Commission Guidelines and Other Risk Scales. *Drug Safety* 16: 1–11.

Bogardus, Sidney T., Eric Holmboe and James F. Jekel. 1999. Perils, Pitfalls, and Possibilities in Talking about Medical Risk. *Journal of the American Medical Association* 281(11): 1037–41.

Bornstein, Brian H., and A. Christine Emler. 2001. Rationality in Medical Decision Making: A Review of the Literature on Doctors' Decision-Making Biases. *Journal of Evaluation in Clinical Practice* 7(2): 97–107.

Bresnick, Jennifer. 2014. Predictive, Clinical Analytics at MGH Turn Data into Insights. Health IT Analytics. http://healthitanalytics.com/2014/08/20/predictive-clinical-analytics-at-mgh-turn-data-into-insights/

Brody, Howard. 1993. *The Healer's Power*. New Haven, CT: Yale University Press.

Burgess Diana J., Michelle van Ryn, Megan Crowley-Matoka and Jennifer Malat. 2006. Understanding the Provider Contribution to Race/Ethnicity Disparities in Pain Treatment: Insights from Dual Process Models of Stereotyping. *Pain Medicine* 7(2): 119–34.

Campbell, Emily J., Arun Krishnaraj, Mitchell Harris, Sanjay Saini and James M. Richter. 2012. Automated Before-Procedure Electronic Health Record Screening to Assess Appropriateness for GI Endoscopy and Sedation. *Gastrointestinal Endoscopy* 17(4): 786–92.

Cookson, Michael S., Gunnar Aus, Arthur L. Burnett, Edith D. Canby-Hagino, Anthony V. D'Amico, Roger R. Dmochowski, David T. Eton, Jeffrey D. Forman, S. Larry Goldenberg, Javier Hernandez, Celestia S. Higano, Stephen R. Kraus, Judd W. Moul, Catherine Tangen, J. Brantley Thrasher and Ian Thompson. 2007. Variation in the Definition of Biochemical Recurrence in Patients Treated for Localized Prostate Cancer: The American Urological Association Prostate Guidelines for Localized Prostate Cancer Update Panel Report and Recommendations for a Standard in the Reporting of Surgical Outcomes. *The Journal of Urology* 177(2): 540–5.

Cousin, Gaëtan, Marianne Schmid Mast, Debra L. Roter and Judith A. Hall. 2012. Concordance between Physician Communication Style and Patient Attitudes Predicts Patient Satisfaction. *Patient Education and Counseling* 87(2): 193–7.

Cousin, Gaëtan, Marianne Schmid Mast and Nicole Jaunin-Stalder. 2013. When Physician-Expressed Uncertainty Leads to Patient Dissatisfaction: A Gender Study. *Medical Education* 47(9): 923–31.

Diem, Susan J., John D. Lantos and James A. Tulsky. 1996. Cardiopulmonary Resuscitation on Television: Miracles and Misinformation. *New England Journal of Medicine* 334(24): 1578–82.

Dong, Li, Amy Donaldson, Ryan Metzger and Heather Keenan. 2012. Analgesic Administration in the Emergency Department for Children Requiring Hospitalization for Long-Bone Fracture. *Pediatric Emergency Care* 28(2): 109–14.

Donohoe, Rachael T., Karen Haefeli and Fionna Moore. 2006. Public Perceptions and Experiences of Myocardial Infarction, Cardiac Arrest and CPR in London. *Resuscitation* 71(1): 70–9.

Eich, Eric, and Joseph P. Forgas. 2003. Mood, Cognition, and Memory. In *Handbook of Psychology, Vol. 4*, edited by Irving B. Weiner et al., 61–83. New York: Wiley.

Evans, D., R. Gareth, Julian Barwell, Diana M. Eccles, Amanda Collins, Louise Izatt, Chris Jacobs, Alan Donaldson, Angela F. Brady, Andrew Cuthbert, Rachel Harrison, Sue Thomas, Anthony Howell, The FH02 Study Group, RGC teams, Zosia Miedzybrodzka and Alex Murray. 2014. The Angelina Jolie Effect: How High Celebrity Profile Can Have a Major Impact on Provision of Cancer Related Services. *Breast Cancer Research* 16(5): 442–7.

Fowler Jr, Floyd J., Patricia M. Gallagher, Julie P.W. Bynum, Michael J. Barry, F. Leslie Lucas and Jonathan S. Skinner. 2012. Decision-Making Process Reported by Medicare Patients who had Coronary Artery Stenting or Surgery for Prostate Cancer. *Journal of General Internal Medicine* 27(8): 911–16.

Fox, Craig R., and Amos Tversky. 1995. Ambiguity Aversion and Comparative Ignorance. *The Quarterly Journal of Economics* 110(3): 585–603.

Galavotti, Christine, and Donna L. Richter. 2000. Talking about Hysterectomy: The Experiences of Women from Four Cultural Groups. *Journal of Women's Health and Gender-Based Medicine* 9(Suppl. 2): S63–7.

Gillotti, Cathy, Teresa Thompson and Kelly McNeilis 2002. Communicative Competence in the Delivery of Bad News. *Social Science and Medicine* 54(7), 1011–23.

Ginwala, Allison. 2014. Breaking the Mold: Four Asian American Women Define Beauty, Detail Identity, and Deconstruct Stereotypes. Honors thesis. Paper 182. Durham, NH: University of New Hampshire.

Halpern, Jodi, and Robert M. Arnold. 2008. Affective Forecasting: An Unrecognized Challenge in Making Serious Health Decisions. *Journal of General Internal Medicine* 23(10): 1708–12.

Han, Paul K.J., Richard P. Moser and William M.P. Klein. 2006. Perceived Ambiguity about Cancer Prevention Recommendations: Relationship to Perceptions of Cancer Preventability, Risk, and Worry. *Journal of Health Communication* 11(S1): 51–69.

Harrison, Yvonne, and James A. Horne. 1999. One Night of Sleep Loss Impairs Innovative Thinking and Flexible Decision Making. *Organizational Behavior and Human Decision Processes* 78(2): 128–45.

Harvey, H. Benjamin, Arun Krishnaraj and Tarik K. Alkasab. 2014. A Software System to Collect Expert Relevance Ratings of Medical Record Items for Specific Clinical Tasks. *JMIR Medical Informatics* 2(1): e3.

Hawley, Sarah T., Jennifer J. Griggs, Ann S. Hamilton, John J. Graff, Nancy K. Janz, Monica Morrow, Reshma Jagsi, Barbara Salem and Steven J. Katz. 2009. Decision Involvement and Receipt of Mastectomy among Racially and Ethnically Diverse Breast Cancer Patients. *Journal of the National Cancer Institute* 101(19): 1337–47.

Hegarty, P., Orla Parslow, Y. Gavriel Ansara and Freyja Quick. 2013. Androcentrism: Changing the Landscape without Leveling the Playing Field? In *The Safe Handbook of Gender and Psychology*, edited by Michelle K. Ryan and Nyla R. Branscombe, 29–44. London: Sage.

Hyde, Janet S. 2005.The Gender Similarities Hypothesis. *American Psychologist* 60(6): 581–92.

Jones, G. Kirk, Kori L. Brewer and Herbert G. Garrison. 2000. Public Expectations of Survival Following Cardiopulmonary Resuscitation. *Academic Emergency Medicine* 7(1): 48–53.

Kahneman, Daniel, and Amos Tversky. 1984. Choices, Values and Frames. *American Psychologist* 39(4): 341–50.

Killgore, William D.S., Thomas J. Balkin and Nancy J. Wesensten. 2006. Impaired Decision Making Following 49 h of Sleep Deprivation. *Journal of Sleep Research* 15(1): 7–13.

Kornbrot, Diana E., Rachel M. Msetfi and Melvyn J. Grimwood. 2013. Time Perception and Depressive Realism: Judgment Type, Psychophysical Functions and Bias. *PLoS ONE* 8(8): e71585.

LeBlanc, Vicki R., Lee R. Brooks and Geoffrey R. Norman. 2002. Believing is Seeing: The Influence of a Diagnostic Hypothesis on the Interpretation of Clinical Features. *Academic Medicine* 77(10): S67–9.

Lim, Julian, and David F. Dinges. 2010. A Meta-Analysis of the Impact of Short-Term Sleep Deprivation on Cognitive Variables. *Psychological Bulletin* 136(3): 375–89.

Lloyd, Andrew J. 2001. The Extent of Patients' Understanding of the Risk of Treatments. *Quality in Health Care* 10(Suppl. 1): i14–18.

Lloyd, Andrew, Paul Hayes, Peter R.F. Bell and A. Ross Naylor. 2001. The Role of Risk and Benefit Perception in Informed Consent for Surgery. *Medical Decision Making* 21(2): 141–9.

Malenka, David J., John A. Baron, Sarah Johansen, Jon W. Wahrenberger and Jonathan M. Ross. 1993. The Framing Effect of Relative and Absolute Risk. *Journal of General Internal Medicine* 8(10): 543–8.

Maly, Rose C., Yoshiko Umezawa, Carl T. Ratliff and Barbara Leake. 2006. Racial/Ethnic Group Differences in Treatment Decision-Making and Treatment Received among Older Breast Carcinoma Patients. *Cancer* 106(4): 957–65.

Martella, Diana, Maria Casagrande and Juan Lupiáñez. 2011. Alerting, Orienting and Executive Control: The Effects of Sleep Deprivation on Attentional Networks. *Experimental Brain Research* 210(1): 81–9.

Meyerowitz, Beth E., and Shelly Chaiken. 1987. The Effect of Message Framing on Breast Self-Examination Attitudes, Intentions, and Behavior. *Journal of Personality and Social Psychology* 52(3): 500.

Moriarty, Orla, Brian E. McGuire and David P. Finn. 2011. The Effect of Pain on Cognitive Function: A Review of Clinical and Preclinical Research. *Progress in Neurobiology* 93(3): 385–404.

Papagrigoriadis, Savvas, and Bob Heyman. 2003. Patients' Views on Follow up of Colorectal Cancer: Implications for Risk Communication and Decision Making. *Postgraduate Medical Journal* 79(933): 403–7.

Philippot, Pierre, and Alexandre Schaefer. 2001. Emotion and Memory. In *Emotions: Current Issues and Future Directions*, edited by Tracy J. Mayne and George A. Bonanno, 82–122. New York, NY: Guildford Press.

Poisson, Sharon N., S. Claiborne Johnston, Stephen Sidney, Jeffrey G. Klingman and Mai N. Nguyen-Huynh. 2010. Gender Differences in Treatment of Severe Carotid Stenosis after Transient Ischemic Attack. *Stroke* 41: 1891–5.

Politi, Mary C., Paul K.J. Han, and Nananda F. Col. 2007. Communicating the Uncertainty of Harms and Benefits of Medical Interventions. *Medical Decision Making* 27(5): 681–95.

Politi, Mary C., Melissa A. Clark, Hernando Ombao, Don Dizon and Glyn Elwyn. 2011. Communicating Uncertainty Can Lead to Less Decision Satisfaction: A Necessary Cost of Involving Patients in Shared Decision Making? *Health Expectations* 14(1): 84–91.

Reaume, Geoffrey. 2002. Lunatic to Patient to Person: Nomenclature in Psychiatric History and the Influence of Patients' Activism in North America. *International Journal of Law and Psychiatry* 25(4): 405–26.

Redelmeier, Donald A., and Robert B. Cialdini. 2002. Problems for Clinical Judgment: 5 Principles of Influence in Medical Practice. *Canadian Medical Association Journal* 166(13): 1680–4.

Reitsma, Welmoed, Marian J.E. Mourits, Merel Koning, Astrid Pascal and Berend van der Lei. 2011. No (Wo)Man Is an Island – The Influence of Physicians' Personal Predisposition to Labia Minora Appearance on Their Clinical Decision Making: A Cross-Sectional Survey. *The Journal of Sexual Medicine* 8(8): 2377–85.

Reyna, Valerie F. 2008. How People Make Decisions That Involve Risk: A Dual-Processes Approach. *Current Directions in Psychological Science* 13(2): 60–6.

Rivera, Semilla M., John P. Hatch, Calogero Dolce, Robert A. Bays, Joseph E. Van Sickels and John D. Rugh. 2000. Patients' Own Reasons and Patient-Perceived Recommendations for Orthognathic Surgery. *American Journal of Orthodontics and Dentofacial Orthopedics* 118(2): 134–40.

Schapira, Marilyn M., Ann B. Nattinger and Colleen A. McHorney. 2001. Frequency or Probability? A Qualitative Study of Risk Communication Formats Used in Health Care. *Medical Decision Making* 21(6): 459–67.

Schouten, Barbara C., and Sanne Schinkel. 2014. Turkish Migrant GP Patients' Expression of Emotional Cues and Concerns in Encounters with and without Informal Interpreters. *Patient Education and Counseling* 97(1): 23–9.

Seminowicz, David A., Timothy H. Wideman, Lina Naso, Zeinab Hatami-Khoroushahi, Summaya Fallatah, Mark A. Ware, Peter Jarzem, M. Catherine Bushnell, Yoram Shir, Jean A. Ouellet and Laura S. Stone. 2011. Effective Treatment of Chronic Low Back Pain in Humans Reverses Abnormal Brain Anatomy and Function. *The Journal of Neuroscience* 31(20): 7540–50.

Siegel, Corey A. 2010. Lost in Translation: Helping Patients Understand the Risks of Infammatory Bowel Disease Therapy. *Inflammatory Bowel Disease* 16(12): 2168–72.

Solomon, Patricia. 2001. Congruence between Health Professionals' and Patients' Pain Ratings: A Review of the Literature. *Scandinavian Journal of Caring Sciences* 15(2): 174–80.

Speed, Ewen. 2006. Patients, Consumers and Survivors: A Case Study of Mental Health Service User Discourses. *Social Science and Medicine* 62(1): 28–38.

Sproten, Alec, Carsten Diener, Christian Fiebach and Christiane Schwieren. 2010. Aging and Decision Making: How Aging Affects Decisions Under Uncertainty. University of Heidelberg Department of Economics. http://www.ub.uni-heidelberg.de/archiv/11361

Steginga, S.K., S. Occhipinti, R.A. Gardiner, J. Yaxley and P. Heathcote. 2002. Making Decisions about Treatment for Localized Prostate Cancer. *BJU International* 89(3): 255–60.

Tobin, Jonathan N., Sylvia Wassertheil-Smoller, John P. Wexler, Richard M. Steingart, Nancy Budner, Lloyd Lense and Joseph Wachspress. 1987. Sex Bias in Considering Coronary Bypass Surgery. *Annals of Internal Medicine* 107(1): 19–25.

Tsui, Jamie, James Lau and Lisa Shieh. 2014. Septris and SICKO: Implementing and Using Learning Analytics and Gamification in Medical Education. EDUCAUSE Learning Initiative. https://net.educause.edu/ir/library/pdf/ELIB1401.pdf

Tversky, Amos, and Daniel Kahneman. 1981. The Framing of Decisions and the Psychology of Choice. *Science* 211(4481): 453–8.

Tversky, Amos, and Daniel Kahneman. 1992. Advances in Prospect Theory: Cumulative Representation of Uncertainty. *Journal of Risk and Uncertainty* 5(4): 297–323.

Van den Bulck, Jan, and K. Damiaans. 2004. Cardiopulmonary Resuscitation on Flemish Television: Challenges to the Television Effects Hypothesis. *Emergency Medicine Journal* 21(5): 565–7.

Veronesi, Umberto, Natale Cascinelli, Luigi Mariani, Marco Greco, Roberto Saccozzi, Alberto Luini, Marisel Aguilar and Ettore Marubini. 2002. Twenty-Year Follow-up of a Randomized Study Comparing Breast-Conserving Surgery with Radical Mastectomy for Early Breast Cancer. *New England Journal of Medicine* 347(16): 1227–32.

Weinstein, Neil D., Kathryn Kolb, and Bernard D. Goldstein. 1996. Using Time Intervals between Expected Events to Communicate Risk Magnitudes. *Risk Analysis* 16(3): 305–8.

Zohar, Dov, Orna Tzischinsky and Rachel Epstein. 2005. The Effects of Sleep Loss on Medical Residents' Emotional Reactions to Work Events: A Cognitive-Energy Model. *Sleep: Journal of Sleep and Sleep Disorders Research* 28(1): 47–54.

Y. Gavriel Ansara completed his Master of Science and PhD at the School of Psychology, University of Surrey, UK. He received the 2011 National Psychology Postgraduate Teaching Award given to one person annually by the UK Higher Education Academy for excellence in teaching, and the 2012 Transgender Research Award from the American Psychological Association for a significant and original research contribution to the field. He is an Associate Editor of the *International Journal of Human Rights in Healthcare* and has worked as Manager of Research & Policy at the National LGBTI Health Alliance, Australia's national peak body for LGBTI health and wellbeing. Some of his research interests include cisgenderism, decision science, endocrinology, health disparities and history of science.

5 Breaking Informed Consent: Strategies for Risk Communication in Surgical Practice

Maria R. Dahm and Israel Berger

5.1 Introduction

In Australia and many other countries, all people have the right to refuse or consent to medical treatment – including life-saving treatment. Four principles underlie valid consent: (1) the patient has the capacity to consent, (2) the patient gives consent voluntarily, (3) the consent includes the procedure(s) that will be performed and (4) the patient is able to make informed choices based on adequate information provided by medical professionals (Consumers Health Forum of Australia 2013).

Patients may react poorly to formal informed consent processes, being presented with forms and other processes in which some kind of progression is expected. Consent forms, a necessary component of modern medical practice, can hinder conversation and contribute to informed consent processes becoming ritualistic, thus reducing the patient's ability to make autonomous, informed choices (Habiba et al. 2004). Therefore, it is not enough for a patient to read and sign a consent form; the health professional must attempt to sit down with them and ensure that they understand the procedure, risks and potential benefits. Sound communication and interpersonal skills are vital in such consultations. Although clinicians may desire more uniform language and communication tools (Edwards et al. 1998), this could interfere with patient autonomy in much the same way as consent forms.

Skilled communication is similarly crucial to informed consent following bad news situations. Patients who have recently received diagnoses of potentially devastating illnesses may be distraught and unable to absorb all but basic details, making the ideal informed consent impossible without distressing them (Tobias and Souhami 1993). It is up to the clinician to judge what is an appropriate level of information for each patient at that time and to schedule follow-up appointments as necessary, potentially with the patient's loved ones present.

Little research has addressed informed consent in the surgical context, and surgeons are, as a whole, neither specifically trained nor competent to guide patients through legally correct informed consent processes (Leclercq et al. 2010). A need for improvement exists especially in discussing risks and uncertainties and in promoting shared decision-making (Levinson, Hudak and Tricco 2013: 15). Kim and colleagues (2013) also found that study quality is generally low and that core informed consent principles and patient emotions often are not addressed. The few studies that have used qualitative methods to explore the informed consent process have utilized interviews (Kim et al. 2013). Informed consent research based on naturally occurring interactions between clinicians and patients seems altogether absent.

In this chapter, we qualitatively examine surgical consultations to identify risk communication strategies used to obtain informed consent. Drawing on recordings of 37 interactions collected in the consulting rooms of a colorectal surgeon, we identified two particular strategies of presenting risk and obtaining informed consent: (1) *set pieces* used to relate risk information about "routine" procedures such as colonoscopies; and (2) *breaking informed consent* – a unique strategy employed by the observed surgeon in more demanding situations such as the discussion of "big", potentially life-changing surgeries. In the following sections, we provide information on common approaches to informed consent, shared decision-making and breaking bad news, and discuss research on communication practices in these areas before addressing our findings and their implications.

5.2   Informed Consent

In a review of malpractice claims and negligence complaints in Australia, Gogos and colleagues (2011) found that between 2002 and 2008, 57 per cent of complaints about informed consent were made against surgeons, with the primary allegation in 71 per cent of cases being failure to mention or properly explain risks. Several barriers exist to obtaining an ideal informed consent, including clinician time (Consumers Health Forum of Australia 2013), confusion about when informed consent is required (ibid.), overestimation of information provided and concerns about providing excessive information (Makoul, Arntson and Schofield 1995), clinicians' poor understanding of statistics (Edwards, Elwyn and Mulley 2002), difficulty communicating risks effectively and without jargon (Jenkins et al. 1999), language barriers (Schenker et al. 2007) and inability to assess patients' comprehension (Penn et al. 2009). A recent review of surgical communication practices also revealed that, amongst other shortcomings, surgeons need to improve their communication for consent processes, especially when discussing risks and uncertainties, and to promote shared decision-making (Levinson, Hudak and Tricco 2013).

Surgeons, however, use a range of communication resources in obtaining informed consent – but do so with varying success. A survey of 330 gynaecologists found that they give detailed descriptions of risks and alternatives to surgery but less detailed descriptions of post-operative course, expected benefits and functional or anatomical changes (Abed et al. 2007). They reported confirming patient understanding most often by asking patients whether they have any questions (a strategy that is likely to miss patients' concerns, Heritage et al. 2007) and rarely by evaluating patient literacy. Sanders and Skevington (2004) found that most patients who had recently been diagnosed with bowel cancer were not actively involved in the informed consent process with oncologists. Active involvement was usually prevented by four communication troubles: (1) conflicting expectations about the most appropriate treatment, (2) unexpected information, (3) issues related to treatment costs and benefits, and (4) lack of a clear treatment recommendation. The authors advise that clinicians should provide not only adequate information but also their own interpretation about the pros and cons of treatment options. Although patients do not necessarily want a paternalistic approach, they are seeking expert opinion. Given that patients who have just received a cancer diagnosis may be unable to process much information themselves, this may be even more important in oncology settings.

5.3   Shared Decision-Making

Both interpersonal communication and systemic processes must be examined to improve informed consent. A prominent alternative to informed consent models is shared decision-making (SDM), which has been shown, along with increased information provision, to be patients' top priority (Schattner, Bronstein and Jellin 2006). SDM is not simply a patient-centred approach in which patients are the "centre" of healthcare, where *clinicians' interpretations* of patients' potential concerns are considered and treatment options are largely decided by clinicians and presented to patients for consent. Instead, in SDM, patients are actively involved in making decisions about their treatment and exploring treatment options with the help of clinicians. Four principles characterize SDM: "(1) that at least two participants – physician and patient – be involved; (2) that both parties share information; (3) that both parties take steps to build a consensus about the preferred treatment; and (4) that an agreement is reached on the treatment to implement" (Charles, Gafni and Whelan 1997: 681).

Based on a literature review of competencies, Towle and Godolphin (1999) used semi-structured interviews with family doctors, patients and health educators to validate their model of *informed* shared decision-making (ISDM) and provide competencies for doctors and patients. While the patient is undoubtedly an equal partner in ISDM, it would be beyond the scope of this chapter to discuss the patient competencies in detail. We therefore concentrate only on the eight competencies identified by Towle and Godolphin (1999) for doctors across five concepts central to ISDM:

- Partnership
  1. Develop a partnership with the patient
- Explicitness
  2. Establish or review the patient's preferences for information
  3. Establish or review the patient's preferences for a role in decision-making and the existence and nature of any uncertainty about the course of action to take
- An informed patient and physician
  4. Ascertain and respond to the patient's ideas, concerns and expectations
  5. Identify choices and evaluate the research evidence in relation to the individual patient
- Shared decision-making
  6. Present evidence, taking into account competencies 2 and 3, framing effects etc. Help the patient to reflect on and assess the impact of alternative decisions with regard to his or her values and lifestyle
  7. Make or negotiate a decision in partnership with the patient and resolve conflict
- Completeness
  8. Agree on an action plan and complete arrangements for follow-up

Towle and colleagues (2006) later tested their model with family physicians and their existing patients, finding that they were able to elicit concerns, ideas and expectations (although, interestingly, not about treatment) and agree on an action plan. Explicit preferences for role and information were not elicited, so perhaps these are best inferred from patient cues. Clinicians also had difficulty integrating the ISDM model into their existing practice by altering these well-established relationships. Despite this, clinicians felt the ISDM model was helpful and should be implemented. Perhaps in the case of existing patients, gradual integration would be smoother than an immediate overhaul of the existing relationship.

Generally, clinicians perceive a number of barriers to SDM: lack of time, physicians' predisposition and skill, and patients' lack of experience in making their own healthcare decisions (Edwards et al. 2005; Towle and Godolphin 1999; Towle et al. 2006). SDM can be conceptualized as a relationship-building approach, as it is regarded as proceeding more smoothly, providing more opportunities for patients to defer decision-making, and being more interactionally balanced (Edwards et al. 2005). However, we are not aware of any studies that have specifically looked at moments within SDM-oriented consultations that can be harnessed to build rapport. Additionally, Epstein, Alper and Quill (2004) found that studies about consent and decision-making have rarely examined clinical communication directly, instead relying on focus groups, interviews, surveys and experiments to examine preferences for different communication strategies. Although this review was conducted over 10 years ago, a similar paucity of direct observation of discussions involving evidence, risk and consent continues today.

5.4   Communicating Risks, Benefits and Uncertainty

The communication of risk is essential for the informed consent process. Risk communication has been described as "a fundamental duty of physicians both to fulfil a role as trusted adviser and to promote the ethical principle of autonomy" (Bogardus, Holmboe and Jekel 1999: 1037). One study found that 80 per cent of patients wanted to be informed of all risks, even those that occur less than 1 per cent of the time, making risk communication not only an important legal and ethical process but also one highly desired by patients (Oosthuizen, Burns and Timon 2012). Risk may be communicated in global terms (e.g., injury, cost, lost time) or in specific terms within one category (e.g., muscle pain, scarring, nausea), termed, respectively, *thick* and *thin* conceptualization of risk (Wachbroit 1991). These may of course be mixed in practice, for example mentioning the possibility of "additional costs" but being specific about physical risks. Patients may express satisfaction with the information received in the moment but be retrospectively dissatisfied upon experiencing the adverse events described, indicating that although theoretical information can be delivered adequately, the experience of personal suffering may not – or perhaps cannot – be adequately conveyed (Little et al. 2008).

The *subjective badness* (Bogardus, Holmboe and Jekel 1999) that a patient places on risks is much more difficult for clinicians to gauge, given that they can never completely operate from another's perspective. It is here that the informed consent principle of communicating risks that might be significant to the individual patient (even if very rare) becomes relevant. Clinicians can work from the perspective of "a reasonable person" only to a degree before taking into account a holistic and often unconscious assessment of the patient's lifestyle and goals. An average reasonable person might not mind an incision being larger than initially planned, but this could be untenable for a swimsuit model, or a certain patient may have concerns that are outside the realm of most people (e.g., fear of urinary catheters). Thus, the clinician needs to explore, know and recall details of the patient's life in order to consider what a reasonable person *in the patient's position* would want to know. In order to do this, they need to have information about the patient and their culture, values and experience. This is related to the idea that risk may be considered acceptable/unacceptable, serious/non-serious, justifiable/unjustifiable, depending on the person, and decisions may be further affected by how avoidable/ unavoidable and rare/common the risk is (Calman 1996).

5.5   Breaking Bad News

Risk communication may be further complicated if informed consent is sought in close temporal proximity to the delivery of bad news, e.g., when a cancer diagnosis is immediately followed by treatment discussions. Just as Towle and Godoplhin (1999) proposed competencies for SDM, several formal protocols have been proposed to aid clinicians in breaking bad news (e.g., Baile et al. 2000; Narayanan, Bista and Koshy 2010; Sparks et al. 2007; Villagran et al. 2010). By providing a structured framework, protocols are intended to ease the distress of the clinician and thereby that of the patient or loved ones (see Harrison and Walling 2010 for a thorough review of breaking bad news protocols). SPIKES (Baile et al. 2000) is one of the more widely used protocols consisting of three phases and various linear steps:

- Preparation
    * Setting up
    * patient's **P**erception
    * obtaining patient's **I**nvitation
- Breaking bad news
    * giving **K**nowledge and information to the patient
    * addressing the patient's **E**motions with empathetic responses
- Prospect
    * **S**trategy and summary
    (Sparks et al. 2007)

Although protocols may aid clinicians' thinking about elements of breaking bad news (BBN), formalization of bad news delivery could lead to greater stress and anxiety about doing it correctly (see, e.g., Persaud and Howell 1993). Other authors have described, instead, broader competencies for BBN. Based on a grounded theory analysis of medical student and simulated patient BBN encounters, Villagran and colleagues (2010) propose the communication- rather than protocol-based COMFORT model, a collection of concrete communication strategies that can be used non-linearly: **C**ommunicating, **O**rientation, **M**indfulness, **F**amily, **O**ngoing support, **R**eiterative messages and **T**eam. Sparks and colleagues (2007) describe more general approaches to BBN based on a grounded theory analysis of written patient narratives. They identify four strategies that clinicians use to break bad news: indirect (with little or no disclosure), direct (open communication, ensuring all parties are working from the same definitions), comforting (attempting to reduce patient distress) and empowerment (emphasizing individual power, self-efficacy and personal control). Although the strategies themselves are inherently neither positive nor negative, they can be used appropriately or inappropriately. For example, if indirect communication, which relies on implied meanings and distancing, is used to break news of a death, the recipient may not understand that the person has died. On the other hand, the recipient may interpret it as giving the news gently.

Another study on medical student interaction with simulated patients has identified several communicative behaviours that have been associated with higher communicative competence ratings in delivering bad news, including, for example: small talk, open questions, restatements and verifying (Gillotti, Thompson and McNeilis 2002: 1018). However, clinicians' use of relational strategies such as attentiveness to seating arrangements, using drawings to help explain, and providing information about what happens next, may depend on experiential learning rather than explicit training (Lamiani et al. 2011), thus bringing into question the use of decontextualized protocols and competencies to teach communication skills for breaking bad news and informed consent.

5.6   Method

5.6.1   Data Collection and Site

Given the lack of studies analysing authentic interaction to study communication strategies used in informed consent consultations, this chapter analyses naturally occurring surgical consultations between a colorectal surgeon (whom we assigned the pseudonym *James*) and his patients. This data was originally collected as part of a pilot study to identify and compare communication strategies commonly used by native and non-native English speaking doctors (see Chapter 3 of this volume; Dahm et al. 2015). During two data collection sessions in October 2011 and June 2012, 37 new and repeat patients aged between their early 20s and 80s consented to having their consultations audio-recorded. Complementary ethnographic data (Wolcott 2008) were collected in the form of observational fieldnotes, and a semi-structured interview with James to elicit his perspective on his communicative style, strategies identified during observations and approach to informed consent was conducted after preliminary data exploration to ensure that the surgeon's perspective was also included in further analysis. All audio data were transcribed, de-identified and assigned a code. The study was approved by the Macquarie University Human Research Ethics Committee.

5.6.2   The Data

In order to compare complex consent consultations with those of a more routine nature, we decided to concentrate on consultations dedicated to discussing colonoscopies (n=6), as this was the most frequently discussed routine procedure, and upcoming bowel cancer surgeries (n=2), as this is a possible surgical path following colonoscopy. Both bowel cancer surgery consultations concentrated on surgical treatment and future management, as James had broken the cancer diagnosis to the patients in previous, unrecorded consultations. Consultation 11_XH involved a 47-year-old male patient accompanied by his mother; consultation 33_NT involved a 79-year-old female accompanied by three of her daughters.

Although colonoscopies were discussed in nearly 20 per cent (n=7) of consultations, we included only consultations that focused solely on the colonoscopy and excluded one interaction focused on a combined colonoscopy and hernia repair procedure. Three patients had already undergone a colonoscopy in the past (03_IL; 10_NN; 16_SM), and it was the first time for the other three patients (01_EN; 18_SCN; 07_OW).

5.6.3 Data Analysis

With the exception of four patients who opted to self-record, one researcher was present during each consultation to observe and take fieldnotes on, for example, nonverbal aspects of the consultation. Utilizing these notes, the researchers immersed themselves in the transcripts and flagged communication strategies for further analysis during repeated readings of the growing data pool. Analysis combined two steps: (1) an iterative process of immersion in the consultation data complemented by the ethnographic fieldnotes and semi-structured interview; and (2) close analysis of selected interactions drawing on a range of communicative frameworks of informed consent and breaking bad news. Standard orthographic transcripts are presented with line numbers and speaker labels.

5.7 Findings

From the iterative analysis, it emerged that James employed different communicative approaches in consent consultations for more routine procedures such as colonoscopies, as compared to those employed for more complex and potentially life-altering surgeries (i.e., bowel cancer resections). The routine procedures were often discussed using *set pieces* that were frequently adjusted to the situation. The more complex interactions, in contrast, did not rely on set pieces but combined communicative strategies found in informed decision-making (Towle and Godolphin 1999) or breaking bad news (Baile et al. 2000; Sparks et al. 2007; Villagran et al. 2010). Drawing on a quote from the semi-structured interview, we refer to this strategy as *breaking informed consent*.

5.7.1   Set Pieces

For colonoscopy consultations, James follows a script that is readily adapted to the individual patient and contingencies of the conversation. In the interview, James referred to such scripts as "little set pieces". The set piece for routine colonoscopies progressed through stages (outlined in detail below and in Figure 5.1). In this set piece, James makes use of relationship-building practices, such as signposts (Robins et al. 2011), diagrams (Paling 2003), self-disclosure (Beach et al. 2004; Dahm et al. 2015), and normalization (Caffi 1999). James's colonoscopy informed consent set piece progresses through various stages: from gathering patients' perceptions about (and experiences of) the procedure, signposting anatomical drawings followed by the actual drawing sequence, describing the procedure and risks, opening discussion for shared decision-making, to providing reassurance or confirming the necessity for the procedure. Despite being somewhat scripted and having been rehearsed in many iterations, his set piece allows him to adjust to the situation and provide additional information depending on the patient. The same basic information is shared each time but with the option to add sequences or change the order to adjust to the background and information needs of an individual patient and thus build further rapport.

James first explores the patient's perception and seeks to find out what they know, expect and want out of the process. This is ordinarily an information-gathering

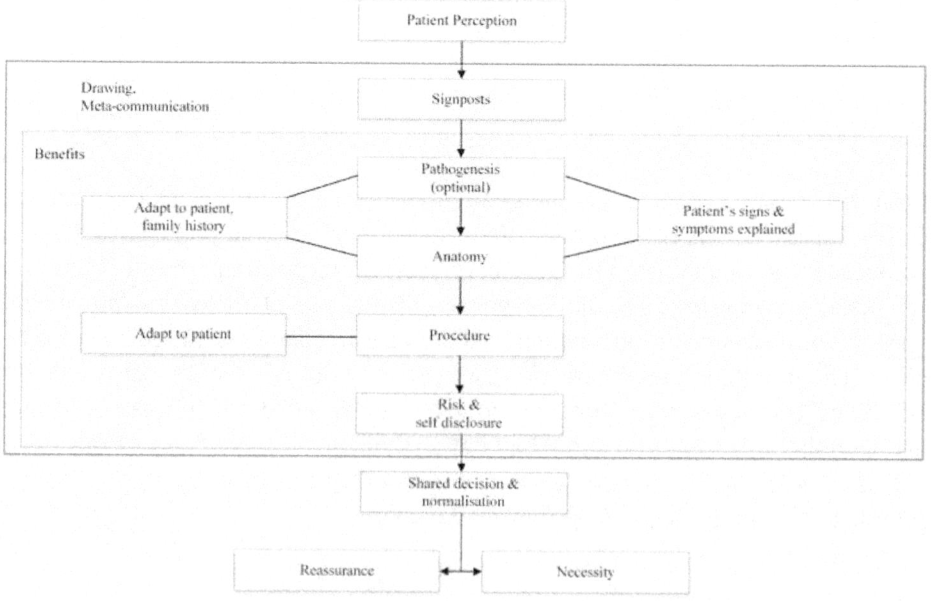

Figure 5.1: James's set piece for colonoscopy

process to enable him to then provide relevant and easily comprehensible information to the patient, but this stage may also involve a perspective display sequence (PDS; Maynard 1989) designed to create an opportunity for the patient to share their opinion. James then signposts the upcoming drawing/demonstration aspect of the discussion. Throughout the drawing phase, there is the potential for meta-talk about the act of drawing and the communication of procedures and risks through drawings. During the drawing phase, a series of topics may be discussed, using the drawing as a reference. The drawing sequence offers an opportunity for James to explain polyp-to-cancer pathogenesis and the patient's actual signs and symptoms as they relate to his description of bowel anatomy. James then moves on to describe the procedure itself, adapting what is said to the patient's presenting concerns and demeanour. As he describes risks, he continues to provide patients with an accessible and portable visual reference.

Interestingly, benefits are not given a phase of their own but rather are embedded in discussions of pathogenesis, anatomy, the procedure or risks (e.g., "If we find a polyp and remove it [benefit], there could be some bleeding [risk]."). After the colonoscopy-associated risks and benefits have been discussed, James creates a space for shared decision-making and provides implicit recommendations. In this space, he may normalize the colonoscopy experience or provide arguments for or against having the procedure. Once patients consent to colonoscopy, James reassures them in their decision, focusing on "peace of mind" after screening or the necessity of the procedure given their symptoms. In this way, he shows that patients have made a good decision and avoids unnecessary patient distress.

5.7.2 Patient Perception

In Extract 1, James issues a standard enquiry into the patient's knowledge followed by a description of the previously unfamiliar procedure. In lines 145–6, James names a test, "CT colonoscopy" (a computed tomography [CT] colonography, or "virtual colonoscopy") followed by "have you heard of those?", to which the patient responds "no" (line 147). Although James does not explicitly describe the procedure as a CT scan of the colon, he alludes to the fact that it involves a bowel preparation and a CT scanner (lines 150 and 152). He describes how the team can do the CT scan immediately after attempting a colonoscopy (lines 149–55).

Extract 1 [16_SM]

```
145 J:  ... and we can do a, a test called a CT colonoscopy. Have you heard
146     of those?
147 P:  No
148 J:  It's not very pleasant, and, and you have it awake, but what we might
149     do is just take the precaution of, um, we'll let the, the imaging – we'll
150     let the CT scanner people know that you're floating around, we'll plan to
151     do a colonoscopy, and if we don't succeed, then we can, on the same
152     bowel prep, so you don't have to go through it all again
```

```
153 P:   Oh ( )
154 J:   We could just get you straight down to the, ah, CT scanner, do the scan
155      then give you a sandwich
156 P:   Yeah
```

5.7.3 Signposts

Extract 2 provides an example of the kind of signpost James uses in relation to drawing a diagram, "I'll draw you a picture" (line 225), a formulation he routinely uses during this phase. This extract also includes an example of meta-communication about the act of drawing for patients. He sets this up by referring back to a previous episode in the consultation that focused on drawing pictures (line 227) and adds "I've got colleagues who have their pictures drawn for them [printable diagrams], but I like to draw my own" (lines 229 and 231).

Extract 2 [18_SCN]
```
225 J:   I'll draw you a picture.
226 P:   Uh-huh.
227 J:   So, um, oh, we were just talking before about drawing pictures.
228 P:   Road maps.
229 J:   Yeah, I've got colleagues who have their pictures drawn for them
230 P:   Oh.
231 J:   But I, I, I like to draw my own.
232 P:   Right
```

During the interview, James explicitly described his use of drawings and orientation as a deliberate strategy for providing tailored information that is also suited to adapting the discussion to individual patients:

I'll say, "right, let me draw a picture of how we'll do that. These are the complications. When we balance, we balance them up." ...I'll mix it up, really finely nuance it, you know, because I tell you, you can tell if you're making them uncomfortable or you go in a slightly different direction...adjusting it...When I draw my pictures of procedures and complications and things, I turn to the patient, even go to some trouble to write upside down so that I'm writing for them, which some of them notice and some of them don't. I say, "it's because it's your information; I know it's a bit clumsy."

5.7.4 Pathogenesis

Extract 3 follows on from James drawing a picture and the intervening discussion. In this extract, James describes the pathogenesis of cancer from polyps (lines 165–8; 174–8). The pathogenesis phase of James's informed consent set piece is optional, and embedded in this example is a benefit declaration "the nice thing is that if you find a polyp when it's like this size and remove it, it's not going to grow into a cancer" (lines 180–1).

Extract 3 [01_EN]

```
158 J:   I'll draw you a- I'll draw you a picture.
         [...]
165 J:   So I don't think you've got bowel cancer but bowel cancer is really
166      common and it starts off...
167 P:   Aha.
168 J:   ...as a little polyp. It's not even a cancer.
         [...]
174 J:   And that, that little polyp thing gets bigger and bigger...
175 P:   Yes.
176 J:   ...and eventually they can turn into a cancer...
177 P:   Yes.
178 J:   ...and that whole process can take five to ten years...
179 P:   Aha
180 J:   ...and the nice thing is that if you find a polyp when it's like this
181      size and remove it, it's not going to grow into a cancer.
```

5.7.5 Anatomy

Extract 4 is an example of James's description of anatomy for patients. In Extract 4, James names parts of his drawing (lines 162, 164, 166, 168). In doing so, he also starts a sequence that allows him to adapt to the patient's individual information needs as linked to her signs and symptoms and explains how her diverticulosis can cause a narrowing of the bowel (lines 168–9). As mentioned above, anatomy, pathogenesis, and their related adaptions to the patient and situation are very closely related.

Extract 4 [16_SM]

```
162 J:   So map of the bowel.
163 P:   Yep.
164 J:   And the appendix is around here.
165 P:   Yep
166 J:   And the small bowel's there. That's the outside world.
167 P:   Right.
168 J:   And this area here is where the diverticulosis normally is, and it, it
169      can narrow down.
```

5.7.6 Procedure

In Extracts 5 and 6, James describes how a colonoscopy is performed, following a basic script of "we wash the bowel out, put you to sleep, put a telescope up" and adapting his description based on the patient's presenting concern. For example, the description in Extract 5 ends in "put a telescope all the way around" (lines 272–3) and a reassuring statement regarding the simplicity of the procedure "that's it really" (line 275). Extract 6 ends in a similar way but also includes benefit declarations: "put this telescope up, and if we find one of these little polyps, we remove it" (lines 204–5) and "that's the good side of all of this" (line 207).

Extract 5 [18_SCN: procedure]

```
272 J:   So we wash the bowel out, put you to sleep, put a telescope all
273      the way around
274 P:   Right, yep
275 J:   And, um, that's it really
276 P:   I'd be happy for that, yeah
```

Extract 6 [01_EN: procedure]

```
204 J:   We wash the bowel out, put you to sleep, put this telescope up,
205      and if we find one of these little polyps, we remove it.
206 P    Yes
207 J    That's the, the, the, the good side of all of this.
```

5.7.7   Risk

In communicating risk, James continues to use drawings but also discloses his
experiences with complications and adjusts the discussion of risk according to individual patients. He usually begins with a signpost to lead into the new topic, "with
some risks" (Extract 7, line 494), and proceeds to give a direct and honest account
of potential complications, "We can poke a hole through the bowel" (line 494).

In Extract 7, following laughter and "that's a bonus" from the patient (line 497),
James produces a joke-to-serious "no" (Schegloff 2001), and says that by telling
patients about the risk, it keeps him aware of it and therefore careful (lines 498–
501). He proceeds to list the next risk, excessive bleeding if polyps are removed,
and discloses that he has caused this before (lines 503–4). He presents a worst case
scenario of excessive bleeding requiring a blood transfusion (line 504), a very real
possibility that James has encountered before.

Extract 7 [03_IL]

```
494 J:   ... with some risks. We can poke a hole through the bowel. I draw this
495      for everybody, but I've never actually poked a hole through the bowel
496      like that.
497 P:   ((laughs)) that's a bonus.
498 J:   No, I've got to tell you, I've got to tell you and I think that.
499 P:   Yes, of course.
500 J:   I think that in telling you, it keeps me, it keeps me likely, it just keeps
501      me aware of it and I stay careful. Removing polyps, if we find any,
502 P:   Right
503 J:   I've certainly injured people doing that and cause bleeding and enough to
504      cause a blood transfusion or you know.
```

This disclosure of professional experience of a complication is similar to, but
quite distinct from, self-disclosure. Take Extract 8 below, for example, where
James discloses that he has had a bowel preparation. In this example, his personal experience of the procedure aids in relational rapport building, whereas
disclosure of having caused a complication is face-threatening. Such disclosure

takes a risk for the sake of honesty and carries the potential benefit of being seen as trustworthy.

Extract 8 [10_NN]

```
260 J:   So we wash the bowel out; you remember what that's like
261 P:   Yes, yes, yes, that's a little bit of fun
262 J:   Yes, I've had it too
263 P:   ((Laughs))
```

5.7.8 Shared Decisions

In the shared decision phase of informed consent, James uses contextual information about the patient's presenting concern and their perception of what constitutes a risk versus a benefit to present implicit recommendations and elicit a decision from the patient. In Extract 9, James presents the patient, whose consultation thus far involved the possibility of polyps following a positive screening test for occult blood in the stool, with an image of weighing risks and benefits on a scale (222–3, 225). He ends this analogy by normalizing two opposing decisions: to have a colonoscopy and get potential polyps removed versus not accepting the risks of a colonoscopy (lines 225–8). He juxtaposes this decision-making with the fact that the patient is having the consultation (lines 228–9), and the patient agrees (lines 230 and 232).

Extract 9 [01_EN]

```
222 J:   Um, but, in any case, you know, we, we, there's like a little scale
223      and we're weighing up the risks on the one hand of this,
224 P:   Yes
225 J:   of this test and the benefits on the other like you might have a
226      polyp and you remove it, and sometimes I'll have this conversation
227      with someone and they'll say, "ooh, no thanks, I don't want to risk
228      that," and that's alright, but I, I, suspect one of the reasons you're
229      here is so we can organise a colonoscopy for you
230 P:   Yes ( )
231 J:   Yes, you do, now um
232 P:   No good deep- putting your head in the sand, is it?
```

In Extract 10, the patient is older and has a family history of bowel cancer, thus making him very likely to develop bowel cancer himself. Rather than presenting himself as neutral here, James weighs up the risks and benefits himself, explicitly stating that the benefits outweigh the risks and which factors support this reasoning (lines 281–2). The patient agrees, "exactly", in line 283.

Extract 10 [10_NN]

```
281 J:   So you weigh up the risks and benefits, and, you know, somebody
282      your age with your family history, the benefits outweigh the risks, so
283 P:   Exactly.
284 J:   Good, we'll do that.
```

5.7.9   Reassurance or Necessity

After a decision has been made to pursue a colonoscopy (in our data, all patients decided to have colonoscopy), James again orients to the patient's presenting concern by referring to the colonoscopy as either for reassurance or a necessity. In Extract 11, following discussion of possible sources of bleeding (lines 187–96), James states that he thinks a haemorrhoid is the most likely source due to the amount and frequency of bleeding (lines 196–8). He explicitly states that he does not think anything needs to be done and that the purpose of the colonoscopy is to rule out any other causes (lines 198–9). In line 204, he explicitly names this purpose as "reassurance".

Extract 11 [16_SM]

```
187 P:   Yeah, fair enough, so with the bleeding, could that be diverticulitis
188      bleeding, or polyp bleeding, or
189 J:   Yeah, look, it, it could be any of those things.
190 P:   Right.
191 J:   Probably not polyp bleeding, cause it would be scantier than that,
192      and it would be mixed in with the stool.
193 P:   No, it wasn't.
194 J:   Diverticular bleeding's often much more torrential than that, and
195      you would just bowel movement after bowel movement that was
196      blood alone. So what I'm thinking is that, that it's more likely to be
197      coming from, from a haemorrhoid, and the fact that there's just been
198      the one episode, I don't think we need to do anything about that
199      except make sure that there's nothing else causing it. Does that
200      make sense?
201 P:   Yeah
202 J:   So...
203 P:   It does.
204 J:   ...reassurance
```

Necessity may be communicated as either a good thing to do (as in Extract 11) or because a serious problem needs to be corrected. In Extract 12, James's orientation to the colonoscopy as absolutely necessary is evident in his description of the patient's symptoms as worrying, "you really shouldn't have bloody mucus" (line 249) and the patient's account demonstrates agreement, "that's what I thought, that's a mm-mm, that's not right" (line 252). James issues a proclamation rather than a recommendation in line 253, "we'll have a look", to which she consents "okay" (line 254).

Extract 12 [07_OW]

```
249 J:   But you really shouldn't have bloody mucus
250 P:   No no.
251 J:   Yeah.
252 P:   That's what I thought, that's a mm-mm, that's not right.
253 J:   We'll have a look.
254 P:   Okay.
```

5.7.10 Breaking Informed Consent: Risks as Bad News

One potential result of colonoscopy is that a cancer may be found. This diagnosis carries with it several life-changing consequences that affect the approach to medical care. Unlike in routine procedures, patients with cancer often do not have the choice to do nothing and continue with a "normal" life. A choice of non-treatment for a cancer patient is an active decision to live with a condition that will most likely become terminal. In addition to being told their diagnosis, patients also learn about a host of potential complications that could befall them with or without treatment. The actual choices are, in effect, to forego any kind of treatment and die, or to choose among the most reliable treatments for their particular cancer and, depending on the severity of their cancer, live or at least be more comfortable.

Bowel cancer is commonly treated by removing the affected section of bowel, a major operation that is fraught with very real risks ranging from relatively minor inconveniences (e.g., numbness near the incision) to the need for re-operation (e.g., leaking where the bowel has been joined together) or even death (e.g., sepsis). Rather than following a set piece as when communicating risk in routine consultations such as for colonoscopies, James trades the rehearsed yet adaptable script for individualized, open and honest communication of risks associated with bowel cancer surgery. James's departure from a standardized approach to informed consent does not imply a departure from patterns altogether, however. Instead of aligning with informed consent (Towle and Godolphin 1999) per se, his style bears many features more commonly associated with breaking bad news. While James is not breaking bad news in the sense of disclosing the original diagnosis, we find that he uses communicative strategies for breaking bad news to relay the major nature of the surgery and the potential for complications as openly and directly as possible. This form of risk communication provides patients with the vital information that they need to be able to make an informed decision. This similarity to breaking bad news is reflected in James's explanation during the follow-up interview and thus our reference to this communicative act as *breaking informed consent*.

In the interview, James explained how he views risk communication in the context of major surgical intervention as a form of breaking bad news:

> It's very important to me that patients understand what they're in for if they're having a big operation, so I don't sugar-coat that. I'll actually, sometimes I'll say "This is the process of informed consent and there are some things you need to know about. In a way, I'm breaking bad news just explaining to you the things that could go wrong with this operation. It'd be great if we could wave a magic wand and the cancer is gone but no, you can get blood clots and infection and the bowel can leak." So that's breaking bad news in a way.

We will examine how James presents benefits and risks in these consultations, and, drawing on communicative frameworks for ISDM (Towle and Godolphin 1999) and breaking bad news (Baile et al. 2000; Sparks et al. 2007; Villagran et al. 2010), we will illustrate how he incorporates breaking bad news strategies into this more complex process of *breaking informed consent.*

5.7.11   Benefits and Risks

As with colonoscopy, benefits are not necessarily mentioned explicitly in cancer surgery consultations. Although the alternative of not doing the operation is mentioned, this is not discussed at length. Rather the patient in Extract 13 explicitly states that there is no option other than to do the surgery. Patients are there to have their cancer removed; that this is a benefit to them is assumed.

Extract 13 [33_NT]

```
649 P:   But you haven't got any option have you?
650 J:   I think so yeah.
651 P:   Really you haven't got an option.
652 J:   No.
653 P:   That's the way it goes, got to go with it...
```

Extract 14 represents the closest thing to an explicit benefit mentioned in these two consultations: James uses the patient's age to make a benefit declaration "you've got another forty years" (line 208), while at the same time using it to illustrate the necessity of the surgery given the patient's current condition, "or not cause you know the way you're going at the moment" (line 210).

Extract 14 [11_XH]

```
207 P:   Forty-seven.
208 J:   Yes you know you've got another forty years.
209 P:   Um.
210 J:   Or not cause you know the way you're going at the moment.
```

Rather than talk about benefits, explicit, direct (Sparks et al. 2007) and often unmitigated mention of risks was far more common in these two consultations, in addition to direct responses to patients' questions or concerns. Risk communication took the form of breaking informed consent, which we will explore in more detail in subsequent sections.

5.7.12   Breaking Informed Consent: Risk Communication

Using congruencies in the communicative strategies associated with obtaining informed consent and breaking bad news offers the surgeon a wide range of communication resources that might not be available otherwise due to constraints in either framework. For example, the main focus in Towle and Godolphin's (1999) framework for ISDM seems to be on explicit discussions of roles and responsibilities, and exchange of information to allow patients to take an active role in decision-making. The *partnership* competency is mostly concerned with the nature of the relationship between clinicians and patients and only mentions "opportunities for partnership building" in passing (p. 767). This stands in stark contrast to the call put out to surgeons almost 30 years ago to realize the relationship-building potential of the informed consent process (cf. Edwards and Yahne 1987). This is where strategies from breaking bad news can make a significant difference.

While the structurally oriented, linear approach to breaking bad news described in SPIKES (Baile et al. 2000) only fleetingly covers making a "connection with the patient" (p. 305), it does make explicit allowance for "addressing the patient's emotions with empathetic responses" (p. 306). On the other hand, the non-linear strategies in the COMFORT model (Villagran et al. 2010) and those described by Sparks and colleagues (2007) offer ample resources to engage with patients and their families by being mindful and comforting, respectively. Villagran and colleagues (2010) even specifically promote mindfulness as an "intrapersonal process that enhances interpersonal connection and patient-centred interactions through both verbal and nonverbal interactions" (p. 228).

Taking advantage of combining strategies from informed consent and breaking bad news allows the surgeon to overcome gaps in communicative strategies, and the wide variety of available resources enables him to fulfil both medical and relational goals in the *breaking informed consent process*. In the following sections, we will illuminate James's communication style by looking at corresponding strategies from the three selected breaking bad news frameworks.

5.7.13 Setting up and Family

Physical preparation, seating arrangements, agenda setting and the inclusion of significant others and family (Baile et al. 2000; Villagran et al. 2010) seem to play a much bigger role in the pre-surgical cancer consultations than in routine informed consent. James again uses communicative strategies like signposts, humorous remarks and colloquial language, and makes his strategies and perspectives known to the patient, thus turning the patient into an equal interaction partner and showing how important the conversation is for all parties involved.

James takes great care in ensuring that the physical setup is conducive to a serious discussion of the gravity of the impending decision regarding surgery. He further ensures that family members are able to attend the consultation or that they are at least known to him. For example, in Extract 15, James seats the patient and her three daughters in what he calls "a healing circle" (line 14). He also signals his interest in the family members through an explicit signpost about getting to know their names (lines 23–5). His casual openness at the beginning of the consultations initiates laughter from the patient and her family and helps to establish a more friendly and patient-centred atmosphere (see Chapter 3 of this volume).

Extract 15 [33_NT]

```
09 J:    And we'll just - actually what we'll do, we'll make a bit of a...
10 D:    Circle. ((patient's daughter))
11 J:    We'll make a...
12       ((laughter))
13 D2:   A pow-wow. ((patient's daughter))
14 J:    A healing circle.
15       ((laughter))
16 J:    There we go.
         [...]
23 J:    Okay. Thank you everybody for coming; that's just great. Who've we
24       got? I tell you what, give me one second. I need to go and get a bit of
25       paper and I'll write down some names and...
```

The physical setting and atmosphere also allows family members to further contribute to the consultation by asking questions (e.g., "So is there one the one um mass in the lungs?" [...] "So within one operation, would you remove those?", 33_NT) or suggesting alternative arrangements (e.g., "So can you not do the um the x-ray or whatever it is today and still do the operation on the bowel tomorrow?", 33_NT). Before turning to explain the risks of a cancer resection, James even explicitly states his preference for involving family members in such consultations:

> And this is the main reason I'm bringing you all...here, is you'd like to think oh, we just remove the cancer with this, you know...[...] Yeah, the wave of a magic wand [...]...but it's not always the case. And sometimes things go wrong and that's a real nuisance and uhm it's the wrong time to meet you guys. So it's better to have met you before the wheels fall off, like we practise talking to each other, rather than after [...] when your mum's potentially really sick [...] and [...] and you're all stressed. (33_NT, lines 499–516, backchannels from patient and family members omitted).

An agenda is usually set early during the consultations and made explicit through signposting as illustrated in Extract 16 (lines 91–2, 94, 96), where the signpost actually triggered one of the patient's daughters to raise an additional contributing concern that should be (and which was later) discussed (lines 97–9).

Extract 16 [33_NT]

```
91 J:    Oh. So but - so we'll talk about that because, in fact, what
92       we're going to do is we're going to talk about the operation...
93 D:    Yeah. ((patient's daughter))
94 J:    ...what I expect to find and what to do about it...
95 P:    Right.
96 J:    ...and what might go wrong with it is the other side.
```

```
97 D:    Mum's a bit worried because dad had died with the bowel cancer.
98       Mum doesn't want to go through what dad did. And so did mum's
99       father... ((patient's daughter))
```

Because of the delicate nature of breaking bad news, doctors are urged to avoid any interruption by turning off pagers or mobile phones (Baile et al. 2000). James extended this sentiment to complex consent consultations, explicitly identifying (line 78) and managing potential interruptions (line 83–4) such as telephone calls with signposts and colloquial language as shown in Extract 17.

Extract 17 [11_XH]

```
78 J:    Did [receptionist] mention that I might have to go to the operating room?
         [...]
83 J:    Now - bugger them they can, well, they can wait for us. This is a very
84       important discussion.
```

5.7.14 Orientation and Reiterative Messages

In breaking bad news, *orientation* refers to providing information about diagnosis and prognosis in language appropriate to the patient and family's levels of health literacy and addressing their ideas about hope or probability in separate statements (Villagran et al. 2010). In these complex consultations, James provided unmitigated disclosure of the possibility of complications in simple language. Although it is likely that the patient will recover as expected, James presented complications and poor outcomes as something that could realistically happen rather than something he had to disclose to everyone for the sake of informed consent (e.g., "the question is, are we going to be able to get this out and leave everything else in your pelvis?", 11_XH; "It would be unusual for them [lung nodules] to be a problem for the bowel cancer but it, it could be. And one of the things that we'll arrange today is yet another sort of an x-ray, which will tell us whether or not we need to, to follow that", 33_NT).

James also relied on reiterative messages, for example to orient patients and family to the sheer gravity of the potential surgeries they were discussing. Reiterative messages are distributed throughout the interaction and reframe or rephrase the same message slightly to help patients better grasp its meaning and implications (Villagran et al. 2010). James did not use reiterative messages for one patient (33_NT), as her most likely initial surgical treatment option was a relatively straightforward bowel resection. For the other patient (11_XH), however, treatment choices were complicated by the position of the tumour and involved either removing only the affected bowel section or removing other organs due to local invasion of the cancer.

Extract 18 [11_XH]

```
137  J:   Um, so the really big decision that, that, well, we have to make together
138        over the next, really over the next day or two, not much longer, is
139        whether when we take this out, we take out only the cancer and the bowel
140        or whether we need to take out the other things too.
           [...]
150  J:   and it can - and so I think that the main idea I wanted to, to implant
151        today, and that's a huge idea.
           [...]
160  J:   That's, that's a big deal.
           [...]
174  J:   [...] you know, it's a, a, a mutilating operation in some ways but the
175        - it's an operation that, if I had to have it, I would give some serious
176        thought as to whether I would have it or not, you know.
```

In this case (Extract 18), James reiterates over multiple instances that they will have to make a "really big decision" (line 137) between the relatively straightforward bowel resection and removing other organs and, through his reiteration, honestly and openly communicates the gravity of the latter option.

5.7.15 Communicating, Giving Knowledge, and Direct and Indirect Strategies

Communicating in the COMFORT model refers to using familiar, unambiguous language to communicate bad news without excessive detail (Villagran et al. 2010). James frequently uses metaphors to provide clear descriptions (e.g., "You know, you've got a narrow little male pelvis with a tennis ball sitting in the middle of it. That's not a lot of room," 11_XH) or in place of drawings when talking about complications (Extract 19, lines 534–5).

Extract 19 [33_NT]

```
531  P:   Where would it leak to
532  J:   Well it leaks into your belly
533  D:   Oh ((Patient's daughter))
534  J:   So it's a little bit like you've had a ruptured appendix when that
535        happens.
```

To deliver easily understandable explanations but also to align more closely with the patients, and to establish and maintain rapport and partnership, James often relies on colloquial language (e.g., "So what Dr [last name] did was he put the telescope in, went all the way around here [...] and took a couple of little bites of this", 33_NT; "No but we'll need to be pretty damned sure of it before we operate on you", 11_XH; "That's why we bring you guys", 33_NT).

As far as patient preferences for information (Towle and Godolphin 1999) are concerned, although James did not solicit the patients' existing knowledge or ideas about the procedure, he did use communicative strategies to achieve a similar level of knowledge regarding patients' *perception* (Baile et al. 2000). For example, by providing a summary of his understanding of their case so far, James provided patients (or family members) with the opportunity to correct him or to add further information from their own personal perspective (see Extract 20, lines 186–7).

Extract 20 [11_XH]

```
177 J:   ...and this is the area of the tumour. You know, that's sort of down there.
178 P:   So it's in the pouch. Is it in the pouch or outside of the pouch?
179 J:   Not sure exactly.
180 P:   Because it don't - feels high and still got all this up here...
181 J:   Yeah, I know.
182 P:   ...where it, at times, it's hard and no movement sort of thing.
183 J:   Yes, I - and I think that's this cancer blocking off.
184 P:   Right.
185 J:   That's, I think what you feel is happening as well.
186 P:   So that's why I'm feeling - obviously seeing it so low that's obviously
187      why I'm feeling full and going to the toilet 20 times a day.
```

In terms of giving information, James frequently uses a direct approach (Sparks et al. 2007), whether stating his concern for the patient ("I – well, I'm – I'm concerned about you", 11_XH), disclosing uncertainty ("and my only concern seeing you today was that they mightn't have the proper result yet", 11_XH), naming the diagnosis ("there is a couple of nodules in the lung", 33_NT) or confirming the risk of complications ("I'm a bit stressed, because I hate it when things go wrong, and they do", 33_NT). His direct approach in disclosing and explaining the risks of the proposed surgeries provides patients with an honest account of the potential complication and makes the possibility of a poor outcome a real rather than theoretical possibility (e.g., Extract 21, lines 542–3, 545).

Extract 21 [33_NT]

```
539 D:   [it can cause] septicaemia.
540 J:   Yeah, it can make you...
541 P:   Oh really?
542 J:   Yeah, it can make you really, really sick. It - it would probably mean
543      another operation.
544 P:   If that happens?
545 J:   Yeah. It could even mean a colostomy bag.
```

In the colonoscopy consultations, benefits are discussed indirectly, but risks are discussed directly. In the cancer surgery consultations, however, James uses indirect communication strategies (Sparks et al. 2007) to discuss prognosis and further treatment ("Um, she may need chemotherapy but again, that's something that we'll weigh up [...] with her general, you know, strength...", 33_NT) as well as recovery. For example, in Extract 22, James draws on his knowledge of the patient's history of "big operations" (lines 253–4) to give an indirect answer to the patient's question about recovery periods.

Extract 22 [33_NT]

```
251 P:   Mmm, and then what is sort of the, um, recovery sort of scenario just
252      so I can get all that into perspective?
253 J:   Yeah, yeah, no, you-you've - you've been through these sort of big
254      operations before, (4.0) so you-you've got a fair idea about that.
```

5.7.16 Emotions and Mindfulness

Mindfulness refers to the need for clinicians to attend to each BBN interaction without regard to scripts or formulaic responses, as James does in departing from his informed consent set piece. The goal of mindfulness is to enhance interpersonal connections to help patients understand and deal with the emotional distress of bad news (Villagran et al. 2010). Included in this are demonstrating that one cares and is empathetic to the patient and their distress and allowing the patient time to sit and digest what they have been told, all of which feature in James's cancer surgery consultations.

James displays attentiveness to the patients' emotions, expressing empathy to alleviate expressed fears, offer reassurance and support each patient's decision. Empathic responses in relation to patient emotions or concerns often take the form of immediate comforting strategies (Sparks et al. 2007). For example, in Extract 23, James reacts to the patient tearing up after he highlights the gravity of the decision ("That's, that's a big deal", line 160) and gives the patient permission to cry by indicating that a "big box" of tissues is available (line 162).

Extract 23 [11_XH]

```
160 J:   That's, that's a big deal.
161 P:   But you won't be 100 per cent sure about that yet, will you?
162 J:   I've got a big box of Kleenex here. Here you go.
163 P:   [Sighs].
```

Yet James is careful to avoid unrealistic or formulaic reassurance when faced with questions that cannot be answered without further tests, an approach that attempts to balance staying focused on the current problem with attending to the patient's fears.

In Extract 24, the patient's daughter has asked about the lesion in the patient's lung that requires further imaging to diagnose (line 699), and the patient recycles James's word "unusual" from earlier in the consultation, "yeah it's unusual isn't it" (line 701). James responds in line 702, "that's a problem for another day really". Without reiteration of the need for further testing, this could easily come across as dismissing the concern. Although the patient's daughter demonstrates recognition of this caveat ("yeah", line 703), the patient takes up the topic, rephrasing her question in line 701 to "is that a common thing?" in line 704. After some discussion of why the lesion might be in the lungs (lines 705–8), the patient's daughter asks "is it common for a smoker, an ex-smoker?" in line 709. James claims inadequate knowledge ("I'm the wrong person to ask...I'm guts", lines 710 and 712), the daughter accepts this (lines 711 and 713), and the participants laugh (line 714). James offers reassurance that "we'll know soon" at this point (line 715). The daughter accepts this with "right okay" at line 716, and James and the patient go on to reiterate the plan to "follow it" (line 718).

Extract 24 [33_NT]

```
697 J:   So the only the only overlay is that thing behind the pectoral
698      muscle...
699 D:   What's in her lungs ((Patient's daughter))
700 J:   ...on the right and the lungs.
701 P:   Yeah it's unusual isn't it.
702 J:   That's that's a problem for another day really.
703 D:   Yeah.
704 P:   Is that a common thing?
705 J:   The lungs? Um, no.
706 D:   But you were a smoker, mum, so it could be to do with the smoking.
707 P:   And probably because I'm ((    ))
708 J:   Yeah
709 D:   Is it common for a smoker, an ex-smoker?
710 J:   I'm the wrong person to ask
711 D:   Yeah right okay
712 J:   I'm guts
713 D:   Right okay
714      ((laughter))
715 J:   And we'll know soon
716 D:   Right okay
717 J:   And it's just one of those things that
718 P:   Well you've just, you've got to go as it happens, you've got to follow it.
```

Rather than having a phase at which the patient makes a decision on available treatment options, the treatment plan has generally been vaguely decided before the consultation. Instead, discussion of the exact plan for treatment is initiated, including any further tests that would aid the surgery, the timing of the surgery and whether the anaesthetist or other surgeons should see the patient before the day of surgery. It is here that treatment negotiation occurs and the final treatment plan is summarized.

5.7.17 Ongoing Support and Teamwork

Ongoing dialogue about care should be directly linked to a need for continuity of care and avoiding abandonment of the patient (Villagran et al. 2010). This may be communicated through words or actions and also creates opportunities for clarification, addresses patient concerns and offers indirect reassurance. James discusses continuity of care explicitly, for example by referring to the hospital's cancer focus and the availability of a single centre for ongoing care ("the hospital's sort of been built with a cancer focus so", 33_NT) and expressing concern at having not seen the other patient for a long time whilst liaising with another hospital ("I thought that I'd lost track of you", 11_XH).

In cancer care especially, the entire healthcare team is actively involved in patient care. Referring to the team and its members builds on the theme of *ongoing support*, that the patient will not be abandoned (Villagran et al. 2010). James mentions the healthcare team, including debates about how to go forward and members who will only be involved for the surgery itself such as the anaesthetist ("and we'll make sure you're in the best shape for anaesthetic. [...] We might get the anaesthetist to look at you [...]", 33_NT). James also expresses the teamwork approach by using the inclusive pronoun "we" (doctor and patient) rather than "I" or "you" when discussing treatment plans and further testing, thereby directly implicating himself, the patient and the rest of the healthcare team.

Extract 25 [33_NT]

```
343 J:   It would be unusual for them [lung nodules] to be a problem for the
344      bowel cancer but it, it could be.
345      And one of the things that we'll arrange today is yet another sort of
346      an x-ray, which will tell us whether or not we need to, to follow that...
347 D:   Yep. (Patient's daughter)
348 P:   Oh right.
349 J:   ...up further.
350 D:   Right.
351 J:   You know, whether that's something we need to deal with.
```

For example in Extract 25, he proposes the scheduling of further testing as a joint action using phrases such as *"we'll* arrange" (line 345), "will tell *us* whether or not *we* need to" (line 346) and "*we* need to deal with" (line 351), and in this way highlights the relevance of the test and its implication for future *joint* actions for the doctor-patient-family team.

5.8   Summary and Implications for Surgical Communication Training

Informed consent and *breaking bad news* are important "set pieces" in the non-technical armamentarium of the proceduralist. In surgery, the former is often considered a legal requirement "obtained" before a procedure, whereas the latter is viewed as a sensitive responsibility where distressing information is delivered to patients and families. Considering their superficial differences, these tasks are rarely contemplated together, yet they share unexpected commonalities. Considering informed consent as a variation of breaking bad news can add depth and meaning to the process and can improve patient safety by fostering a trusting relationship with patients and their families. In fact, it allows all parties to better manage the regrettable but inevitable risks of surgery.

The surgeon in this study included the patient's family at an early stage, aiming to build resilient relationships to better manage both success and mishap. The presence of key relatives in pre-surgical discussions allowed everyone to practice talking with each other. The surgeon was able to explain that surgery does not mean waving a magic wand and that there might be "bad news" later. This idea of potential bad news needs to be broken as carefully and deliberately as any other bad news. For patient's relatives, this means that initial consultations take on the aura of a "first date" or a "team-building exercise" such that if surgical complications arise, they will not have to form a team under difficult circumstances – they are already a team that is committed to the patient's wellbeing.

It is especially the importance and appreciation that the *breaking informed consent* process places on relationship-building, empathy and rapport that define it as a relational *and* medical tool and distinguish it from the purely goal-oriented consent process that is often considered a mere formality. In this respect, *breaking informed consent* can potentially provide a practical answer to the plea Edwards and Yahne (1987: 578) made to surgeons nearly 30 years ago:

> We hope that surgeons can learn to look at the informed consent process as a wonderful opportunity to communicate their personal concern for the patient as a person, not just a sick gallbladder to remove, and that this process can become the channel through which the wounded relationship of the patient and the physician can be healed.

The management of surgical complications is an important aspect of medical training, yet the skills of obtaining informed consent and breaking bad news are usually taught formally (and separately) using protocols and guidelines. We acknowledge that educational views and habitual beliefs framing informed consent as a legal necessity rather than a communicative opportunity need to be addressed before the breaking informed consent technique can be incorporated into medical education and professional development. However, we feel that the first step towards realizing the relationship-building potential of informed consent lies in reflective engagement with the actual practice of *breaking informed consent* through the close study of discourse of the kind presented in this chapter. Guided examination, reflections and discussion of the interactional work achieved by the surgeon by breaking informed consent can offer valuable tools for trainee and professional development (O'Grady 2011) and provide a sustainable alternative to the more prescriptive and linear protocols that have traditionally been used in teaching informed consent and breaking bad news. We hope that by making experienced surgeons and trainees critically aware of a wide range of communication resources available from both informed consent and breaking bad news frameworks, they may be encouraged to establish rapport and trust early on and to build a strong relationship with patients and their families "before the wheels fall off".

5.9   Concluding Remarks

While this study has focused only on the practices of one colorectal surgeon in two types of consultations, it highlights that language and communicative strategies used while obtaining informed consent greatly influence patients' engagement in the understanding of the risks involved in a procedure as well as the character of the relationship formed between surgeon and patient. Combining communicative strategies from informed consent and breaking bad news into an approach dubbed *breaking informed consent* can help to build trusting relationships with patients and their families and can thus provide a strong foundation to prepare patients for and to manage potential future complications. By illustrating the relational potential of the informed consent process, our study makes a contribution to expanding surgeons' understanding of the consent process beyond being a mere legal prerequisite to surgery and provides practical advice on the communicative resources that surgeons can use to enhance their relationships with patients during risk communication. Understanding of this phenomenon could be enhanced by further research examining how informed consent, breaking bad news and diagnostic testing interact in other surgical specialities, non-surgical specialities and diagnoses that are not life-threatening.

Transcription Notation

See Chapter 3, this volume.

Acknowledgements

The authors wish to thank the surgeon and patients who participated in the project, and the staff at the Macquarie University Hospital Clinic.

References

Abed, Husam, Rebecca Rogers, Deborah Helitzer and Teddy D. Warner. 2007. Informed Consent in Gynecologic Surgery. *American Journal of Obstetrics and Gynecology* 197(6): 674.e1. doi: 10.1016/j.ajog.2007.08.066

Baile, Walter F., Robert Buckman, Renato Lenzi, Gary Glober, Estela A. Beale and Andrzej P. Kudelka. 2000. SPIKES – A Six-Step Protocol for Delivering Bad News: Application to the Patient with Cancer. *The Oncologist* 5(4): 302–11.

Beach, Mary Catherine, Debra Roter, Susan Larson, Daniel E. Ford, Wendy Levinson and Richard Frankel. 2004. What Do Physicians Tell Patients about Themselves? A

Qualitative Analysis of Physician Self-Disclosure. *Journal of General Internal Medicine* 19(9): 911–16. doi: 10.1111/j.1525-1497.2004.30604.x

Bogardus Jr, Sidney T., Eric Holmboe and James F. Jekel. 1999. Perils, Pitfalls, and Possibilities in Talking about Medical Risk. *JAMA* 281(11): 1037–41.

Caffi, Claudia. 1999. On Mitigation. *Journal of Pragmatics* 31(7): 881–909.

Calman, Kenneth C. 1996. Cancer: Science and Society and the Communication of Risk. *BMJ: British Medical Journal* 313(7060): 799–802.

Charles, Cathy, Amiram Gafni and Tim Whelan. 1997. Shared Decision-Making in the Medical Encounter: What Does It Mean? (or It Takes at Least Two to Tango). *Social Science & Medicine* 44(5): 681–92. doi: 10.1016/S0277-9536(96)00221-3

Consumers Health Forum of Australia. 2013. Informed Consent in Healthcare: An Issues Paper. Barton, ACT.

Dahm, Maria R., Catherine O'Grady, Lynda Yates and Peter Roger. 2015. Into the Spotlight: Exploring the Use of the Dictaphone During Surgical Consultations. *Health Communication* 30(5): 513–20. doi: 10.1080/10410236.2014.894603

Edwards, Adrian, Glyn Elwyn and Al Mulley. 2002. Explaining Risks: Turning Numerical Data into Meaningful Pictures. *BMJ: British Medical Journal* 324 (7341): 827–30.

Edwards, Adrian, Glyn Elwyn, Fiona Wood, Christine Atwell, Lindsay Prior and Helen Houston. 2005. Shared Decision Making and Risk Communication in Practice: A Qualitative Study of GPs' Experiences. *The British Journal of General Practice* 55(510): 6.

Edwards, Adrian, Elaine Matthews, Roison Pill and Michael Bloor. 1998. Communication about Risk: The Responses of Primary Care Professionals to Standardizing the "Language of Risk" and Communication Tools. *Family Practice* 15(4): 301.

Edwards, W. Sterling, and Carolina Yahne. 1987. Surgical Informed Consent: What It Is and Is Not. *The American Journal of Surgery* 154(6): 574–8. doi: 10.1016/0002-9610(87)90219-4

Epstein, Ronald M., Brian S. Alper and Timothy E. Quill. 2004. Communicating Evidence for Participatory Decision Making. *JAMA* 291(19): 2359–66.

Gillotti, Cathy, Teresa Thompson and Kelly McNeilis. 2002. Communicative Competence in the Delivery of Bad News. *Social Science & Medicine* 54(7): 1011–23. doi: 10.1016/s0277-9536(01)00073-9

Gogos, Andrew J., Richard B. Clark, Marie M. Bismark, Russell L. Gruen and David M. Studdert. 2011. When Informed Consent Goes Poorly: A Descriptive Study of Medical Negligence Claims and Patient Complaints. *Medical Journal of Australia* 195(6): 340.

Habiba, Marwan, Clare Jackson, Andrea Akkad, Sara Kenyon and Mary Dixon-Woods. 2004. Women's Accounts of Consenting to Surgery: Is Consent a Quality Problem? *Quality & Safety in Health Care* 13(6): 422.

Harrison, Mark Eldon, and Anne Walling. 2010. What Do We Know about Giving Bad News? A Review. *Clinical Pediatrics* 49(7): 619. doi: 10.1177/0009922810361380

Heritage, John, Jeffrey D. Robinson, Marc N. Elliott, Megan Beckett and Michael Wilkes. 2007. Reducing Patients' Unmet Concerns in Primary Care: The Difference One Word Can Make. *Journal of General Internal Medicine* 22(10): 1429.

Jenkins, Val A., Lesley J. Fallowfield, Anna Souhami and Mary Sawtell. 1999. How Do Doctors Explain Randomised Clinical Trials to Their Patients? *European Journal of Cancer* 35(8): 1187–93. doi: 10.1016/s0959-8049(99)00116-1

Kim, Sara, Sinan Jabori, Jessica O'Connell, Shanna Freeman, Cha Chi Fung, Sahrish Ekram, Amruta Unawame and Gail Van Norman. 2013. Research Methodologies in Informed Consent Studies Involving Surgical and Invasive Procedures: Time to Re-Examine? *Patient Education and Counseling* 93(3): 559–66. doi: 10.1016/j.pec.2013.08.018

Lamiani, Giulia, Serena Barello, David M. Browning, Elena Vegni and Elaine C. Meyer. 2011. Uncovering and Validating Clinicians' Experiential Knowledge when Facing Difficult Conversations: A Cross-Cultural Perspective. *Patient Education and Counseling* 87(3): 307–12. doi: 10.1016/j.pec.2011.11.012

Leclercq, Wouter K.G., Bram J. Keulers, Marc R.M. Scheltinga, Paul H. Spauwen and Gert-Jan van der Wilt. 2010. A Review of Surgical Informed Consent: Past, Present and Future – A Quest to Help Patients Make Better Decisions. *World Journal of Surgery* 34(7): 1406–15.

Levinson, Wendy, Pamela Hudak and Andrea C. Tricco. 2013. A Systematic Review of Surgeon-Patient Communication: Strengths and Opportunities for Improvement. *Patient Education and Counseling* 93(1): 3–17. doi: 10.1016/j.pec.2013.03.023

Little, Miles, Christopher F.C. Jordens, Catherine McGrath, Kathleen Montgomery, Wendy Lipworth and Ian Kerridge. 2008. Informed Consent and Medical Ordeal: A Qualitative Study. *Internal Medicine Journal* 38(8): 624. doi: 10.1111/j.1445-5994.2008.01700.x

Makoul, Gregory, Paul Arntson and Theo Schofield. 1995. Health Promotion in Primary Care: Physician-Patient Communication and Decision Making about Prescription Medications. *Social Science & Medicine* 41(9): 1241–54. doi: 10.1016/0277-9536(95)00061-b

Maynard, Douglas W. 1989. Perspective-Display Sequences in Conversation. *Western Journal of Speech Communication* 53(2): 91–113. doi: 10.1080/10570318909374294.

Narayanan, Vijayakumar, Bibek Bista and Cheriyan Koshy. 2010. "BREAKS" Protocol for Breaking Bad News. *Indian Journal of Palliative Care* 16(2): 61–5. doi: 10.4103/0973-1075.68401

O'Grady, Catherine. 2011. Teaching the Communication of Empathy in Patient-Centred Medicine. In *English Language and the Medical Profession: Instructing and Assessing the Communication Skills of International Physicians*, edited by Barbara J. Hoekje and Sara M. Tipton, 43–72. Bingley: Emerald.

Oosthuizen, Johannes C., Paul Burns and Conrad Timon. 2012. The Changing Face of Informed Surgical Consent. *The Journal of Laryngology & Otology* 126(3): 236–9. doi: 10.1017/S0022215111003021

Paling, John. 2003. Strategies to Help Patients Understand Risks. *BMJ: British Medical Journal* 327(7417): 745–8.

Penn, Claire, Tali Frankel, Jennifer Watermeyer and Madeleine Müller. 2009. Informed Consent and Aphasia: Evidence of Pitfalls in the Process. *Aphasiology* 23(1): 3–32. doi: 10.1080/02687030701521786

Persaud, Raj, and John B.L. Howell. 1993. Breaking Bad News. *The Lancet* 341(8848): 832–3. doi: 10.1016/0140-6736(93)90611-J

Robins, Lynne, Douglas Brock, Saskia Witteborn, Lanae Miner, Larry Mauksch and Kelly Edwards. 2011. Identifying Transparency in Physician Communication. *Patient Education and Counseling* 83(1): 73–9. doi: 10.1016/j.pec.2010.05.004

Sanders, Tom, and Suzanne Skevington. 2004. Participation as an Expression of Patient Uncertainty: An Exploration of Bowel Cancer Consultations. *Psycho-Oncology* 13(10): 675–88. doi: 10.1002/pon.779

Schattner, Ami, Alexander Bronstein and Navah Jellin. 2006. Information and Shared Decision-Making Are Top Patients' Priorities. *BMC Health Services Research* 6: 21. doi: 10.1186/1472-6963-6-21

Schegloff, Emanuel A. 2001. Getting Serious: Joke→Serious "No". *Journal of Pragmatics* 33(12): 1947–55.

Schenker, Yael, Frances Wang, Sarah Jane Selig, Rita Ng and Alicia Fernandez. 2007. The Impact of Language Barriers on Documentation of Informed Consent at a Hospital with On-Site Interpreter Services. *Journal of General Internal Medicine* 22(Suppl 2): 294–9. doi: 10.1007/s11606-007-0359-1

Sparks, Lisa, Melinda M. Villagran, Jessica Parker-Raley and Corey B. Cunningham. 2007. A Patient-Centered Approach to Breaking Bad News: Communication Guidelines for Health Care Providers. *Journal of Applied Communication Research* 35(2): 177–96. doi: 10.1080/00909880701262997

Tobias, Jeffrey S., and Robert L. Souhami. 1993. Fully Informed Consent Can Be Needlessly Cruel. *BMJ: British Medical Journal* 307(6913): 1199–201.

Towle, Angela, and William Godolphin. 1999. Framework for Teaching and Learning Informed Shared Decision Making. *BMJ: British Medical Journal* 319 (7212): 766–9.

Towle, Angela, William Godolphin, Garry Grams and Amanda Lamarre. 2006. Putting Informed and Shared Decision Making into Practice. *Health Expectations: An International Journal of Public Participation in Health Care and Health Policy* 9(4): 321.

Villagran, Melinda, Joy Goldsmith, Elaine Wittenberg-lyles and Paula Baldwin. 2010. Creating COMFORT: A Communication-Based Model for Breaking Bad News. *Communication Education* 59(3): 220–34. doi: 10.1080/03634521003624031

Wachbroit, Robert. 1991. Describing Risk. In *Risk Assessment in Genetic Engineering. Environmental Release of Organisms*, edited by Morris A. Levin and Harlee S. Strauss, 368–7. New York: McGraw-Hill.

Wolcott, Harry F. 2008. *Ethnography: A Way of Seeing*. 2nd ed. Langham, MD: AltaMira.

Maria R. Dahm completed an Early Career Research Fellowship in Linguistics at Macquarie University, Sydney, and is currently working with the Australian Institute of Health Innovation at Macquarie where she combines her passion for patient-centred health research with her expertise in qualitative and mixed methods research. Her PhD (completed in 2012) examined the impact of medical terminology on English-medium consultations involving non-native speakers. Her research interests include communication and culture in intercultural health and other workplace contexts, health informatics and English for Specific Purposes.

Israel Berger completed his PhD in psychology at the University of Roehampton, London. He is a final year medical student at Sydney Medical School, University of Sydney, with a view toward surgery. He has taught research methods to undergraduate and postgraduate students in the UK and Australia. In his own research, he uses a variety of qualitative and quantitative methodologies to explore public health and service provision issues and is interested in healthcare interactions as a conversation analyst.

6 Do Surgeons Want to Operate? Negotiating the Treatment Plan in Surgical Consultations

Maria Stubbe, Sarah J. White, Lindsay Macdonald, Anthony C. Dowell, Rod Gardner and Kevin Dew

6.1 Introduction

The so-called surgeon's law or surgeon's creed – *"if in doubt, cut it out"* – reflects a stereotypical perception that surgeons will generally "want to operate" rather than recommending less invasive treatments. Whilst this is clearly an apocryphal saying, there is nevertheless some empirical evidence that suggests surgeons may indeed orient to surgery as a "default option". Recent observational studies of decision-making processes in North American orthopaedic consultations, for instance, have found that recommendations in favour of surgery were usually presented in more simple and direct terms than proposals *not* to operate which required more extended negotiation (Hudak, Clark and Raymond 2011, 2012). Other research has shown that, although surgeons are encouraged during training to provide patients with treatment options including discussion of risks and benefits (Tongue, Epps and Forese 2005), surgeons vary in the amount of information they provide, and such discussions do not always occur (Keating et al. 2003; Pleat et al. 2004; Brezis et al. 2008). Traditional models of the medical consultation also assume that patients typically defer to the medical authority of the doctor in reaching treatment decisions (Heritage and Clayman 2010), and that patients are relatively passive participants in consultations, with doctors initiating most actions and proposals (Robinson 2003). The prevailing view of surgical consultations, then, has been one that depicts surgeons as using their specialized clinical reasoning to "rule in" a possible diagnosis and determine whether the patient would benefit or not from a surgical procedure to resolve the presenting problem, with the patient taking these professional judgements largely on trust.

Recent decades have seen a progressive shift away from paternalistic physician-centred models like these to more patient-centred approaches, both in training and medical curricula (Silverman, Kurtz and Draper 2013) and in actual practice (Salzburg Global Seminar 2011; Stewart et al. 2003). This shift is reflected in a large and growing body of research on shared decision-making (Charles, Gafni and Whelan 1997; Collins et al. 2007; Elwyn et al. 2012). Contemporary patient-centred models of the medical consultation emphasize mutuality and a "view of the ideal patient as one who actively participates in his or her health" (Cegala and Post 2006: 855). This view is predicated on a presumption that enhanced patient partic-ipation will improve outcomes by encouraging patient understanding and involve-ment in their care (Collins et al. 2007) and there is some evidence that patients in primary care settings increasingly do seek to engage in this way with their doctors (Costello and Roberts 2001; Robinson 2001). As yet however, there is no clear consensus on exactly what "patient participation" in a consultation means or how this might be measured, or indeed what level of participation in decision-making patients themselves actually want (Collins et al. 2007; Hudak et al. 2008). One common conception is of different degrees of participation or different levels of involvement ranging from simpler or lower level activities such as seeking infor-mation, to higher level participation in medical decision-making (Street et al. 2009; Thompson 2007). Another common focus is on shared decision-making along a continuum from relatively unilateral decisions (by either physician or patient) to more bilateral processes (Collins et al. 2005; Makoul and Clayman 2006).

Research evidence now starting to emerge shows that, as in primary care, surgical patients also frequently exert a greater degree of agency than traditional models of the consultation would suggest. Patients can and do influence decision-making, with treatment recommendations in particular shown to be a joint interactional achieve-ment by surgeon and patient (Clark and Hudak 2011 and Chapter 7, this volume; Hudak et al. 2010; White 2011). At the same time, these and other studies continue to highlight the inherent asymmetries arising both from the surgeon's very special-ized medical knowledge and expertise, and from the patient's lack of familiarity in most cases with this type of consultation setting. Because such asymmetries are inevitably greater than in the primary care context, achieving a genuine partnership approach to decision-making in surgical consultations is arguably more challenging, with real limits on patients' capacity and/or willingness to engage with the clinical complexities involved (Etchells et al. 2011; Janz et al. 2004; Sinding et al. 2010). At this point therefore, it remains unclear to what extent or in what ways contemporary patient-centred models of the consultation emphasizing mutuality and shared deci-sion-making can be said to be reflected in surgical clinic interactions.

The focus of this chapter is on the naturally occurring interactional processes by which surgeons and patients negotiate and reach decisions about treatment plans in consultations where a surgical or other invasive procedure is discussed, and how surgeons' recommendations align (or not) with expressed patient wishes and concerns. Our exploration of these issues is based on analysis of surgical consultations from a range of specialties, video-recorded between 2005 and 2010 in New Zealand hospital outpatient clinics (see below). The next section briefly reviews some recent research relating to decision-making during the treatment recommendation phase of health interactions, including surgical consultations. We then provide a brief description of our data and methods, before summarizing the general patterns identified in our analysis alongside more detailed examination of representative extracts from individual cases.

6.2　Previous Research

A small but growing body of research on the detail of surgeon-patient communication provides evidence that the reality of surgical consultations is much more varied and multi-layered than that implied by the traditional and rather stereotypical view outlined in the opening paragraph. This real-life complexity relates to overall consultation structure and the range of activities carried out in surgical interviews, and is also reflected in the nature of patient agency and participation in the surgical consultation, particularly during the "interactional negotiation" of treatment plans.

Surgical consultations, like medical consultations more generally, are constructed from a more or less linear series of interdependent activities which together form the basis of a recognizable "interactional project" (Robinson 2003; and as discussed in Chapter 2, this volume). The specific activity structures seen in particular consultations can and do vary depending on the purpose of the visit; not all activities are seen in every consultation, but the overall sequence of activities remains fairly constant. The structure of surgical consultations also differs in some important ways from the typical trajectory found in primary care consultations. For example, one important feature of many surgical consultations (other than routine follow-up visits) is that for the consultation to proceed satisfactorily, mutual agreement must be reached right at the start on the fact that the patient has been referred (and sometimes on the reason for referral), and this is not always a straightforward matter (White et al. 2013, 2014). Moreover, the referring doctor is at least implicitly an additional party to the decision-making process (Charles, Gafni and Whelan 1997).

The past two decades have seen the development of a substantial body of research that closely examines the fine interactional detail of doctor-patient consultations using conversation analysis and related methodologies, though once again, until recently most of this work focused on primary care visits (Heritage and Maynard 2006). Activities core to the consultation such as problem presentation, history taking, diagnosis, and openings and closings have received a great deal of attention, but less work has been done thus far on the activity of "proposing next steps" or treatment recommendation, especially in surgical consultations. One aspect that has received attention is the way in which patient participation during this stage interacts with the "progressivity" of the consultation (Schegloff 2007).

In the case of other activities such as diagnosis, simple acknowledgement by the patient is generally sufficient for the consultation to progress to the next stage. However, the treatment stage presents a sequential constraint in that the consultation cannot proceed to closure in the usual way unless and until the patient accepts a treatment proposal or some other course of action is mutually agreed upon. The treatment recommendation stage thus provides a built-in opportunity for patients to participate in decision-making, and patient resistance has the potential to influence the doctor's treatment recommendations or even to change an already made proposal or decision (Koenig 2011; Stivers and Robinson 2006).

For example, a study of antibiotic prescribing in paediatric primary care settings (Stivers 2005) found that while doctors generally framed their treatment recommendations either as a proposal *for* or *against* treatment, patients offered greater resistance to recommendations *against* treatment. Conversation analytic research has shown that such resistance is often passive in nature, with patients withholding acceptance and responding to a treatment proposal with minimal responses or even silence. More active forms of resistance can also occur where patients overtly contest the doctor's recommendation. In either case, clinicians need to pursue acceptance of an agreed treatment plan to allow the consultation to progress to the next stage. Accordingly, clinicians typically structure their recommendations so as to avoid resistance and encourage acceptance by the patient. Doctors may pursue acceptance through various means such as modifying the treatment recommendation, reiterating their evidence for the proposed treatment, restating their recommendation or using devices such as tag questions to encourage an aligning response.

Several recent empirical studies of surgical consultations have concluded that surgeons orient to surgery as a "default option", reflecting what is claimed to be an institutional bias towards "for surgery" recommendations. The main evidence for this thus far has come from conversation analytic research on a large set of recorded consultations between patients and orthopaedic surgeons in Canada (Hudak, Clark and Raymond 2011, 2012). Close analysis of these consultations revealed the influence of patients on decision-making, with treatment decisions shown to be a skilfully negotiated joint achievement by surgeon and patient.

However, the researchers also observed a consistent pattern of asymmetry across the data set in the way treatment recommendations were constructed and delivered by the surgeons. Recommendations *"for surgery"* usually came early in the advice-giving sequence, and were framed in simple and straightforward terms as the most obvious or realistic option. In conversation analytic terms, they were therefore "designed" for acceptance. By contrast, *"not for surgery"* recommendations (i.e., those where surgery at this time was ruled out and an alternative or no treatment was proposed) were usually more complex in an interactional sense and required more extended negotiation than "*for surgery*" decisions. "*Not for surgery*" recommendations tended to be delayed, were expressed in more indirect and mitigated ways, and often included some discussion of risk or other proposed treatment options. These characteristics are markers of a "dispreferred" conversational action – namely, one that is not the structurally "preferred" or expected response (Maynard 1992). As noted above, in the Canadian studies this pattern is interpreted as support for the hypothesis that surgery is oriented to as a default option. However, it is also worth bearing in mind the possibility that where "*not for surgery*" cases are more complex clinically (which they could well be), this may also result in the interaction being more extended and/or complex.

In addition, non-surgical treatments in these consultations were almost always presented along a continuum in relation to surgery. The researchers concluded that this resulted in surgery becoming "omni-relevant" throughout the consultation – providing an implicit context for the discussion – and that surgery was thus accorded a privileged status as the "last best resort" (Hudak, Clark and Raymond 2012; Chapter 7, this volume). Hudak and colleagues thus claim that the observed asymmetries between "*for surgery*" and "*not for surgery*" recommendations in their data cannot be fully accounted for by simple alignment or misalignment of preferences between patients and surgeons. They suggest there is also an underlying interactional tension between an hypothesized bias on the part of surgeons towards surgery versus consideration of individual patient needs or preferences in deciding upon next steps in their orthopaedic surgical consultations. The remainder of this chapter explores whether and to what extent similar tensions can be observed to play out in a smaller but more diverse cross-specialty set of surgeon-patient consultations recorded in New Zealand outpatient clinics.

6.3   Data and Methods

6.3.1   Context

In the New Zealand public hospital system, access to elective surgery is by means of referral to a surgical outpatient clinic by the patient's general practitioner (GP) or by another specialist. Patients with private medical insurance may instead choose to be referred to a private clinic for certain procedures. In the public system, elective surgery is rationed and access to a procedure depends on the patient reaching a threshold score determined by means of a specialty-specific clinical prioritization protocol. In some of the cases analysed for this study therefore, even where surgery may have been the surgeon's preferred treatment option, the patient would not necessarily have been guaranteed to qualify at the time of the recorded consultation.

6.3.2 Participants and Settings

The data set discussed in this chapter comprises recordings of 47 surgical consultations involving 39 patients and 16 surgeons, collected between 2003 and 2007 by the Applied Research on Communication in Health (ARCH) group[1] in the course of successive studies of doctor-patient interaction in New Zealand primary and secondary care settings. This data includes the 35 consultations discussed in Chapter 2 (this volume) and an additional 12 surgical consultations collected as part of a later study (see below).

Table 6.1 summarizes the number of participants and consultations recorded in the different specialties. Patients were reasonably evenly split in terms of gender (22 women and 17 men), but most of the surgeons (all but two) were male and five were registrars,[2] including one of the female surgeons. The majority of the consultations were recorded in hospital outpatient clinics except for two pre-operative assessments and one standard consultation which took place in a ward setting. Consultation length ranged from just over three minutes for a very straightforward referral to 40 minutes for a complex first assessment; the average consultation length overall was 13:35 minutes. The objective was to obtain a reasonably diverse sample, and in total, nine surgical specialties are represented in the data, with the largest number of consultations recorded in general surgery clinics. Forty of the recorded consultations took place in public hospital clinics, with seven (involving two different doctor-patient pairs) recorded in private clinics.

Table 6.1: Overview of recorded consultations

Clinics	Doctors	Patients	Total Consultations	Private Clinic Consultations
General	5	21	21	–
Vascular	1	2	2	–
Orthopaedic	1	2	2	–
Cardiothoracic	1	3	3	–
Breast Cancer	2	7	7	–
Colorectal	2	2	3	2
Otolaryngology	1	1	5	5
Neurosurgery	1	1*	1	–
Ophthalmology	2	1*	3	–
Totals	16	39	47	7

* One patient had four separate consultations with three surgeons from two different specialties.

---

1   http://www.otago.ac.nz/wellington/research/arch/
2   A registrar in New Zealand is a doctor who has completed their postgraduate training and has entered into specialist training.

6.3.3   Data Collection

For the 35 consultations from the original data set, the data collection methodology was as follows. On agreed days a researcher attended the clinic, having previously recruited the clinicians involved, approached patients attending the clinic that day who fitted the inclusion criteria, and invited them to participate. Patients were excluded where conditions were acute and if they were under 18 years of age. The remaining 12 consultations were recorded in a similar manner, but the patients had already given consent prior to attending the appointment – this additional data is drawn from four case studies collected for a subsequent project in which individual patients were tracked through a series of hospital consultations resulting from a single referral by a general practitioner. In the case of one patient, this included first assessments with two different surgeons (a neurosurgeon and an ophthalmologist) plus a pre-operative assessment and post-surgical follow-up with a different ophthalmologist. A second case came from a private clinic and involved two consultations prior to nasal/sinus surgery and three follow-up appointments which also included minor post-operative procedures. The third case involved a first assessment and post-operative follow-up with a colorectal surgeon also in a private clinic, while the fourth included a routine follow-up appointment in the public hospital for a chronic condition which had required surgery in the past. For all recordings, the researcher set up the recording equipment immediately prior to the start of each consultation and then left the room. All participants were debriefed immediately after each encounter and any medical notes or letters relating to that consultation were also collected where consent to do so was granted by the patient.

6.3.4   Data Analysis

Once recorded, all consultations were logged by a researcher for clinical content (type/purpose, topics discussed, activities, outcomes), and were then independently transcribed and cross-referenced to all other related data such as interviews, field-notes and clinical documentation. A subset of consultations where surgical treatment recommendations occurred or could potentially have occurred were identified for further in-depth analysis. Micro-analysis of these interactions was undertaken using conversation analysis as the main methodological framework.

The focus of conversation analysis is on those features of talk-in-interaction that can be seen to be salient to the participants themselves as an interaction proceeds (Drew and Heritage 2006). This has become a common methodological approach in research on healthcare interactions, including research looking at encounters between patients undertaking chemotherapy and their doctors (Díaz 2000), consultations related to antibiotic medication (Heritage and Stivers 1999) and psychiatric consultations (Seale et al. 2007). Conversation analysis is an appropriate tool to shed light on the nature of clinical decision-making because it focuses on the sequences and unfolding of talk as these occur turn by turn in social interaction. This approach does not rely on the imputed thoughts, rationales and justifications of those involved, but instead looks to the rules of interaction itself. The term "rules" here does not refer to a rigid set of prescriptive norms but, rather, is used in the sense of accepted "standards that determine what constitutes an activity of that kind, whether the activity has been performed correctly and so on" (Hutchinson, Read and Sharrock 2008: 41). In a consultation about possible elective surgery, the relevant activity is to determine whether someone is willing to and/or should undergo surgery.

6.4   Consultation Types and Outcomes

All 47 consultations in the data set were surveyed to identify and describe any instances of treatment activity and "next steps" discussion and decision-making that occurred. This analysis revealed a variety of recommended treatments including but not limited to surgical procedures, and also two consultations in which no treatment activity occurred. The treatment recommendation activity could include description and discussion of treatment options, explanation of risks, instructions on how to prepare for treatment, description of the procedure and recovery process, and discussion of administrative processes. In this section we provide a summary overview of the data set, including the consultation type and purpose, and the range of outcomes in terms of treatment decisions made.

6.4.1   Consultation Types

Discussion of certain kinds of treatment options, and surgical procedures in particular, is clearly not equally relevant for all visit types. Three different consultation types were identified in this data: first or initial visits, check-up visits and follow-up visits (White et al. 2014). In New Zealand, the first two both require a letter of referral from another doctor, and as referred visits, the overall activity structures for both initial and check-up visits are very similar (see Chapter 2, this volume). Follow-up visits are quite different from the other two visit types in terms of structure and purpose as they do not require a referral, and do not necessarily share a common structure or purpose with the first two types.

A *first* or *initial visit* was defined as a referred consultation where the patient had not seen a surgeon in this particular clinic about this problem before. A *check-up visit* was one requested by the patient or the referring doctor where the patient had either seen the surgeon before, or where the patient had received surgery for a particular problem. A *follow-up visit* was one where the surgeon him- or herself had requested that the patient see him/her again after a specified period of time. In this data set there were 24 referred first or initial visits, four referred check-up visits and 19 follow-up consultations, five of which involved patient-surgeon pairs already recorded previously. The sub-types of follow-up visit in this data included post-diagnostic testing, pre-surgical assessment, post-operative check-up, post-emergency admission and routine follow-up.

6.4.2 Outcomes

A variety of different treatment recommendations and outcomes occurred during the "deciding next steps" or treatment discussion phase of the 47 surgical consultations in our data, as shown in Table 6.2. The outcome was not always a "treatment" in the traditional sense of a surgical procedure or prescription of medication in order to cure or ameliorate a problem. These kinds of treatment recommendation did occur in over half of the consultations, but treatment decisions also commonly included referrals for diagnostic testing or other kinds of investigative procedure, suggested lifestyle changes, or an explicit decision to undertake no further tests or treatment. A treatment recommendation could also be a proposal to continue follow-up visits for a specific period (which may or may not include diagnostic testing) or referral to a different specialist. Non-surgical recommendations that encompassed further investigations (or in some cases follow-up appointments), could perhaps more accurately be described as *"not yet (but possibly) for surgery"*. Such recommendations arise at an earlier stage of the overall decision-making process, and as such may well prove subsequently to be *"for surgery"* outcomes in embryo.

In addition, more than one decision or treatment recommendation could be made in any one consultation. For example, a referral for diagnostic testing would usually be accompanied by making an appointment either with a surgeon in the clinic or with the patient's general practitioner, and lifestyle advice generally occurred along with other recommendations. There were also two consultations in the data set where there was no treatment activity sequence at all – these were both post-surgical follow-ups and treatment (including further follow-up) was not broached by either the patient or the surgeon.

Surgery was both the recommended treatment and the agreed decision outcome in 18 of the 47 consultations considered here. In six of these consultations, surgery had already been at least provisionally decided upon as the most appropriate treatment prior to the recorded interaction. This once again highlights the observation above that the decision-making process often extends beyond a single consultation. There were five cases where surgery was discussed but a definite decision was made *not* to operate. In one of these, the surgeon proposed surgery but this was declined by the patient (see Case 6 below). In the other four cases, the doctor recommended against surgery because the risks were seen to outweigh potential benefits – two of

Table 6.2: Outcomes of treatment activity

Decision or outcome	Number
"For surgery" – decision made to operate	18
Referral for diagnostic tests or other specialist investigation	17
Diagnostic procedure performed during consultation	8
Follow-up appointment(s) made	20
Prescription or advice about use of medication	8
Lifestyle change(s) recommended	8
Decision not to refer for further tests or treatment	6
No treatment discussion	2

these patients aligned with the doctor's *"not for surgery"* recommendation, but two resisted it and (unsuccessfully) pursued a possible surgical option.

The remaining 27 consultations in this data set had various non-surgical treatment outcomes in the first instance. Seven cases were post-operative or routine follow-ups resulting in discharge where discussion of further surgery was not relevant, though other treatment discussion of some kind did occur in five of these. Diagnostic testing or referral to another specialist was recommended in 17 consultations where surgery was not (as yet) the recommended treatment, and a diagnostic procedure was performed during the consultation in a further eight cases. In many of these, and in all other consultations where a surgeon explicitly recommended against surgery or further diagnostic testing, or where no other treatment was offered, arrangements were made for a follow-up visit or referral to another doctor.

6.5   Interactional Analysis of Treatment Discussions

This section describes patterns observed across the data set in how recommendations for or against surgery were framed and discussed, and explores some ways in which any tensions between the surgeon's recommended treatment and the patient's preferences or reservations were resolved. These observations are illustrated with extracts from the treatment discussions in several "telling cases" (Mitchell 1984) that were selected to provide further insight into the interactional details of how different treatment decisions were negotiated.

6.5.1   "For Surgery" Decisions

Surgery was the recommended treatment and agreed outcome in 18 of the consultations considered here. In all of these cases the doctor framed surgery as the preferred treatment option, and in most cases delivered the recommendation directly and simply without hedging or delay. The description of the procedure was often optimized – that is, expressed in such a way as to emphasize the positive aspects and downplay possible negatives. Patients usually quickly aligned with the surgeon's recommendation, with patient/carer resistance to a *"for surgery"* recommendation only occurring in one case. (We do not know of course to what extent these patients may have previously formed an expectation that surgery was the desired outcome through, for example, discussion with their general practitioner at the time of referral.) In addition, surgeons did not generally initiate discussion of any non-surgical alternatives. The patterns in these cases are largely consistent with the findings of Hudak and colleagues discussed earlier. There were also six instances where surgery had already been discussed and decided upon in a previous consultation. In these cases, surgeons were observed to focus on discussing the procedure and the recovery process, and sometimes the risks (see below), but the decision itself was not revisited.

Case 1 (TS-SP19-01)

This case provides a typical illustration of the straightforward delivery and acceptance of an optimized *"for surgery"* recommendation as described above. In this consultation with an ophthalmology registrar, an older patient has presented with deteriorating vision and a history of falls which has also been the subject of investigations by other specialists. The patient's wife (WF) is in the consulting room along with a caregiver (CR); the latter often speaks on behalf of the patient who has a degree of intellectual impairment.

The doctor (SG) begins by asking *"what's the problem with your eyes"* and the caregiver provides an account of the patient having problems walking and the GP finding that *"he was really blind in one eye"* from a cataract. The surgeon then enquires into specific aspects of the patient's health, medications, living circumstances and ability to understand, before performing an eye examination to confirm the cause of the reported problems: *"could be the cataract doing it that's the most likely thing but we need to make sure that there's nothing al– else going on in the back of the eye"*.[3] After the eye examination the sequence in Extract 1 occurs.

Case 1, Extract 1

```
01 SG:   there are definitely cataracts there and that's the
02       main reason why you can't see so well (1.5)
03 PT:   mmmm
04 SG:   they're just (  ) as i can see um the cataract's
05       definitely much worse on the right hand side than the
```

---

3   A transcription key is provided at the end Chapter 2. All personal and place names used are pseudonyms.

```
06        left hand side and th- the type is the one that (striates)
07        light quite a bit so you know that would count that w-
08        that goes with the vision changes that er we've noticed today
09        uumm the question is whether (0.5) you were keen
10        for us to do something about that Barry (0.5) would
11        you like us to fix that if w- if y- if if you:: (0.5)
12        er if we can› (.) would you like us to do that (.)
13 PT:    oh yes plea[se]
          ((lines omitted))
17 CR:    ((aside to WF)) said to have have the operation to
18        fi[x        his        eyes]
19 SG:     [cos this will invol]ve an an operation to: u:m
20        to replace the um the cloudy lens (in the) eye with
21        an artificial lens and it's quite a safe procedure
22        um and most people get good vision afterwards
23 CR:    do you want to have the operation for Barry to
24        have the operation
25 WF:    yeah
26 CR:    yeah
27 SG:    if possible you know we'll put you on the list
          ((lines omitted))
28 SG:    so i-i guess (0.5) the only question left is
29        whether we are keen to do it under local or general
30        have you got any (.) you know feelings about that
31        so i'll just - we just need to do some paperwork now
```

After confirming the diagnosis of cataracts (line 1), the surgeon immediately offers the possibility of doing something to "*fix*" the problem (lines 11–12), though this solution is not yet identified as surgery. This offer is in the form of a question, but is framed as "good news" in that the problem (by implication something that needs to be "*fixed*") has now been identified and can be corrected. The surgeon's questions in lines 9–11 ("*whether you were keen for us to do something*" and "*would you like us to fix that*") are formulated so that Barry is more likely to agree.[4]

This offer is followed by a more negative "*if we can*" (lines 11–12). The surgeon's delivery here is marked by hesitation and stuttering shifting from "*if w–*" to "*if y– if if you::*" before returning to "*if we*", but these dysfluencies appear to relate to possible (though unlikely) uncertainty around the patient's prioritization for surgery, not to the decision to operate itself. Having received a positive response (line 13), the surgeon goes on to explain that this will involve an operation which is "*quite safe*" and one that has a positive outcome for "*most people*" (lines 19–22), and by line 27 the decision has clearly been made. The "*only question left*" (line 28) is whether a local or general anaesthetic would be preferred before ("*if possible*") the "*paperwork*" for putting the patient on the list for surgery is completed, and the decision is rubber-stamped.

---

4 In technical terms, the positive polarity of their grammatical structure is designed to seek an agreeing response.

<u>Case 2</u> (IS-SP04-04)

This second consultation provides a particularly clear example of how the activities of diagnosis and proposing next steps are inextricably linked, another dynamic that must be taken into account when interpreting the way a treatment proposal is delivered and received. Here we can see the same pattern of direct and straightforward delivery of a *"for surgery"* recommendation at the point where treatment is first discussed, along with an eventual unproblematic alignment to the proposal by the patient. However, getting to this point has entailed a great deal of extra interactional "work" by the surgeon because the patient is initially unaware she has a problem that may require surgical intervention.

This patient has been referred by another specialist but is happy in her belief that she now experiences good health, a stance that is endorsed by her adult son who has accompanied her to the appointment. The surgeon clearly understands that her test results tell a different story, but cannot move on to proposing next steps until the patient acknowledges the diagnostic news that there is a problem that needs to be addressed. Maynard's (2003) research on the delivery of good news and bad news provides a useful framework for understanding what occurs in this case. He argues that clinicians typically employ the format of the "news delivery sequence" found in everyday conversation prior to delivering a diagnosis, by first asking questions that encourage patients to display their understandings in a type of sequence known as a "perspective display series". This helps to expose and manage any potential mismatch between the patient's expectations and the doctor's conclusions. If interactional "work" like this is not done, then patients may misapprehend or even reject diagnostic "news", and ultimately fail to align with the doctor's treatment proposal.

Extract 1 represents a repeating pattern in this consultation. The surgeon asks about the patient's health and receives invariably positive responses, to which he in turn makes non-committal responses like "yeah" (lines 3, 5, 15, 18), followed by a questioning of her self-assessment. In total the surgeon queries the patient's self-assessment nine times. The patient maintains her "no problem" responses no matter how the surgeon builds his questions to elicit a perceived problem, which is the "preferred" response (Maynard 1992).

Case 2, Extract 1

```
01 SG:    so how are you now
02 PT:    good
03 SG:    yeah
04 PT:    good
05 SG:    yeah¿ that was-it was fairly um (2) um (.) the
06        ((other hospital)) doctors have been on to us about
07        you and (.) that you'd had this obstruction of the
08        bile duct and (.) you've been unwell there and they put
09        a (.) um a um a a um sort of small internal tube there
10        to help the bile (.) [drain]
11 PT:                         [yeah ] i was very fluorescent
12        yellow for [thre::e ]
13 SG:               [were you]
```

```
14 PT:   months (.) so
15 SG:   (.) yeah (.) yeah (.) yeah a- a- an-and prior to that
16       how have you been as far as your general health goes
17 PT:   it was good wasn't it for Christmas very good
18 SG:   o:h yeah
19       ((lines omitted))
20 SG:   in the normal sequence of things (.) are you
21       reasonably active or (.)
22 PT:   very [active     ]
23 SG:        [active yeah]
```

In Extract 2, the surgeon finally breaks this cycle by asking if the other doctors had explained that a blockage such as hers in the bile duct is "*normally*" a growth. The patient now recognizes that the surgeon has foreshadowed some bad news, although her first response (lines 32–3) is to again assert a no-problem reading: "*but they also said that there was no trace of (.) cancer*". The surgeon then delicately elaborates in such a way that the patient herself preemptively ends his sentence on lines 38–40 with its serious import: "*you'd normally...get an answer*" but past tests are not "*conclusive*". There is a slight stress on the word "*normally*" here which signals that the inconclusiveness of the result is *not* normal. This leaves the surgeon able to repeat the patient's ending (line 41) and to elaborate further to deliver the bad news (i.e., that such a blockage usually indicates a malignancy). At this point the patient finally realizes what is being discussed, as indicated by her "*oh*" (line 45) which indicates a moment of recognition (Heritage 1984). Such "news receipts" are not a regular response to medical assessments, but do occur when the doctor's assessment contrasts with the patient's understanding (Heath 1992). The diagnosis, unexpected as it was, has been delivered by the surgeon with such competent attention to the patient's orientation that she is highly aligned with the surgeon by the end of the process.

Case 2, Extract 2 (3 minutes into the consultation)

```
24 SG:   so um did the ((SUBURB)) doctors explain that the (.)
25       blockage of the bile duct we'd (1) normally expect that to
26       be a um through a-rather than- a (.) (g- growth) either
27       in the p- pancreas or the bile duct itself
28 PT:   mm [mm ]
29 SG:      [did] they explain that?
30 PT:   yes
31 SG:   yeah
32 PT:   but they also said that there was no trace of (.)
33       cancer in the(0.2)specimen that they [took in]
34 SG:                                         [y-yes ] ye:s
35       well (.) which isn't unusual (.) you know it's just um
36       (.) they (.) they can - they just draw out some
37       cells from the bile duct itself (though) you'd
38       norm-you'd normally get (.) (should) get an answer
39       on that so the-the-fact that ( ) isn't you know-
40 PT:   conclusive
41 SG:   it isn't conclusive and I think we'd-you know we'd (.)
42       usually have to (.) a-assu:me that a blockage of the
43       bile duct in that position is um through a malignancy. (.)
```

```
44          [mm]
45 PT:      [oh]
46 SG:      u- u- usually in the pancreas (.) but sometimes in the
47          bile duct yeah
48 PT:      mm
```

The surgeon can then finally initiate his treatment proposal for *"a small opera-tion"*, as seen in Extract 3. He introduces this indirectly using a hypothetical for-mulation: *"if we were going to take this further..."* (lines 49–50). There is some further discussion to clarify what is being proposed and answering questions posed by the patient and her son, before the patient herself suggests the course of action of further investigation (line 56) that the surgeon has suggested, in the upshot to an apparently successful process of shared decision-making.

Case 2, Extract 3

```
49 SG:      so (.) um if we were (.) if we were going to take
50          this further then the next step would be just to do
51          to do a small operation (.) to look um (.) in your
52          abdomen through some small holes and (.) some
53          instruments just to try and get more information er
54          as to whether it's localized or not
55          ((lines omitted))
56 PT:      could we go ahead and [do that mister((name)) and]
57 SG:                            [y-yeah   okay   yeah   yeah]
58          an-an-and then after that we'll know y-you know a bit more
```

This example illustrates the point that while diagnostic news of a serious con-dition is unlikely to be welcome, the way the interaction is managed may make patients more ready or less ready to realize and cope with the diagnosis and thus genuinely able to engage with discussion of possible treatments.

Case 3 (SS-SP08-02)

In the third illustrative case, an otherwise healthy 80-year-old woman has presented with a problematic hip. It is the one consultation in the data set involving a *"for surgery"* recommendation and outcome where the surgeon does provide details of treatment options other than surgery. The consultation begins with the patient pre-empting the treatment recommendation; she makes it very clear that she wants the surgeon to *"fix"* her *"worn out"* and *"pretty painful"* hip, thus implying that she expects an operation will be the likely outcome. Clearly this patient is unlikely to need much persuading if the surgeon does deem surgery to be the best option.

Case 3, Extract 1

```
01 SG:      alright no::w (.) how can i help you
02 PT:      well i hope to get my hip fixed [hah hah]
03 SG:                                      [do  you]
04 PT:      (h)y(h)es hah hah .hhh (.) i had a x ray but i you know i dunno what
05          the s- story was that they was worn out my hip they tell me (.) been
06          pretty painful mind you
```

After stating that the x-rays confirm the diagnosis of arthritis, the surgeon then runs through several non-surgical management options (medication, homoeopathy, physiotherapy, alternative medicine), commenting that these *"are obviously some of the things you're already doing"* and discounting them one by one before moving to his treatment recommendation, as shown in Extract 2. The surgeon here explicitly invokes his clinical expertise to single out and promote surgery, describing it in lines 31–3 as *"the only way...in MY opinion"* for the patient to *"make a big leap in mobility"*. Having briefly acknowledged the surgeon's dismissal of each non-surgical option as he presented it, the patient then, with no further discussion, immediately agrees to the proposal to operate with the comment *"yes...that's fine by me"*. The doctor's response *"is it?"* in line 37 is produced as a somewhat ironic confirmation question, possibly echoing his gently ironic reaction to the patient's pre-emptive remarks at the beginning of the consultation, an interpretation supported by the patient's laughing response. Given the prior context, it is possible that the surgeon has chosen to set out the clinical reasoning behind his *"for surgery"* recommendation quite explicitly in order to underline his professional authority – he *is* recommending surgery, but for good reason, not simply because the patient was expecting it to be offered.

Case 3, Extract 2

```
25 SG:   uh all those interventions are designed to be to relieve pain.
26       (0.4) they don't improve function very much (1.0) and the final
27       thing is to put a new hip in. (1.4) now (0.4) e- >the choice of
28       course is ultimately you:rs¿< [.hhh] uh:m
29 PT:                                [mm ]
30       (0.8)
31 SG:   but if you want to make a big leap in your mobility (0.4) the
32       only way you're going to do that in MY opinion is to have a new
33       hip put in.
34 PT:   mm mm
35 SG:   mm
36 PT:   (h)y(h)es mm (1.8) that's that's fine b(h)y m(h)e(h),
37 SG:   is it?
38 PT:   ha ha yes
```

Unlike the first two cases, this consultation does not fit the general interactional pattern described earlier, in that, here, the alternatives to surgery are canvassed first. However, these options are set up as "straw men", and it is very clear that the surgeon considers surgery to be the "last best option" (Hudak, Clark and Raymond 2012), although he does emphasize that the choice is the patient's (lines 27–8). Once the patient has formally agreed to the option of surgery, the doctor spends some time discussing practical arrangements and what to expect afterwards. There is however no discussion of surgical risks (see below) and no further negotiation before the decision to proceed is finalized and the consultation ends with an agreement to go ahead.

6.5.2   Risk Discussions and Resistance

Risk discussions occurred in all four cases where surgery was explicitly ruled out, and in the three pre-surgery assessment visits. However, the risks of surgery were discussed in only half the consultations where a *"for surgery"* decision was first made. As in Cases 1–3 above, discussion tended to focus instead on details of the procedure and recovery process, along with administrative concerns involving scheduling and waiting lists. In some cases risks may already have been discussed in a previous consultation, but in general, risk discussions in our data took place either immediately prior to surgery, or where there was some ambivalence about surgery on the part of either doctor or patient.

A close analysis of how surgeons typically presented the risks of a given procedure reveals just how challenging this particular aspect of treatment discussions could be to negotiate. In such interactions, we can see surgeons performing a delicate balancing act between the need to relay risk information accurately, attending to the fear and associated reluctance to proceed that such possibilities might engender in the patient, while at the same time constructing and justifying their own clinical assessment of the potential risks and benefits involved in the proposed procedure. This is not dissimilar to the interactional dilemmas we observed in a previous study of primary care consultations where medication side-effects were being discussed (Dew et al. 2012).

Case 4 (IS-SP03-02)

This is the risk discussion from the consultation discussed in Chapter 2 (Extract 13, p. 24). Surgery has been strongly recommended and readily agreed to by the patient, but the stakes are high if something goes wrong, especially as this is a fairly young patient. Prior to the risk discussion, the surgeon has already downplayed the extent of the surgery being proposed: *"at this stage we would t– it you know if we're talking about surgery we'd be (.) talking about doing a limited op-operation to deal with the bit of bowel that's causing the trouble"*. After describing the procedure, the surgeon begins the risk discussion with an optimized assessment of the surgery as *"a fAIrly straightforward operation?"*, though with the caveat that *"l:ike (0.4) every operation ↓there there are (sort of) risks"*, before he goes on to briefly describe the expected scenario of going home within a few days and the bowel recovering normally. The surgeon details a variety of risks arising from *"any:: (.) bowel surgery when we're sort of joi:n the two ends of the bowel together"*. He starts with the most serious possible risk, that *"the two ends don't heal"*; this is described as *"the most important... risk"* and potentially *"a serious complication"* where *"you get what's called a leak"*. However the delivery is quite matter of fact, and this possibility is juxtaposed with the assessment that it is very rare: *"now that would happen in may:be: (0.5) something in the order of one percent of people?*

(0.3) >undergoing this surg-=(a) one in a hundred,<" by comparison with the best case scenario of healing *"absolutely perfectly"*. This reframes the most likely risk as being both improbable and not catastrophic, only "less than perfect" healing.

The surgeon ends his risk explanation by restating the expected "no problem" outcome and the positive benefits of the surgery: *"we can't totally abolish the risk okay so (.) but but er (.) you know the the as i said the expected outcome is that (.) you know you'd (.) somewhere round about five days you'd be able to go home (.) your bowels would be working a lot easier and it'll prevent occurrence of these (.) twistings"*. Later in the consultation, the surgeon reconfirms the patient's decision to proceed, asking if he has any questions, and recaps the risk discussion saying *"the most important thing is just th= the sma:ll risk which (.) o- o- of an anastomotic leak, ah:: the OTHer complications would be pretty uncommon, apart from wound infection"*. These contrasting characterizations appear designed to minimize the potential concern and possible resistance to surgical treatment that a risk discussion may invoke, while at the same time *not* diminishing the seriousness of the possible risks involved. The consultation then proceeds unproblematically to making arrangements for the operation.

Case 5 (IS-SP02-01)

The next case also includes a risk discussion, but contrasts with the preceding example in two ways. Firstly, here it is the patient and not the surgeon who raises the possibility of a particular surgical procedure. Secondly, in doing so he questions the non-surgical options of diagnostic testing and lifestyle changes that have just been recommended by the surgeon. Although the patient has aligned with the surgeon's plan by the end of the consultation, the question of surgery is at least theoretically left open for further discussion after a recommended ultrasound scan. The surgeon is quite assertive throughout, making it clear that he would not be happy to recommend this procedure; the risk discussion here thus functions to support the doctor's *"not for surgery"* stance.

Extract 1 begins with the patient asking about a possible surgical treatment (removal of a rib) and the surgeon answering that this procedure is *"controversial"* – the hedging and dysfluency here display the doctor's awareness that his response may not align with the patient's perspective that this procedure might be worthy of consideration.

Case 5, Extract 1

```
01 PT:   °uh:m no i don't think i had any other questions.° (3.4) what
02       (0.4) so you got any more thoughts on whether that first rib
03       needs to come out or;
04 SG:   .hhuh:m (0.8) yeah i mean that- th- th- (.) the the situation
05       with taking the first rib out it- it's (.) it's a very sort of
06       controversial (0.8) area in you know in in in this particular
07       problem.
```

The doctor then goes on to set out a series of additional arguments to support his no-surgery stance, starting with evidence that the procedure is no more beneficial than medication. This is followed by a detailed evaluation of risks, beginning with a "worst case" narrative from the surgeon's personal experience, contrasted with the patient's own situation which is much less serious, thus making such a risk unjustifiable in the surgeon's opinion.

Case 5, Extract 2

```
16 SG:   a few years ago when i was working in ((CITY)) we tried that on a
17       young person who had a stroke for (example) had a bleed in the brain
18       and you know um (.) it wasn't a very pleasant situation so it's it's
19       sort of made me much more cautious about recommending that sort of
20       treatment (.) and er (.) you know if if your arm was extremely
21       swollen and uncomfortable (.) and you we- you were going to have
22       developed (venous) gangrene in y- in your fingers that's a different
23       matter that's [a ]=
24 PT:                 [mm]=
25 SP:                    =serious situation we would have done that
26       treatment for you (.) but for you y- you really weren't affected
27       very much you had a little bit of swelling and your veins were a bit
28       prominent but apart from that you were pretty much okay (.) and i could
29       see that your arm was going to settle settle down and get back to
30       normal pretty smartly (.)
```

The surgeon concludes the risk discussion with the statement that he doesn't think there is any reason to take the first rib out. He proposes reviewing this decision after the scan but makes it clear he is unlikely to change his recommendation: *"my personal philosophy is that if you're getting better on the current treatment then that's great we just keep on going as is (.) and you d– you don't subject yourself to any further risk"*. The patient continues to resist the *"not for surgery"* recommendation, invoking the authority of a doctor at his mother's workplace whom he quotes as saying *"oh (.) the rib's gotta come out"*. After some brief further discussion, the doctor offers to refer the patient for a second opinion. The patient declines this offer, the original treatment plan of diagnostic testing is re-accepted and the sequence is closed. The surgeon has successfully dissuaded the patient from surgery by leaving the option on the table for future discussion.

6.5.3   Resistance to "For Surgery" Recommendations

Overall there was little patient resistance to treatment recommendations, including surgery, in this data set. Resistance occurred in only seven out of the 47 consultations, though several patients did raise other potential treatments that they thought might be considered once diagnostic tests had been carried out. There was one consultation where the patient (and support persons) resisted a recommendation *"for surgery"*. This final case provides an interesting example of the forms such resistance can take and how surgeons manage the resulting interaction, and at the same time further exemplifies several of the other points made above.

Case 6 [IS-SP02-02]

The elderly patient in this consultation has reduced capacity as a result of a stroke, so it is mainly his wife who interacts with the surgeon. The consultation focuses on how to manage a large aortic aneurysm which has grown above the site where a previous one was recently repaired. There is no attempt by this surgeon to elicit the patient's or carer's perspective, as was seen in Case 2. The surgeon here is also much more tentative in his recommendation for surgery than in the other *"for surgery"* cases discussed above, although the proposal to consider a procedure does still come early in the consultation.

The doctor begins by reviewing the notes and then briefly summarizes the situation, including the risk of kidney failure if the standard *"surgical treatment to fix this"* were to be used in this particular case, thus effectively discounting this as a realistic possibility. The surgeon then describes a *"new technique"* (a stent), which he presents as a less invasive alternative: *"so there's a possibility that we could consider something like that as well"*. Although worded quite tentatively, the surgeon optimizes this option, describing it as one which is *"designed for elderly frail people who have lots of other medical problems...and who wouldn't come through surgery all that well"*. This suggestion receives only a brief acknowledgment *"mm"* from the wife. Extract 1 begins at the point where the surgeon again suggests that this is a possible option and one he would be prepared to look at more closely.

Case 6, Extract 1

```
01 SG:   a- and (0.6) and so (2.8) it it it certainly
02        would be possible to (0.4) to think to to look at these films a
03        bit more closely=
04 WI:                    =mm=
05 SG:                       =than i- i've looked at them [today.>   ]and (.)
06 WI:                                                    [yeah yeah]
07 SG:   think about doing something like that.
08 WI:   um
09        (2)
10 SG:   [a- a- ]
11 WI:   [big de]cision isn't it.
12 SG:   it is a big decisi:on¿ [uh:m ]
13 WI:                          [°mm.°]
```

The way the surgeon words this suggestion again implies a degree of ambivalence about performing any kind of procedure – it is something that it is *"possible to...think about doing"* (lines 2–7), and thus falls short of a clear recommendation to proceed. The stent proposal is once again resisted passively by the patient, his wife and his daughter, none of whom offer any kind of positive uptake. The patient's wife then responds with a delaying *"um"* which is followed by a two-second pause

and an assessment of the decision-making process (line 11) rather than an acceptance or non-acceptance of the recommendation itself.

There is further discussion about the diagnosis, then the surgeon once again
pursues the less invasive procedure, commenting that it should go ahead as soon as
possible *"if we a:re thinking about fixing it"*. The patient's wife begins her active
resistance at this point. In Extract 2, she and the daughter state the patient is unwill-
ing to undergo further treatment, which the patient himself later emphatically confirms. The surgeon does not continue to pursue surgery in light of this resistance.

Case 6, Extract 2

```
14 WI:   i- it's mark's decision
15 SG:   oh of course.
16 WI:   [and]
17 DA:   [mm ]
18 SG:   absolutely.
19 WI:   °i don't [think] he's° (°°going to be [prepared to [have]°°)=
20 SG:            [yeah ]                      [mm:.            ]
21 WI:   =(°°an [oper]ation°°) he's been [through] a [great] dea:l.
22 SG:          [yeah]                   [yeah  ]   [mm:. ]
23 SG:   mm:.
24 DA:   okay.
25 SG:   °mm°
26 WI:   he really has,
         ((40 lines omitted))
67 DA:   dad dad has said to us no:.
68 SG:   yeah [yeah]
69 WI:        [yeah] he has mm
70 SG:   .hh and and and that's a very reasonable (.) [thing ]
71 WI:                                                [yeah i] think it is too
```

However, the surgeon does not withdraw his *"for surgery"* advice completely,
advising that it would be reasonable to monitor the situation, and that it may become
necessary to reconsider if the patient's condition worsens to the point where the
aneurysm becomes painful. This could be interpreted as an example of "defensive
medicine" – if the doctor had to justify a *"not for surgery"* decision to his peers,
ongoing monitoring would be justifiable in terms of evidence-based practice, but
not to the point of withdrawing an operative option completely. After discussion
about what symptoms to look out for, the surgeon lays out the worst case scenario: *"when they rupture it's extremely painful and most people will die when that
happens"* (though he later estimates the actual risk of a rupture to be in the order
of *"10–15 per cent per annum"*). Towards the end of the consultation the daughter asks: *"knowing that it's dad's decision...but what's your recommendation"*, and
the surgeon reiterates that *"keeping an eye on things would be very reasonable
actually"*. The final decision is to book a scan and a follow-up appointment in six
months.

The treatment discussion in this consultation does not follow the pattern described
above of a directly worded *"for surgery"* recommendation delivered early in the
treatment sequence; on the contrary it is more typical of the way *"not for surgery"*

recommendations have been described in previous studies. However, it is a good example of active negotiation between the parties in a situation where the optimal course of action is at best uncertain. The doctor has a limited range of options to offer and there is relatively little to choose between them in this case. If nothing is done, the aneurysm will grow and eventually bleed resulting in the patient's death, and if the surgeon operates with the standard procedure, the likely outcome is renal failure. The stent option is presented as the best option, but is acknowledged to be a relatively new procedure with unknown risks. It is therefore unsurprising that the doctor's advice is formulated somewhat tentatively.

The surgeon is also aware that this is a "preference-sensitive" decision (Mullan 2004), one where the particular value the patient places on his quality of life may override what the doctor sees as the most effective treatment in clinical terms, something that is made quite explicit by the patient and his accompanying family members. Although the surgeon does appear to favour an immediate surgical intervention, in the light of the patient's reluctance to undergo a further procedure, he keeps this option in play for the future as a "last best resort" (Hudak, Clark and Raymond 2012).

6.6   Discussion and Conclusions

This chapter set out to describe the decision-making processes observed during treatment discussions in a collection of consultations between surgeons and patients in New Zealand. A survey of the data set revealed that where surgical treatment of some kind was a possible outcome, the most frequent decision was either to proceed with surgery, or to undertake further investigation or follow-up, thus leaving the way open to discussing surgery again at some point in the future, or perhaps as part of a planned prelude to surgery. Where surgeons explicitly recommended against surgery, recommended further testing or concluded no treatment was required, they generally spent time making their diagnostic reasoning explicit, and in all these cases some kind of follow-up was offered. More detailed analysis of treatment and risk discussions confirmed a consistent asymmetry between the parties. In these consultations, the surgeon's recommendation usually prevailed, and alignment between surgeon and patient was achieved with little resistance in most cases. In the few cases where this was not true, the doctor would offer a compromise and/or the final decision might be deferred pending further investigations. Our study thus broadly supports the conclusions of previous research that surgeons (and patients) tend to orient to surgery as a normative or "default" outcome.

This finding is perhaps not altogether surprising. From the patient's perspective, when a person is referred by their GP or another doctor to a surgical specialist for a yet-to-be resolved problem, it is not unreasonable to assume that they will orient to surgery as at least one possible outcome (Hudak, Clark and Raymond 2012).

Moreover, in the data considered here, the consultations where *"for surgery"* proposals were delivered in a more straightforward and optimized way also seemed to be those where there seemed little doubt on the part of the surgeon at least that this was the generally agreed best (or only possible) treatment, as in Case 1 above.

However, by contrast with previous research, in our data the more complex and extended discussions tended to occur in those cases where the "best" treatment option was less clear-cut or the decision was more negotiable for one reason or another, not just those where there was a *"not for surgery"* proposal. Possible scenarios could include a lack of alignment between surgeon and patient as to the need for surgery (Case 2), patient resistance to the surgeon's recommendation (Cases 5 and 6), the patient taking the initiative and making a treatment proposal (Cases 3 and 5), cases with more complex risk-benefit equations (Cases 4, 5, 6) and "preference-sensitive" decisions (Case 6).

Several of the case studies discussed here also show clearly that patients may view risk (and potential benefits) differently to the way surgeons do, and that they do not necessarily surrender their own perspectives and agendas in the face of medical authority. Patients may or may not wish to undergo an invasive procedure, even if it is offered, or they may be intent upon pursuing a particular kind of treatment even where this is contrary to the doctor's advice. One factor that may complicate the progress of a surgical consultation, then, is the patient's willingness (or not) to accept a particular treatment recommendation.

Resistance to a proposed plan will delay the progress of the consultation to its conclusion, as the patient's acceptance is a structural requirement at this stage of a consultation, and as in Cases 5 and 6 above, can result in the surgeon making concessions to accommodate patient preferences. In addition, a particular diagnosis or a proposed treatment plan may have been expected, as in Cases 1, 3 and 4 above, but equally could come as a surprise to the patient, as in Case 2. If unexpected, the diagnosis and/or treatment proposal may be conceptualized (by one or both participants) as constituting either "bad news" or "good news". As this chapter has illustrated, the way such "news" is perceived and responded to by patients also influences in various ways how diagnostic and decision-making processes unfold in the course of the consultation. It is also perfectly possible that a patient does not have any particular expectation or preference – in this respect the treatment discussion represents "architecture not archaeology" for the patient (Stiggelbout 2014).

In this data set, a combination of often quite subtle communicative strategies was used by surgeons to skilfully steer patients through a discussion of their diagnosis and treatment options and towards acceptance of what the surgeon thought best, whilst also allowing some space for discussing patient preferences and concerns. With some exceptions, the surgeons in this study most often followed the pattern reported in the Canadian research of presenting the surgical option early and directly in those cases where surgery was unambiguously the recommended treatment. In such consultations the option of surgery was generally presented as "good news" for the patient in the sense that it offered a solution to their problem, and was framed variously as the only or most effective option available, or as being essential (there being no other realistic choice). Case 1 provides a clear example of how such sequences typically played out, resulting in an unproblematic alignment between surgeon and patient on the treatment decision. The success of this strategy of course depends on a shared understanding of what the presenting problem is, and that this could or might need to be addressed by a surgical procedure. This was usually quickly established in the opening stages of a consultation, but if not, as in Case 2, the surgeon would first elicit the patient's perspectives and expectations.

As discussed in several of the cases above, once a surgical recommendation was made, it was very common for descriptions of the procedure itself as well as possible risks and outcomes, to be formulated in an "optimized" way so as to minimize resistance and encourage acceptance of surgery as the preferred treatment option. This is consistent with another observation, namely that risk discussions did not always occur in the consultation where the initial decision to proceed with surgery was made. Discussions of surgical risk or undesirable outcomes occurred more frequently and tended to be more extended in preference-sensitive cases where the "best outcome" in a clinical sense appeared to be less clear-cut and/or where the patient's preferences did not immediately align with what the surgeon thought best.

Another strategy, as already noted, was to keep surgery "in play" as a possible option in cases where the surgeon was recommending against surgery or where the patient was resisting the recommendation either for or against surgery. This strategy does appear to minimize resistance from patients, but it may also be a way to offer an alternative option with "face validity" if the patient's problem remains unresolved, or to ensure that a "compromise" solution still meets accepted clinical standards.

However, none of this means that a recommendation *"for surgery"* is a foregone conclusion in any given case. Surgeons in New Zealand, as elsewhere, typically act as a gateway to operative intervention, a point that also emerged very clearly from analysis of the interaction in several of the cases discussed above, especially Cases 1, 3 and 5. However, even where surgery is ruled in as a possible option, a patient may still not meet the qualifying criteria or they may not be a suitable candidate for elective surgery at the time of consultation. Factors such as availability of resources, timing, level of risk and cost-benefit ratios all need to be weighed up, especially in publicly funded healthcare settings where care is rationed (Dew et al. 2010). Further information may also be needed before a decision can be made. As a result, the treatment recommendations provided in the surgical consultations in this study encompassed a range of options instead of or in addition to surgery, including further investigations, referral for other treatments, medication, lifestyle advice, planned monitoring or some kind of palliative or other long-term care, as well as recommendations against surgical treatment.

In conclusion, this study has highlighted the extremely complex nature of treatment discussions in surgical consultations. Not surprisingly, surgery is often oriented to by one or both parties as the starting point for treatment discussions in surgical clinic consultations, though, as this analysis has shown, this certainly does not mean that surgeons necessarily "want to operate" in all cases. However, inevitably the surgeon's expertise and recommendations carry huge weight, and the possibility of surgery remains the elephant in the room. Patients will also vary greatly in their confidence and ability to articulate their own perspectives and questions and thus to engage meaningfully in the often unfamiliar setting of a specialist consultation. These realities make it challenging for patients to share equally in the decision-making process. The successful negotiation of next steps therefore requires a high level of interactional competence on the part of surgeons who have to balance the integrity of their own clinical judgements with the needs and preferences of their patients. Further work remains to be done to explore and identify specific interactional strategies that can be used by surgeons (and patients) to achieve mutual understanding and alignment on treatment decisions within and across consultations and at different points along the trajectory of the decision-making process.

Acknowledgements

This research was funded by the New Zealand Health Research Council, the Royal Society of New Zealand Marsden Fund and the University of Otago. The authors thank all participants for generously allowing their consultations to be recorded, and acknowledge the input of colleagues and research assistants from the Applied Research on Communication in Health (ARCH) group to the research projects for which the data was originally collected.

Contributions

MS, SJW, KD and RG designed the study. SJW and LM undertook the fieldwork and data collection. SJW, MS, KD, RG, LM and AD all provided analytic input at various stages. MS and SJW drafted the manuscript and all authors read and approved the final manuscript.

Transcription Notation

See Chapter 2, this volume.

References

Brezis, Mayer, Sarah Israel, Avital Weinstein-Birenshtock, Pnina Pogoda, Ayelet Sharon and Renana Tauber. 2008. Quality of Informed Consent for Invasive Procedures. *International Journal for Quality in Health Care* 20(5): 352–7. doi: 10.1093/intqhc/mzn025

Cegala, Donald J., and Douglas M. Post. 2006. On Addressing Racial and Ethnic Health Disparities: The Potential Role of Patient Communication Skills Interventions. *American Behavioral Scientist* 49(6): 853.

Charles, Cathy, Amiram Gafni and Tim Whelan. 1997. Shared Decision-Making in the Medical Encounter: What Does It Mean? (or It Takes at Least Two to Tango). *Social Science & Medicine* 44(5): 681–2. doi: 10.1016/S0277-9536(96)00221-3

Clark, Shannon J., and Pamela L. Hudak. 2011. When Surgeons Advise against Surgery. *Research on Language & Social Interaction* 44(4): 385–412. doi: 10.1080/08351813.2011.619313

Collins, Sarah, Nicky Britten, Johanna Ruusuvuori and Andrew Thompson. 2007. *Patient Participation in Health Care Consultations: Qualitative Perspectives*. Maidenhead, UK: McGraw-Hill International, Open University Press.

Collins, Sarah, Paul Drew, Ian Watt and Vikki Entwistle. 2005. "Unilateral" and "Bilateral" Practitioner Approaches in Decision-Making about Treatment. *Social Science and Medicine* 61(12): 2611–27.

Costello, Brian A., and Felicia Roberts. 2001. Medical Recommendations as Joint Social Practice. *Health Communication* 13(3): 241–60.

Dew, Kevin, Maria Stubbe, Lindsay Macdonald, Anthony Dowell and Elizabeth Plumridge. 2010. The (Non) Use of Prioritisation Protocols by Surgeons. *Sociology of Health and Illness* 32(4): 545–62.

Dew, Kevin, Maria Stubbe, Anthony Dowell and Lindsay Macdonald. 2012. Side Effects Talk in General Practice Consultations. In *Medical Communication in Clinical Contexts*, edited by Benjamin R. Bates and Rukhsana Ahmed, 95–126. Dubuque, IA: Kendall Hunt.

Díaz, Félix. 2000. The Social Organisation of Chemotherapy Treatment Consultations. *Sociology of Health and Illness* 22(3): 364–89.

Drew, Paul, and John Heritage. 2006. Editors' Introduction. In *Conversation Analysis: Turn-Taking and Repair, Volume 1*, edited by John Heritage and Douglas Maynard. London: Sage.

Elwyn, Glyn, Dominick Frosch, Richard Thompson, Natalie Joseph-Williams, Amy Lloyd and Paul Kinnersley. 2012. Shared Decision-Making: A Model for Clinical Practice. *Journal of General Internal Medicine* 27: 1361–7.

Etchells, Edward, Michel Ferrari, Alex Kiss, Nikki Martyn, Deborah Zinman and Wendy Levinson. 2011. Informed Decision-Making in Elective Major Vascular Surgery: Analysis of 145 Surgeon–Patient Consultations. *Canadian Journal of Surgery (Journal Canadien de Chirurgie)* 54(3): 173–8. doi: 10.1503/cjs.047709

Heath, Christian. 1992. The Delivery and Reception of Diagnosis in the General-Practice Consultation. In *Talk at Work: Interaction in Institutional Settings*, edited by Paul Drew and John Heritage. Cambridge: Cambridge University Press.

Heritage, John. 1984. A Change-of-State Token and Aspects of Its Sequential Placement. In *Structures of Social Action: Studies in Conversation Analysis*, edited by J. Maxwell Atkinson and John Heritage, 299–345. Cambridge: Cambridge University Press.

Heritage, John, and Steven Clayman. 2010. Talk in Action: Interactions, Identities, and Institutions. In *Language in Society*, edited by P. Trudgill. West Sussex: Wiley-Blackwell.

Heritage, John, and Douglas W. Maynard. 2006. *Communication in Medical Care: Interaction between Primary Care Physicians and Patients*. Cambridge: Cambridge University Press.

Heritage, John, and Tanya Stivers. 1999. Online Commentary in Acute Medical Visits: A Method of Shaping Patients' Expectations. *Social Science and Medicine* 49: 1501–17.

Hudak, Pamela L., Shannon J. Clark and Geoffrey Raymond. 2011. How Surgeons Design Treatment Recommendations in Orthopaedic Surgery. *Social Science & Medicine* 73(7): 1028–36. doi: 10.1016/j.socscimed.2011.06.061

Hudak, Pamela L., Shannon J. Clark, and Geoffrey Raymond. 2012. The Omni-Relevance of Surgery: How Medical Specialization Shapes Orthopedic Surgeons' Treatment Recommendations. *Health Communication* 28(6): 533–45. doi: 10.1080/10410236.2012.702642

Hudak, Pamela L., Richard M. Frankel, Clarence III Braddock, Rosane Nisenbaum, Paola Luca, Caitlin McKeever and Wendy Levinson. 2008. Do Patients' Communication Behaviors Provide Insight into Their Preferences for Participation in Decision-Making? *Medical Decision-Making* 28: 385–93.

Hudak, Pamela L., Virginia Teas Gill, Jeffrey P. Aguinaldo, Shannon Clark and Richard Frankel. 2010. "I've Heard Wonderful Things about You": How Patients Compliment Surgeons. *Sociology of Health & Illness* 32(5): 777–97. doi: 10.1111/j.1467-9566.2010.01248.x

Hutchinson, Phil, Rupert Read and Wes Sharrock. 2008. *There Is No Such Thing as a Social Science: In Defence of Peter Winch*. Aldershot: Ashgate.

Janz, Nancy K., Patricia A. Wren, Laurel A. Copeland, Julie C. Lowery, Sherry L. Goldfarb and Edwin G. Wilkins. 2004. Patient-Physician Concordance: Preferences, Perceptions, and Factors Influencing the Breast Cancer Surgical Decision. *Journal of Clinical Oncology* 22(15): 3091–8. doi: 10.1200/jco.2004.09.069

Keating, Nancy L., Jane C. Weeks, Catherine Borbas and Edward Guadagnoli. 2003. Treatment of Early Stage Breast Cancer: Do Surgeons and Patients Agree Regarding whether Treatment Alternatives Were Discussed? *Breast Cancer Research and Treatment* 79: 225–31

Koenig, Christopher J. 2011. Patient Resistance as Agency in Treatment Decisions. *Social Science and Medicine* 72: 1105–14. doi: 10.1016/j.socscimed.2011.02.010

Makoul, Gregory, and Marla L. Clayman. 2006. An Integrative Model of Shared Decision-Making in Medical Encounters. *Patient Education and Counseling* 60(3): 301–12.

Maynard, Douglas W. 1992. On Clinicians Co-Implicating Recipients' Perspective in the Delivery of Diagnostic News. In *Talk at Work: Interaction in Institutional Settings*, edited by Paul Drew and John Heritage, 331–59. Cambridge: Cambridge University Press.

Maynard, Douglas W. 2003. *Bad News, Good News: Conversational Order in Everyday Talk and Clinical Settings*. Chicago: The University of Chicago Press.

Mitchell, Juliet. 1984. Producing Data: Case Studies. In *Ethnographic Research: A Guide to General Conduct*, edited by Roy Ellen, 237–41. London: Academic Press.

Mullan, Fitzhugh. 2004. Wrestling with Variation: An Interview with Jack Wennberg. *Health Affairs* October: 73–80.

Pleat, Jonathan M., Christopher S.J. Dunkin, Charlotte E. Davies, Ruth M. Ripley and Michael P.H. Tyler. 2004. Prospective Survey of Factors Affecting Risk Discussion during Consent in a Surgical Specialty. *British Journal of Surgery* 91: 1377–80.

Robinson, Jeffrey D. 2001. Asymmetry in Action: Sequential Resources in the Negotiation of a Prescription Request. *Text – Interdisciplinary Journal for the Study of Discourse* 21(1–2). doi: 10.1515/text.1.21.1-2.19

Robinson, Jeffrey D. 2003. An Interactional Structure of Medical Activities during Acute Visits and Its Implications for Patients' Participation. *Health Communication* 15(1): 27–59. doi: 10.1207/S15327027HC1501_2

Salzburg Global Seminar. 2011. Salzburg Statement on Shared Decision-Making. *BMJ* 342: 1745.

Schegloff, Emanuel A. 2007. *Sequence Organization in Interaction: Volume 1.* Cambridge: Cambridge University Press.

Seale, Clive, Robert Chaplin, Paul Lelliot and Alan Quirk. 2007. Antipsychotic Medication, Sedation and Mental Clouding: An Observational Study of Psychiatric Consultations. *Social Science & Medicine* 65(4): 698–711.

Silverman, Jonathan, Suzanne M. Kurtz and Juliet Draper. 2013. *Skills for Communicating with Patients.* 3rd ed. Oxford: Radcliffe Publishing.

Sinding, Christina, Pamela Hudak, Jennifer Wiernikowski, Jane Aronson, Pat Miller, Judy Gould and Donna Fitzpatrick-Lewis. 2010. "I Like to Be an Informed Person but...": Negotiating Responsibility for Treatment Decisions in Cancer Care. *Social Science & Medicine* 71(6): 1094–101. doi: 10.1016/j.socscimed.2010.06.005

Stewart, Moira, Judith Belle Brown, W. Wayne Weston, Ian R. McWhinney, Carol L. McWilliam and Thomas R. Freeman. 2003. *Patient-Centered Medicine: Transforming the Clinical Method.* 2nd ed. Oxford: Radcliffe Medical Press.

Stiggelbout, Anne. 2014. Shared Decision-Making: Past, Present, and Future. Plenary, EACH International Conference on Communication in Healthcare, Amsterdam.

Stivers, Tanya. 2005. Parent Resistance to Physicians' Treatment Recommendations: One Resource for Initiating a Negotiation of the Treatment Decision. *Health Communication* 18(1): 41–74. doi: 10.1207/s15327027hc1801_3

Stivers, Tanya, and Jeffrey D. Robinson. 2006. A Preference for Progressivity in Interaction. *Language in Society* 35: 367–92.

Street, Richard L., Gregory Makoul, Neeraj K. Arora and Ronald M. Epstein. 2009. How Does Communication Heal? Pathways Linking Clinician–Patient Communication to Health Outcomes. *Patient Education and Counseling* 74(3): 295–301. doi: 10.1016/j.pec.2008.11.015

Thompson, Andrew. 2007. The Meaning of Patient Involvement and Participation in Health Care Consultations: A Taxonomy. In Sarah Collins, Nicky Britten, Johanna Ruusuvuori and Andrew Thompson, *Patient Participation in Health Care Consultations: Qualitative Perspectives*, 43–64. Maidenhead, UK: McGraw Hill International, Open University Press.

Tongue, John R., Howard R. Epps and Laura L. Forese. 2005. Communication Skills for Patient-Centred Care: Research-Based, Easily Learned Techniques for Medical Interviews that Benefit Orthopaedic Surgeons and Their Patients. *Journal of Bone and Joint Surgery* 87: 652–8.

White, Sarah J. 2011. A Structural Analysis of Surgeon-Patient Consultations in Clinic Settings in New Zealand. Unpublished PhD thesis, University of Otago.

White, Sarah J., Maria H. Stubbe, Kevin P. Dew, Lindsay M. Macdonald, Anthony C. Dowell and Rod Gardner. 2013. Understanding Communication between Surgeon and Patient in Outpatient Consultations. *ANZ Journal of Surgery* 83(5): 307–11. doi: 10.1111/ans.12126

White, Sarah J., Maria H. Stubbe, Lindsay M. Macdonald, Anthony C. Dowell, Kevin P. Dew and Rod Gardner. 2014. Framing the Consultation: The Role of the Referral in Surgeon-Patient Consultations. *Health Communication* 29(1): 74–80. doi: 10.1080/10410236.2012.718252

Maria Stubbe, PhD, is Research Director in the Department of Primary Health Care and General Practice and co-directs the Applied Research on Communication in Health (ARCH) group at the at the Wellington School of Medicine and Health Sciences, University of Otago, Wellington. She has a background in interactional sociolinguistics and analysis of workplace/institutional discourse. Current research interests include shared decision-making in clinical encounters, communication in interpreter-mediated health encounters and patient experiences of health and illness.

Sarah J. White is a qualitative health researcher and linguist with a particular interest in using conversation analysis to understand communication in surgical practice. She is a Senior Lecturer at the Faculty of Medicine and Health Sciences at Macquarie University, Sydney. Sarah was awarded her PhD from the University of Otago, Wellington in 2011 and has professional and academic experience in clinical communication, quality and safety in healthcare, and medical education.

Lindsay Macdonald, MA, is a Research Fellow in the Department of Primary Health Care and General Practice and co-directs the ARCH group, at the Wellington School of Medicine and Health Sciences, University of Otago. She is a registered nurse with a postgraduate degree in nursing and linguistics. Her research interests include aspects of health communication particularly in relation to managing long-term conditions, and how everyday communication can affect health outcomes.

Anthony C. Dowell, MBChB, is Professor of General Practice and Primary Health Care at the Wellington School of Medicine and Health Sciences, University of Otago, where he also co-directs the ARCH group. He is a General Practitioner at the Island Bay Medical Centre, Wellington, and a member of a WHO panel exploring classification issues in mental health for the ICD11 classification of disease. His current academic interests include research in mental healthcare, health services research, quality in healthcare, and communication in healthcare consultation settings.

Rod Gardner, PhD, is Associate Professor in the School of Languages and Cultures at the University of Queensland in Brisbane. His academic and research interests include conversation analysis, second language interaction, indigenous Australian conversation and conversation analysis for classroom interaction and learning.

Kevin Dew, PhD, is Professor of Sociology at Victoria University of Wellington and before that was a senior lecturer in the Department of Public Health at the Wellington School of Medicine and Health Sciences. He is a founding member of the ARCH group. Current research activities include studies of interactions between health professionals and patients, cancer care decision-making in relation to health inequities, the social meanings of medications and the role of public health in contemporary society.

7 Negotiating Treatment Decisions in Orthopaedic Surgery Consultations

Shannon J. Clark and Pamela L. Hudak

7.1 Introduction

People generally consult medical professionals for diagnosis and treatment of their health concerns. Depending on the nature of their problem, patients may be referred to or seek out an appropriate specialist. Orthopaedic surgeons are medical specialists with expertise in assessing musculoskeletal ailments and can perform operative interventions (i.e., surgery) as well as recommend non-surgical treatment options.

The specialization of orthopaedic surgeons is consequential for the interactional organization of consultations between surgeons and patients. Previously, we described how there is an asymmetry between treatments in orthopaedic surgery consultations (Clark and Hudak 2011; Hudak, Clark and Raymond 2011, 2013). Surgery is treated by participants as being omni-relevant; that is, the consultations are organized around and towards surgery as a treatment consideration. Surgery is the treatment option against which other interventions are described, calibrated and considered. It is treated as the "last-best resort": surgery is positioned in relation to other treatments as the "last" option, the treatment reserved for instances when other, less invasive treatments have not been successful in resolving the patient's problem. It is often also talked about as the treatment most likely to offer a relatively lasting solution to the patient's problem (and in this sense, "the best"). However, as an invasive procedure, surgery carries inherent risks and, as such, is not entirely good news.

This chapter draws on our previous work and extends it to consider in greater detail what can happen when patients actively resist surgeons' recommendations. What we show is how patients: (1) invoke aspects of their life experience and their medical history when negotiating treatments with surgeons; and (2) are demonstrably oriented to balancing risks and benefits of surgery. As well, we consider how the omni-relevance of surgery and its mixed nature (i.e., "neither wholly good nor wholly bad") adds interactional complexity to the negotiation of treatment recommendations in this institutional context.

7.2   Methods, Data and Research Setting

Our data were audio recordings of routine clinical visits between 14 orthopaedic surgeons and 121 patients in two metropolitan hospitals in a major Canadian city. Patients had a range of musculoskeletal problems, including arthritis, torn cartilage or ligaments, bunions, injuries and sciatica, and were at various stages in the history of their problem, from seeing the surgeon for the first time, to follow-up review consultations after surgery.

In Canada's predominantly publicly funded healthcare system, consultations with orthopaedic surgeons require referral from another professional, such as a family physician or rheumatologist. As such, even if the patient has not seen the surgeon before, she or he will have discussed the problem with at least one other medical professional. If the surgeon and patient decide on surgery, arrangements are made for the patient to go on a waitlist to undergo the procedure.

The data were transcribed[1] and analysed drawing on the principles of conversation analysis. Our analysis of treatment recommendations drew on a subset of 79 of the 121 consultations in which a treatment decision was made (Clark and Hudak 2011; Hudak, Clark and Raymond 2011, 2013). We observed that surgery was referred to in all but one case, even when surgery was not being recommended. We then built collections of types of recommendations. We identified three basic patterns: recommendations *for* surgery, recommendations *not for* surgery, and recommendations in which the surgeon presented a range of treatment options (including surgery). Some practices and patterns we identified were shared across the three different types of recommendations while others contributed to the unique nature of their particular group. This chapter builds on the practices and patterns that were identified in the data and uses them to undertake four single case analyses of examples in which the patients resist the treatment recommendations (*for* and *not for* surgery).

7.3   The Omni-Relevance of Surgery

In orthopaedic surgery consultations, there is evidence of an asymmetry towards surgery in the organization of treatment recommendations (Clark and Hudak 2011; Hudak, Clark and Raymond 2011, 2013). Specifically:

---

1   See Chapter 2 for Transcription Notation.

(1) Surgery is an organizing axis around which other treatment recommendations are delivered, organized and calibrated;

(2) There is an asymmetry between recommendations *for* surgery vs *not for* surgery whereby recommendations *not for* surgery are typically longer, accounted for and positioned in relation to surgery; and

(3) The asymmetry between recommendations *for* surgery vs *not for* surgery remains even when the recommendation is designed to take the patient's treatment expectations and/or preferences into account. That is, the asymmetry is not solely attributable to alignment between the surgeon and patient when surgery is being recommended and misalignment when it is not.

A further complicating aspect of the negotiation of treatment recommendations in orthopaedic surgery is that neither surgery nor other treatments are seen as unilaterally positive. Of the treatments available to surgeons, surgery is the most drastic – recommending surgery is "bringing in the big guns". However, it also inflicts a trauma on the body, carries risks of infection and complications, and can involve side-effects from anaesthesia, analgesia and antibiotics, pain, scarring as well as substantial life disruption involved with recovery and rehabilitation. As such, surgery is reserved for cases where other treatments would not be or have not been effective and when the benefits of the likely outcome of surgery outweigh the risks of complications. Alternatives to surgery, for example, medication or physiotherapy, may avoid some of the associated risks and negatives of surgery, but may involve the continuing commitment and labour-intensive efforts of the patient while only managing the condition rather than resolving it. Thus, treatment options in surgery have complex cross-cutting facets. The complexity and inherently mixed character of surgery as neither wholly good nor wholly bad, is not only consequential for how surgeons deliver treatment recommendations, but also for how patient preferences and resistance are heard and negotiated.

Before examining patient resistance to treatment recommendations, we first show examples in which patients accept surgeons' recommendations, and also show the asymmetry between deliveries of recommendations *for* surgery (Extract 1) and *not for* surgery (against surgery and/or for something else; Extract 2).

Extract 1 – 10006

```
 1 R:     °I can help you up (by the way).°
 2        (0.7)((rustling in background))
 3 R:     okay.=↑so_ (3.2) ↑the onl- ↑>you know<
 4        you know the answer to: (0.3) helping you
 5        with your pai:n.
 6        °in your hip.°
 7        (Pt: mmm.)
 8 R:     °°you obviously (    ); need a hip replacement.°°
 9        [°°right?°°
10 Pt:    [unfortunately yeah.
11 R:     okay. SO_ (1.4) uhm:_ (3.7) what we can do
12        is we can fill out the paper:s¿
13        for a hip replacement¿
```

In this extract, an orthopaedic surgery fellow (R) sees the patient before the surgeon. In this example, the fellow provides the treatment recommendation. The treatment recommendation is delivered soon after the participants move out of the physical examination phase (lines 1–2). The recommendation: "°°you obviously ( ); need a hip replacement°°" (line 8) identifies a hip replacement as a single, specific treatment and is designed as a direct, unambiguous statement. In line 10, the patient indicates her agreement with "unfortunately yeah", treating the information as something she already knows, but is not particularly happy about. The fellow moves immediately to making arrangements for surgery (lines 11–13).

Extract 2 shows a recommendation *not for* surgery whereby the surgeon recommends against surgery (for now) and offers the patient a referral to another specialist for further advice about medications. Compared with Extract 1, the delivery of this recommendation against surgery is longer and forecast by a number of features.

Extract 2 – 50010

```
 1 Sg:    you do: have a:h (1.0) what I would say >would< (.) >to< be
 2         mild or moderate arth[ritis] in your knee:s okay?
 3 Pt:                          [yes. ]
 4         (1.0)
 5 Sg:    AND AHH: unlike ↓a:h the old wives tales in fact this is not
 6         ↓a: (0.6) occupational hazard for you:,=
 7 Pt:    =m[m hm]
 8 Sg:      [ oka]y it just it comes becau:se (1.1) a lotta people in hh.
 9         thheir sixties and seventies start to develop this t[ype     ]=
10 Pt:                                                          [ye(p/s).]
11 Sg:    =of knee arthritis.
12         (0.8)
13 Sg:    THE U:H_ (0.7) I'm gla:d that you're feeling better with the
14         treatment¿ [that you]'re having,
15 Pt:               [°mm hm° ]
16         (0.4)
17 Sg:    certainly you don't ha:ve ↓a: <surgical pro[blem> ] with=
18 Pt:                                               [mm hm, ]
19 Sg:    =your knee:s, (0.3) it may well be that in the ↑futu:re,
20         (0.3) this tends to be a progressive illne[ss¿ over] ti:me¿
21 Pt:                                               [yes:.   ]
22 Sg:    a:nd (0.5) in the future you ma:y need an op[era]tion °but you°=
23 Pt:                                               [yes]
24 Sg:    =°certainly do not need an operation° No:w.
25         .hh I'M QUITE PREPARED TO A:H_ (.) arra:nge for you °to see one
26         of the arthritis specialists he:re? if you'd like¿°
27 Pt:    yes:.
28 Sg:    they can give you some advice, °with regard to other
29         medications that you might be able to take, a[nd so] on,=okay?°
30 Pt:                                                  [yes:.]
31 Pt:    okay.
32 Sg:    I think that °would be well worth your whi:le.°=
33 Pt:    =mt! okay.=
34 Sg:    =OKAY?
35 Sg:    =OKAY?
36         (0.2)
37 Sg:    SO I'LL DO THA:T¿ you just wait he:re, a::uh we'll get
38         the appointment made for you,
```

The surgeon undertakes extra work in the delivery of the recommendation *not for* surgery, forecasting the recommendation, laying bare the evidential case for it, and anticipating and managing potential resistance (Clark and Hudak 2011). After a negative recommendation – that is, a recommendation against surgery (lines 22, 24) – the surgeon offers the patient a positive next action, referral to another specialist (lines 25–6). While the patient does not provide verbal uptake of the recommendation *against* surgery (Stivers 2005b [discussed further below], 2006), he does provide positive responses to the surgeon's offer of referral (lines 27, 30). The participants reach agreement and move to making arrangements for the referral.

In both Extracts 1 and 2, the patients accept the treatment recommendation, the treatment activity phase is complete (see Robinson 2003) and participants move to the next activity, making arrangements. When patients *resist* recommendations, movement to the next activity is deferred until participants reach consensus. Below, we turn to examine how patients resist surgeons' treatment recommendations in orthopaedic surgery consultations. In particular, we consider how patients actively resist surgeons' recommendations and the grounds on which they challenge or call into question those recommendations. We also consider if and how patients advocate for a particular treatment.

7.4 Resisting Treatment Recommendations

Patients and medical professionals orient to treatment decisions as a joint responsibility (Stivers 2002, 2005a, b, 2007). This stands in contrast to diagnoses, which patients typically treat as the domain of the physician (Heath 1992; Peräkylä 1998, 2002). In paediatric encounters, physicians and parents orient to parent acceptance as normatively relevant on completion of the treatment recommendation (Stivers 2005b, 2006). This orientation means that withholding acceptance, for example, through silence or continuers, constitutes *passive* resistance of the recommendation. In contrast, *active* resistance is a stronger type of resistance in that it is both a responsive and an initiating action; that is, active resistance makes relevant a next action from the physician. "Active resistance includes an action that questions or challenges the physician's treatment recommendation, including proposals of alternative treatments" (Stivers 2005b: 52). Thus, parents initiate negotiation of the treatment recommendation by either withholding acceptance or actively resisting the recommendation.

Participants need to reach agreement before they can close the treatment activity phase. Both passive and active resistance put the physician in the position of pursuing parent acceptance, for example, through convincing the parent/patient to accept the proposed treatment or offering alternatives or concessions. Physicians' pursuit of acceptance can include "offering a rationale for the treatment recommendation, offering evidence for the underlying diagnosis, returning to the examination findings, and offering the parent a concessionary future action" (Stivers 2005b: 47).

Reaching consensus can result in protracted negotiation sequences. We have elected to present long extracts of the four cases of resistance that follow in order to convey a sense of the protracted nature of these negotiations as they unfold and to capture some back and forth of the exchanges between surgeons and patients. The long extracts also allow us to track how participants balance the risks and benefits of surgery against the severity and discomfort of patients' conditions over multiple turns at talk.

Extract 3 shows the patient resisting the surgeon's recommendation, initially passively and then more actively. The patient is consulting the surgeon about a cyst in her thigh which developed after being hit by a car several years earlier. The cyst has become painful and has recently begun to drain. The surgeon diagnoses the cyst as a hardened fat deposit and recommends massage to soften and disperse it.[2]

Extract 3 – 050007

```
 1 Sg:    i-it's just become hard; and what happens is
 2        the fat becomes ↑ha:rd?
 3        and it forms >a little bit of< scar ↓tissue.
 4        .hh so what you should do is massage it.
 5        (0.9)
 6 Sg:    oka:y?
 7        (0.2)
 8 Sg:    and you have to massage it to try and make it ↑soft?
 9        (0.5)
10 Pt:    >yeah but< ↑y'kno:w¿ ↓uh::: it's been ha:rd
11        fo:r for over since the ↑accident?
12 Sg:    yea:h.
13 Pt:    they ↑did- [the:::_     ]
14 Sg:              [and one he-] and one right he:re.
15 Pt:    °yeah I (know but uhm/have one);°=[↑it- it wasn't big;=
16 Sg:                                     [°yea:h.°
17 Pt:    =>and y'know- and< it was good. (with the ti:me?)
18 Sg:    ye[ah.
19 Pt:      [it was going away.=.hh but then it started hurting.
20        (.)
21 Sg:    [°yeah.°
22 Pt:    [uh:m:_ they gave ultra-↑sou:nd¿ for::_  (0.5)
23        (bery soffa) but it >never did.<
24 Sg:    yea:h. [.hh
25 Pt:           [°it's been ( ).°
26 Sg:    it's- it's nothing ba:d.
27        (.)
28 Sg:    it's just- it's just fat that's become ha:rd.
29        .hh so: (.) over time if you massage ↑it?
30        (0.4) it's gonnu slowly get *softer and softer.*
31        m.hhh and what's gonna happen over time
32        is the body's gonna create what's called a <bur↑sa?>
```

---

2 This example has been discussed previously as a deviant case in that it shows a recommendation not for surgery which is neither forecasted nor positioned (at least initially) in relation to surgery (Clark and Hudak 2011).

```
33 Pt:    °°mm hm¿°°
34 Sg:    and it's gonna:, (0.2) create a bursa to make it
35        smoo:th over ↑top? .hh and it'll_ (0.3) the pai:n should_
36        (0.4) slo:wly start *to go awa:y,*
37        (0.4)
38 Pt:    uhm:_>let me ask you because<↑it never has (0.3)
39        before (and why now).
40        >ee an'< y'know it started leakin' ↑(a lot);
41        (0.4)
42 Sg:    m.hh YEAH; IT'S GOOD [QUESTION.
43 Pt:                        [( ).
44 Sg:    SOME HAVE_ sometimes the fa:t starts to: (.) ↑liquify?
45        (0.4)
46 Sg:    after the trauma? and that's why it starts to ↑leak
47        a ↑little ↑bit? .hhh uhm_ (0.3) but it's nothing bad;
48        like it's not (.) cancer >right?<
49        that's the most important [thing.
50 Pt:                              [mm hm;
51 Sg:    .hh coz we wanna make sure that it's not cancer.
52        .hhh so on the MRI¿ (0.5) it does not appear
53        to be cancer¿
54        (0.3)
55 Sg:    a:nd_ (.) from the story you're telling me
56        it doesn't sound like cancer?
57 Pt:    °mm hm.°
58 Sg:    and looking at your leg today; it doesn't look like *cancer.*
59        .hhh so:_ (0.6) the good news is I don't think it's cancer.
60 Pt:    °°mm hm.°°
61 Sg:    mt!.hh uhm:_ (.) but in general_(0.4) I would just
62        leave it ↑alone?
63        (0.5)
64 Sg:    °okay¿° and just (.) massage ↑it? try to make it ↑soft?
65        (0.5)
66 Sg:    it's nothing bad.= if it was ↑cancer then we'd have to talk
67        about taking it out.
68        (.)
69 Pt:    °°mm hm.°°
70 Sg:    but_ it's no:t.
71        (0.6)
72 Sg:    so that's good °*ne:ws.*°
73 Pt:    (well because) I can't lean on this si::de;
74        °an'° (0.6)
75 Sg:    mt!.hh it's gonna take some time to get ↑better;=
76        =it's gotta get soft right?=
77        so you're gonna have to massa:ge i:t_
78        a:nd .hh do all sorts of things;
79        but_ .hh °the° the important thing
80        >is we have to make sure it's not_<
81        (0.6) °can[cer.°
82 Pt:              [>mm hm.<
83 Sg:    so it's not cancer.
84 Pt:    [°°mm:.°°
85 Sg:    [.hh so:_ y'know; give it some ti:me;
86        massa:ge i:t; °and° >y'know.<=
87        =see how it >does;=.hh< now that
88        it's been drai:ned >maybe it'll< start to
89        feel better;
90 Pt:    but they sa:y ( ) the MRI?
91 Sg:    mm h:mm:;
92 Pt:    they told the doctor and she s- >THEY they< gave
93        her two options; one was the: °the orthopaedic surgeon?°
```

```
94        and the other option was (draining)¿
95        (0.2)
96 Pt:    (by a ologist¿ draining¿)
97        (0.3)
98 Sg:    NO NO; IT'S NOT_ [*e*IT'S NOT something
99 Pt:                    [( )_
100 Sg:   .hh if you put a drain in it¿ (0.4)
101       things are just gonna (.) continue to collect.
102       fluid will just re-collect.
103       .mhhh it's gonna take some time for it to go away.
104       (0.3)
105 Sg:   I don't recommend that you have anything
106       °↓done to it.↓°
107       0.3)
108 Sg:   °okay¿°
109 Sg:   every time somebody (.) puts a kni:fe;
110       tries to cut it_ tries to drain it_ .hh (0.5)
111       if it's not infected no:w; you can make it infected.
112 Pt:   °mm hm.°
113 Sg:   °oka:y,° and if you make it in↑fected?
114       you've got a much bigger *problem.*
115       (0.6)
116 Sg:   >°okay?°<
117       (0.2)
118 Sg:   so:; (0.4) °leave it alone.°
119       (0.5)
120 Sg:   that's the best thing to do.
121 Sg:   .hh try to ignore it¿
122       (0.4)
123 Sg:   and then massa:ge i:t_ and try to make it ↑soft?
124       .hh and over time the pain will °↑get ↑less.°
125       (0.5)
126 Sg:   °okay¿°
127 Pt:   °okay.°
```

The surgeon's recommendation, ".hh so what you should do is mass<u>age</u> it" (line 4) is met with passive resistance from the patient in the form of silence (lines 5, 7, 9). The surgeon pursues agreement with an upward intoned "oka:y?" (line 6), and restating the recommendation (line 8). The patient subsequently upgrades her resistance, actively resisting both the non-serious nature of the diagnosis and treatment recommendation. The patient resists the recommendation by citing the duration of the problem (lines 10–11), emphasizing changes and symptomology in the cyst over time (lines 15–19), including the development of pain ("it was going aw<u>ay</u>.=.hh but then it started hurting", line 19), and previous (ineffective) treatments (lines 22–3). The surgeon pursues acceptance, offering further explanation of his diagnosis, the treatment, the healing process and prognosis in relation to pain (lines 28–36). The negotiation of the treatment recommendation continues with the patient questioning the reason for recent developments (lines 38–40). She subsequently cites her experience with the problem, and its impact ("I can't lean on this si::de", line 73), and challenges the recommendation by reporting previous medical investigations (the MRI, line 90). She also introduces surgical treatment as potentially relevant by reporting previous medical informings (lines 92–6). The surgeon is now in the position of disputing the treatment ("draining") indirectly proposed by the patient (lines 98, 100–1).

The surgeon pursues the patient's acceptance by utilizing resources like those noted by Stivers (2005a, b, 2006). These include: accounting for the recommendation and ruling out alternative diagnoses, "it's nothing bad" (lines 26, 47, 66) and "it's not cancer" (lines 48, 51–6, 58–9, 66, 80–1, 83); restating the recommendation (e.g., lines 64, 77, 123–4); reformulating the recommendation, in this case invoking the relevance of surgery by ruling it out (e.g., "but in general_(0.4) I would just leave it ↑alone?", lines 61–2), and explaining the conditions under which surgery would be offered: "if it was ↑cancer then we'd have to talk about taking it out" (lines 66–7); and explicitly pursuing acceptance through "okays" and intonation.

Through the patient's active resistance to the recommendation and her introduction of an invasive intervention (i.e., "draining"), the patient treats the recommendation as threatening the legitimacy of her problem and decision to consult the surgeon. In cases of upper respiratory illness in children, Stivers (2005a) argues that recommending prescription medication implicitly legitimizes the patient's decision to seek medical care; and conversely, recommending against antibiotics can delegitimize the visit (2005a: 960). In orthopaedic surgery consultations, surgery is the treatment that wholly legitimizes the patient's visit. The surgeon's suggestion of massage – a treatment which does not utilize the extent of the surgeon's specialization, which the patient will most likely undertake herself, and which will require the patient's continued efforts over time – does not implicitly validate the legitimacy of the patient's problem and leaves her without a resolution in the near future. The surgeon, in his pursuit of the patient's acceptance, works to display that he has taken the patient's problem seriously, by ruling out a relevant and extremely serious diagnosis, cancer.

While in Extract 3 the patient's introduction of "draining" indirectly pursues the possibility of a surgical intervention via a third-party report, the patient in Extract 4 more explicitly advocates for a course of action as her own preference. The patient is a 49-year-old woman with advanced hip arthritis. The surgeon recommends against surgery for now ("delay surgery"), and proposes a vague treatment ("do something") for managing the patient's condition. This is subsequently specified to be a steroid injection.

Extract 4 – 10005

```
1 Sg:    and >y'know< hips:_ (0.6) we don't think hips
2        will last forty-eight years.=
3        =anymore than your °car'll last forty-eight years.°
4 Pt:    °mhm hhm;°
5 Sg:    an' so as a result we tend to: (0.4) try to de↑lay surgery.
6 Pt:    mm [hm.
7 Sg:       [for the younger °patient; >but not< for the older patient.°
8        (1.0)
9 Sg:    °°you see¿°°
10 Pt:   °°mm hm.°°
```

```
11          (.)
12 Sg:   so:_ (1.2) if ↑we c'n:_ (.) help you:
13        to get your hip more comfortable,
14        (1.0) °you know° you can live with arthritis as long as
15        it's not s:o °painful°; maybe we can do something
16        to make your left hip more comfortable
17        and delay your °>surgery<°.
18        (1.0)
19 Sg:   °that's the thinking.°
20        (0.9)
21 Pt:   mm[hmm,
22 Sg:     [>whaddu-< what do you think about tha:t.
23        (0.7)
24 Pt:   uhm:_ I'm thinking if somethin:g (0.6) ↑did do that
25        (.) that would be ↑fi:ne; .hh however
26        .h I: I would think (.) maybe ↑no:t,
27        but I would [think that] at (0.3) age seventy
28 Sg:               [  gghhm   ]
29 Pt:   I: I wouldn't be as uhm:_ (0.2)
30        ((knock on door))
31        (0.5)
32 Pt:   important;=uhm:_=
33 Ns:   =ah the chaplain's he:re¿
34        I've got a the patients in the roo:m¿
35 Sg:   ok[ay.
36 Ns:     [you wa:nt to talk to the chaplain?
37 Sg:   I- I wanna speak to the chaplain; I'm gonna come.
          ((136 lines removed – 3min56sec))
174       ((surgeon re-enters room))
175 Sg:  SO:>whaddou you think abouth (.) about an injection.
176       (1.0)
177 Pt:  uhm::_ (0.4) i- injections scare ↑me¿ but hhh. hhheh.
178 Sg:  °yea:h.°
179 Pt:  but I- uh I mean I would be: >willing to< go:, (0.9)
180       °u:h° that wa:y_ certainly,=I ↑guess what I'm (0.7)
181       what uh:m_ (0.3) ts! .hh huhhh.
182       ↑>how would I know when_<↑ when when (0.5) it's >time< ts!.hh
183       I- i- it jus- a- a- a:t the mome:nt;
184       uhm_ °what I'm- >I guess what I'm saying is< is u:hm°
185       (0.2) °.hhh I can't do thi:ngs with my ↓kids;°
186 Sg:  [right
187 Pt:  [>and I'm< (0.4) °I mean° I can't do: ↑things:_
188       .hh [things that I'm (0.6) ts! that a:re (0.8) that=
189 Sg:      [right
190 Pt:  I'm USEful fo[::r right ↑no:w,
191 Sg:              [right.
192 Pt:  °and I hate t(h)o s(h)ay i(h)t° but mhaybe (0.4)
193       >might not be quite so ↑↑useful< [for when I'm-
194 Sg:                                    [right.
195 Pt:  when I'm ol:der.
196 Sg:  °yeah.°
197 Pt:  so I'm wondering >if if< (0.9) if anything_
198       a major [thi:ng if that's something I should do=
199 Sg:          [yeuh.
200 Pt:  =while I:'m uh:m_ (1.4)
201 Sg:  well I [to-
202 Pt:        [still a viabl:e_
203 Sg:  I tota[lly under-
204 Pt:       [kind of person.
205 Sg:  I totally understand that and you make a point.
206       (0.7)
```

```
207 Sg: so we're not gonna leave you
208     for a long period of [ti:me;=
209 Pt:                      [ye:ah
210 Sg: =in a bad state.
211 Pt: ye:ah.
212 Sg: what- I'm just simply sug[gesting    ]
213 Pt:                          [that's all I] wanted to kn[o:w;
214 Sg:                                                     [that
215 Sg: we try injections,=[>see if it gets you back]=
216 Pt:                    [ ma k e s s e n c e ;   ]
217 Sg: =on your feet;=
218 Pt: =yeah.
219     (0.7)
220 Sg: a:nd u:h_ if it does then fabulous.
221     (0.5)
222 Sg: and if it doesn't, (0.4) then you'll be back here soon,
223     (0.4) >you can- we c'n h-< make an appointment for you
224     to come back and see me in: [six ] weeks;
225 Pt:                             [yes.]
226 Sg: .hh and you can tell me, if you tell me that
227     you're not doing well and you need the surgery
228     then we:'ll start talking about the surgery.
229     (1.0)
230 Pt: ohkay.
```

In the surgeon's forecasting of his recommendation *not for* surgery, he builds an evidential case for the recommendation (see Clark and Hudak 2011). The surgeon's reasoning for delaying a hip replacement is the likely longevity of the joint if replaced versus the patient's age and life expectancy; that is, the patient would likely outlive the replaced joint ("we don't think hips will last forty-eight years", lines 1–2). The patient begins resisting the treatment recommendation passively by withholding acceptance (see lines 18, 20, 23). When the surgeon explicitly seeks the patient's opinion at line 22 with ">whaddu-< what do you think about tha:t", her resistance to the recommendation becomes more active. After a pause, the patient formulates her resistance initially by echoing the surgeon's use of "thinking" and the conditional "if" format: "uhm_ I'm thinking if somethin:g (0.6) ↑did do that (.) that would be ↑fi:ne" (lines 24–5). Although it is designed as a quasi-agreement, the patient casts doubt on the adequacy of the unspecified treatment (note the stress on "did" which projects an upcoming contrast [Schegloff 1998]). The patient further resists the recommendation by picking up on the surgeon's own reasoning basis of her age as problematic and presenting a counter argument: that at age 70 she would not be as "important" (lines 26–7, 29, 32). The consultation is interrupted by another matter for the surgeon to attend to, and the surgeon delegates discussion of steroid injections to the attending fellow (not shown).

The surgeon explicitly seeks the patient's opinion about steroid injections on his return (line 175). Here, the patient indicates reservations ("injections scare ↑me¿", line 177) but willingness for the procedure ("but I- uh I mean I would be: >willing to< go:, (0.9) °u:h° that wa:y_ certainly", lines 179–80) before returning to account for her previous (and still relevant) resistance. Again, the patient invokes the surgeon's reasoning basis of age to challenge the recommendation. The patient indicates the limitations and life disruptions that her arthritis is causing to her current life ("I can't do thi:ngs with my ↓kids", line 185), and questions the comparative benefit of surgery when she is older. The patient then poses an indirect request for surgery: "so I'm wondering >if if< (0.9) if anything_ a major thi:ng if that's something I should do=while I:'m uh:m_ (1.4) still a viabl:e_ kind of person" (lines 197–204).

Working towards gaining consensus, the surgeon acknowledges the patient's point, and reiterates the proposed treatment as an interim attempt (i.e., "try" and "see if", line 215) to manage the patient's condition and ability to function ("gets you back on your feet", lines 215, 217). He also offers concessionary assurances, positioning the patient within a continuum of care and assuring monitoring of the outcome of injections with a specific time frame ("six weeks", line 224). The surgeon also formulates the decision as being in the patient's hands in the future ("and you can tell me", line 226) as well as a promise that: "if you tell me that you're not doing well and you need the surgery then we:'ll start talking about the surgery" (lines 226–8). This concession retains surgery as relevant in the future, but staves it off for now with another treatment. After a one-second pause, the patient accepts with "ohkay" (line 230).

Both patient and surgeon in Extract 4 can be seen to be oriented to surgery as the last-best resort. They are both oriented to the "big" nature of surgery as an invasive, major treatment which requires consideration and balancing of risks to benefits. While the surgeon displays his reasoning of the recommendation against surgery for now as based on age and the likely longevity of the joint replacement, the patient also uses age to resist the recommendation and advocate *for* the *current* relevance of surgery (as opposed to at a later stage of her life). The patient works to shift the balance of her pain, life disruption and life-stage against the risks of the longevity of the joint to advocate for the appropriateness of a major intervention.

In both Extracts 3 and 4, the patients resist the surgeons' recommendations *not for* surgery. Patients resist on grounds of their lived experience with their problem/s, for example, the severity and duration of their symptoms, life impact, prior medical investigations, diagnoses and treatments, and the perceived likely success of the non-surgical interventions proposed. Recommendations *not for* surgery can threaten the legitimacy of the patient's problem by potentially minimizing the severity of the problem. However, just because a patient resists a recommendation *not for* surgery, does not necessarily mean that she or he *wants* surgery. The next section considers how the cross-cutting facets of surgery are managed interactionally.

7.5 Surgery as Neither Wholly Good nor Wholly Bad

As noted earlier, neither surgery nor other treatments are wholly good news in orthopaedic surgery consultations. Surgery carries the inherent risks and potential complications of an invasive procedure; and while non-surgical treatments such as physiotherapy or medication are not as risky, they may only manage symptoms rather than resolve the underlying problem. This neither wholly good nor wholly bad nature of treatments adds a complicating element to the negotiation of treatment recommendations, as well as to how resistance is managed and patient preferences are heard. In the following two examples, the patients' active resistance is complicated by the both omni-relevance of surgery and the neither wholly good nor wholly bad nature of these recommendations.

Extract 5 shows a recommendation with notable similarities to Extract 4, involving the same surgeon and a patient of a similar age (a 48-year-old woman) facing the same problem, advanced hip osteoarthritis. The surgeon again recommends against surgery for now, and proposes a treatment for managing the patient's pain, this time medication. However, in this consultation, the patient actively resists the affirmative aspect of the recommendation (i.e., medication) rather than specifically resisting the negative aspect of the recommendation (i.e., no surgery). Although the patient resists medication, she subsequently backs away from the implication that her resistance is due to wanting surgery.

Extract 5 – 10001

```
 1 Sg:    [IF YOU WERE seventy-fi:ve
 2        I'd be telling you; (0.2)
 3        ↑let's get this thing done no:w while
 4        you're °healthy.°
 5        (0.3)
 6 Sg:    °and- and [youthful.°°
 7 Pt:              [°'kay.°
 8        (0.4)
 9 Sg:    but at forty-eight I would sa:y_ (0.9)
10        if you're learning to manage it¿
11        so much the better.
12        (0.4)
13 Sg:    °and we'll just delay it.°
14        (0.6)
15 Sg:    now that doesn't mean that you'll:
16        (0.9) be forced to suffer_ (0.5) terrible_
17        ↓u:h disability before we will agree to
18        do your hip=it's not like that at ↑all.
19 Pt:    t! °'kay.°
20        (0.4)
21 Sg:    but >ah< my advice would be to just try to manage it.
22        (0.9)
23 Sg:    have you tried tylenol¿
24        (1.8) ((possibly an inbreath in the pause))
25 Pt:    if you knew what I took advil wise¿
26 Sg:    yeah;
27        (0.4)
```

```
28 Pt:   you'd string me up.
29       (0.5)
30 Sg:   but even so:; [(you see) that's why that's] why I=
31 Pt:                 [ pHHh HH. ↑hhh .hh hhh .hh ]
32 Sg:   =[asked you:.]
33 Pt:    [it do e s  ]n't- it didn't eve:n_ (0.7)
34 Sg:   but (0.4) did you try ↑tyleno:[l¿
35 Pt:                                 [I tried °everything.°
36 Sg:   [°okay.°
37 Pt:   [°I: have tried extra strength;
38       I tried [advil;°
39 Sg:           [°okay.°
40 Pt:   oh >no no no no< [that
41 Sg:                    [did you try full doses
42       of a- of tylenol¿ like [eight tab]lets a day
43 Pt:                          [°°I was°°]
44 Pt:   how bout °°six at a ti:me.°°
45 Sg:   okay. well now yo[u      m]ustn't °do tha:t.°
46                       [((clap))]
47 Pt:   dHH s(h)ee th(h)at's wh(h)y I t(h)old y(h)ou;
48       y(h)ou $DON'T wanna know what I did.=[.HH but=
49 Sg:                                        [okay.
50 Pt:   =[it- it-
51 Sg:    [do you know why it's important not to [do that¿
52 Pt:                                           [°stomach;°
53       (0.5)
54 Sg:   well it's:_ (0.6) ADvil is the stomach.
55       but (0.3) ↓uhm_ (0.2) *a:h_* (0.9) it's one thing
56       to burn a hole in your stomach; but (0.3) if you
57       overdo it with the tylenol you can damage your
58       kidneys.
59 Pt:   yeuh;
60       (0.4)
61 Pt:   no I know.
62       but y'know like_ (0.5) becu- but y'know ↑I was
63       (.) tryin' to get in and ↑see you [guys for eight=
64 Sg:                                      [°yeah.
65 Pt:   =and ten ↑m[onths. .hh and my family doctor=
66 Sg:              [°right.°
67 Pt:   =kept prescribing ↑drugs that were having no impact.
68       .hh no:w (.) y'know meloxica:m see:ms to:: .hh have
69       taken me:_ >y'know I was<on my way ↑anyway¿
70       [but it seems t'have taken me into eve:n (.) just=
71 Sg:   [yeah.
72 Pt:   =a slightly be:tte:r_ (0.2)
73 Sg:   °yeah.°
74 Pt:   zone. .hhh but_ °y'know like w- I: couldn't ↑sleep.°
75       °y'know,° I have four kids;
76       [I had to     sur]vi:ve.
77 Sg:   [°I understand.°]
78 Pt:   [ri:ght?
79 Sg:   [°I understa:nd.°=
80 Pt:   =and nothing I was ↑doing worked.
81       (1.1)
82 Sg:   Now >I have to say< I just got a page
83       that I have to answer.
84 Pt:   °that's okay.°
         ((38 lines removed - 58sec))
123      (0.4)
124 Sg:  oka:y; s[o:_
125 Pt:          [so that's fi:ne; no I'm no:t (.) like
```

```
126       I'm not ↓terribly kee:n about having
127       a hip replacement.↓
128 Pt:   [I mean in] the s(h)ense th(h)at_=
129 Sg:   [  n o :.  ]
130 Sg:   yeah.=
131 Pt:   =like_ .hh y'know I'm no:t uhm_ (0.4) I mean I know
132       that_ (.) °and I understand enough about surgery
133       and surgical risk°=and then afterwards
134       I'm sure there's certain:: things that (.)
135       you're- are changed forever too right¿=
136       because you have this prosthetic ( ) thing
137       in your leg;=my [son by] the way looked at it=
```

The recommendation against surgery (for now) is again mitigated and forecast in its delivery. The surgeon has implied that surgery will not be recommended by presenting the counter-to-reality conditions under which surgery would be offered, if she were 75 (line 1). Although not immediate, the patient produces a quiet acceptance token (line 7) after the hypothetical surgery recommendation. The surgeon then returns to patient's present age of 48 to present the alternative to surgery – managing the condition (line 10). At this point, the recommendation, although vague and mitigated, is potentially complete. The patient passively resists (line 12) and the surgeon begins to pursue acceptance by reformulating the recommendation (lines 13, 21), offering assurances of the availability of surgery in the future, and that the patient will not be "forced to suffer' (lines 15–18).

At the end of the surgeon's restated recommendation, "but >ah< my advice would be to just try to manage it" (line 21), the patient further passively resists. The surgeon now moves from vague treatments to something more specific and it becomes clear that the treatment for "managing" is medication. The surgeon seeks to establish the relevance for a subsequent recommendation for Tylenol with a "pre"-question (Schegloff 2007), "have you tried tylenol¿" (line 23). The patient now begins to actively resist, working to block the relevance of the projected recommendation. She alludes to substantial past experience with not just the medication named by the surgeon ("Tylenol"), but the class of analgesics more broadly ("Advil-wise"), and at a non-recommended level ("you'd string me up", line 28). While the surgeon pursues the same line of treatment by seeking confirmation of her use of Tylenol specifically (line 34) and at a specific dosage ("full doses", "eight tablets a day", lines 41–2), the patient resists further, providing extreme case formulations ("I tried °everything°", line 35), listing alternative brands, and strengths, and extreme doses ("how bout °°six at a ti:me°°", line 44). The patient accounts for the multiple medications tried and extreme dosing as a matter of desperation due to the long wait to get in to see the surgeon (lines 63, 65), repeated experience of ineffectual treatments ("my family doctor kept prescribing ↑drugs that were having no impact", lines 65, 67), and the pressures of her family life ("I: couldn't ↑sleep.° °y'know,° I have four kids; I had to sur]vi:ve" and "nothing I was ↑doing worked", lines 74–6, 80).

The consultation is interrupted when the surgeon breaks off to answer a page. When the surgeon and the patient re-engage, the patient accepts the surgeon's recommendation against surgery ("so that's fi:ne; no I'm no:t (.) like I'm not ↓terribly kee:n about having a hip replacement.↓", lines 125–7) and disclaims having a strong preference for it. She accounts for her preference as based on knowledge of surgery, associated risks and permanent changes to the body that are entailed by the procedure. Subsequently, the participants discuss further the process and procedure for a hip replacement, recovery time as well as the conditions under which the patient would know and decide that she "needs an operation" (not shown).

The design of the treatment recommendation in Extract 5 above to include both a negative (i.e., against surgery for now) and affirmative treatment recommendation (i.e., for medication) is consequential for the patient's resistance in that her resistance to medication is potentially hearable as seeking surgery. The patient orients to and disclaims this hearing explicitly. Later in the consultation, the patient supports her claim of not being "keen" for surgery when she reports having seen a surgeon at another facility who was "ready to sign her up right away", in other words, offering her surgery immediately, and her not having accepted it.

The final example is somewhat different from those above in that the patient resists *surgery* rather than a non-surgical treatment. The surgeon presents surgery as an appropriate and available treatment for the patient's bunions; however, the final decision the participants reach is not to have surgery now, but for the patient to get a prescription for orthopaedic shoes. With the benefit of hindsight, an audio recording and a transcript, it can be seen that the patient is angling towards this treatment from the beginning of the consultation; however, the cross-cutting facets of surgery in this institutional environment complicate the way the patient's proffered treatment preferences can be heard and understood. An earlier part of the consultation is provided to contextualize the patient's subsequent resistance.

Extract 6a – 50006

```
1 Sg:    tell me about your foot.=
2        >what-< what's: [about your foot is [troubling you no:w.
3 Pt                     [.hh                [well doctor clements has
4        had had (0.4) has suggested I come to see you:;
5        (.) because you're the: (0.2) foot expert¿=and .H
6        it's due to the >misshapen=I asked< him actually;
7        to: .hh ah [for a (0.8) a:h for a prescription fo:r
8                   [(( sound of paper, pen click
9        ortho- orthopaedic] shoe:s¿
10       movement         ))]
11 Sg:   ri:ght¿
12 Pt:   because it's getting really difficult to find a shoe
13       that will fit that_ .hh knobby toe and the knobby:
14       °uhm°_ (0.9) [bunion.
15 Sg:                [you got- you got too many bumps on your f[(
16 Pt:                                                          [YEA::H;
17 Sg:   (hh   )]
18 Pt:   yea::h;]
19 Sg:   °°alright. ok[ay.°°
20 Pt:               [yeah.
```

```
21         I'm into the boxes instead of the shoe:s.
22  Sg:    yeuh.
23         (0.6)
24  Pt:    s[o:_
25  Sg:     [well¿
26         (.)
27  Pt:    he suggested coming to see [you: °°(seeing as:)°°
28  Sg:                               [sure.
29  Pt:    [I'M not anxious to have surgery neces[sarily¿
30  Sg:    [w-                                   [I don't-
31         I don't blame you¿
32         (0.2)
33  Sg:    [oka:y¿
34  Pt:    [but but it's only because of the MRSA
35         °which I f::eel-=>it's<° right now .hh I'm clea:r
36         for eighteen months and I just don't want to push:;
37         [(my body).
38  Sg:    [okay.
39         (0.6)
40  Sg:    No:w_  (0.8) is this the biggest problem¿
41         (.)
42         [or is this the biggest problem; or are they both equal.
43  Pt:    [no- ↑well- hhh.
44  Pt:    they're equal.
45  Sg:    okay.
46         (0.7)
47  Sg:    AHM_  (0.3) ↑you can have an operation on your foot;
48         (.)
49  Pt:    yea::h.=
50  Sg:    it's not particularly complicated¿ sur[gery¿
51  Pt:                                          [no::.
52         (0.4)
```

The extract begins with the surgeon eliciting the patient's version of the problem (see White et al. 2014) (lines 1–2). The patient incorporates into her answer the source of her referral ("Doctor Clements", line 3) (ibid.); and an account for why this surgeon in particular was suggested ("because you're the: (0.2) foot expert¿", line 5); the nature of the problem (her "misshapen" feet, line 6); as well as a report of her request to the previous doctor, a prescription for orthopaedic shoes (lines 7, 9). The patient then accounts for this request, explaining: "because it's getting really difficult to find a shoe that will fit that_ .hh knobby toe and the knobby: °uhm°_ (0.9) [bunion" (lines 12–14). In this account, the patient also reaches her characterization of the problem, which the surgeon reformulates as "too many bumps" (line 15). In line 27, the patient returns to her referral from her doctor, accounting for her presence at the surgeon as being at the suggestion of her doctor, and spelling out her own stance towards surgery: "I'M not anxious to have surgery neces[sarily¿" (line 29) while orienting to its omni-relevance.

In a number of ways, the patient has already proffered her treatment preferences. She has expressed wanting a specialized shoe prescription and stated that she is not anxious to have surgery. However, her preferences are presented in a shrouded and ambiguous way. Her presence at the surgeon's office, reported request for a prescription from a previous doctor, alongside a possible compliment (see Hudak et al.

2010), ("because you're the: (0.2) f<u>oo</u>t expert¿", line 5) could be taken as indicating the prior request to now be inadequate, and a need for escalation of treatments. Alternatively, it could be that the previous doctor did not fulfil the request and the patient is now seeking the prescription from the surgeon. Similarly, the patient's account for the current visit as being at the suggestion of her doctor could be understood in different ways. The patient may be downplaying her own role in the decision to consult the surgeon in order to counteract the implication that her presence inherently indicates an expectation or desire for surgery. However, returning to the source of her referral could also be taken as a routine aspect of framing the surgery consultation (White et al. 2014). The surgeon treats the patient's turn as being self-evident and non-accountable ("s<u>u</u>re", line 28). Finally, the patient's statement that she is "not <u>a</u>nxious to have surgery neces[sarily¿" could be taken as expressing that she does not want surgery, *or* as presenting herself as an informed patient who has an understanding of the risks of surgery. The surgeon treats it as prudent, warranted cautiousness towards surgery with his acknowledgement "I don't blame you¿" (line 31). Hearing the patient's reticence for surgery as a display of being an informed and responsible patient could be further supported by the patient's subsequent turn in which she attributes her reluctance to her medical history, she has had MRSA (line 34) – Methicillin-resistant *Staphylococcus aureus*, an infection resistant to common antibiotics.

In line 47, the surgeon moves to deliver treatment advice. His statement, "AHM_ (0.3) ↑you can have an operation on your f<u>oo</u>t" presents surgery as an available treatment for the patient's problem, and endorses the relevance of the patient's introduction of it. The formulation with "can" presents it as an open possibility, without being strongly prescriptive. In response, the client produces an agreement token "yea::h" (line 49). Here, both the surgeon's formulation of the treatment proposal, and the patient's response, treat the matter as an informing, rather than as a decision point. The surgeon then goes on to provide information about the surgery, setting it up as "not particularly c<u>o</u>mplicated" (line 50).

In the asymmetrical institutional environment of medical consultations (Pilnick and Dingwall 2011; Robinson 2001; ten Have 1991), patients have limited opportunities and means through which they can express their wishes for treatment. Utilizing turns that are institutionally relevant, for example, orienting to the referral source, prior health history and previous treatments, as vehicles to present treatment preferences may be ambiguous ways to navigate the constraints of the environment (see also Hudak et al. 2010). However, the downside to such ambiguity is that it carries the risk of not being recognized. In this case, while the surgeon's proposed treatment is couched in a tentative, non-prescriptive, informational format, surgery is nonetheless the treatment that is named and identified. The patient's possible shoe prescription preference has not been picked up. The surgeon goes on to provide information about the surgery process, time in hospital, recovery time and requirements (not shown).

After two minutes (107 lines), Extract 6b begins with the surgeon introducing a decision point. He presents the patient with two alternatives which, depending on the response, project different trajectories for making arrangements.

Extract 6b – 50006

```
160 Sg: WELL WHY DON'T UH- do you want to go ahead with this¿
161     or do you want to think about it,
162 Pt: it's not a bit deal?
163     (0.6)
164 Sg: [i-uh hhh
165 Pt: [>if- I mean of<
166     (.)
167 Pt: I shouldn't say that.
168 Sg: [ev(h)ery o(h)pera(h)tion's a b(h)ig d(h)e(hh)al.]
169 Pt: [hh   hh   hh   hh   hh   hh   hh   hh]
170 Sg: [o(hh)k(h)ay?
171 Pt: [.hhh
172 Pt: NO::; I'm- I'm just uhm my- my concern again was
173     the MRSA¿=[.hh
174 Sg:          =[no; if you'(d)
175     [if you've been negative¿]
176 Pt: [         activating;       ]
177     (0.2)
178 Sg: if you've been [negative,
179 Pt:                [I don't know whether I'm negative;
180     my [blood   hasn't    been] checked.
181 Sg:    [well you'll be tested.]
182 Sg: you'll be tested when you come to the a::h (0.7)
183     when you come to the pre-admission facility¿
184     and if everything's normal¿ then you can-
185     sh:ould be able to go ahead safely.
186     (0.3)
187 Sg: okay? [.hhh and there's no:_
188 Pt:       [well that'd be wonderful.=
189 Sg: =there's no implants¿
190 Pt: [no:.
191 Sg: [°in your- in your feet?°
192     (0.4)
193 Sg: so::_ (0.2) if you do get an infection it's much easier
194     to treat, coz there's no:: [foreign        mate]rial in [there.
195 Pt:                            [yeah; there's no:_]          [I
196     understand.=[there's no-] no prosthetic at all in there.
197 Sg:             [okay?      ]
198 Sg: exactly.=
199 Pt: =.HHH What about uhm_ .hh now_ (0.5) because my (.) right leg
200     is two inches shorter [or so;
201 Sg:                       [°mm hm, mm hm,°°
202 Pt: .hh (0.6) of that just becoming like that a↑gain.
203 Sg: ah (.) no:, coz what we do when we do this operation,
204     we not only take the bump away,
205     (0.6) but we make a cut in the bone and move the bone over¿
206 Pt: right.
207 Sg: so that the °bump can't come back.°
208 Pt: oh okay.
209 Sg: °°okay, so it's go-°° °↑it's a good operation¿ ↑°
210 Pt: yeah.
211 Sg: °°(yeup,)°°
212     (0.3)
213 Pt: if it were your wife would you be suggesting it for your:
```

```
214 Sg: yep¿ [I would actually,
215 Pt:       [signif(h)ic(h)ant oth(h)er¿ hh hh
216 Pt: [wouldja?
217 Sg: [depends_
218 Sg: o'l it depends how much ↑trouble you're having [( ).
219 Pt:                                                [↑we:ll_
220     (0.3) [it's not-
221 Sg:       [y'know if your f- if your foot hurts you¿
222     [a::ll the time¿
223 Pt: [no::. it doesn't.
224 Sg: then I wouldn't ↑do it.
225 Pt: [yea:h.
226 Sg: [°if it doesn't hurt¿°
227     [((PA in background    ))
228 Pt: that's- that's the curious part for the disfiguration.
229     [it really doesn't hurt.
230 Sg: [yeah.
231 Sg: if [your foot isn't-
232 Pt:    [my ankles ache. [but my- my feet [(is a      )
233 Sg:                     [yeah.           [if your foot isn't
234     painful I wouldn't_ °I wouldn't°
235     [°°(have an oper]ation      ).°°
236 Pt: [      no:::;     ]
237 Pt: °yea::h.°
238     (0.6)
239 Pt: °°yea:h.°°
240     (0.3)
241 Sg: so why don't we leave it and [see what (you like)=
242 Pt:                              [can we-
243 Pt: =can we leave it [for a bit;
244 Sg:                  [absolutely. [(yes).
245 Pt:                               [o- only because I was going
246     to ask you for your advice about .hh orthopaedic shoes=knowing
247     I was coming to see you.=
248 Sg: okay,
```

In Extract 6b, the patient is given a choice between making a decision about
the surgery now ("do you want to go ah<u>ea</u>d with this¿", line 160), or delaying the
decision ("or do you want to th<u>i</u>nk about it", line 161). The patient co-implicates
the surgeon in the decision-making process through a series of questions. They
eventually reach a joint decision to "leave it for a bit" and the patient returns to talk
about orthopaedic shoes.

Before providing a response to the surgeon's question, "do you want to go
ah<u>ea</u>d with this¿ or do you want to th<u>i</u>nk about it" (lines 160–1), the patient
initiates a provisory, pre-second question (Schegloff 2007), "it's not a bit deal?"
(line 162). The surgeon, however, cannot provide such assurance: "ev(h)ery o(h)-
pera(h)tion's a b(h)ig d(h)e(hh)al" (line 168). The patient respecifies her question to relate to her specific situation and previous medical history with MRSA.
The surgeon minimizes this concern as a barrier by referencing the patient's
current "well" status (see Extract 6a, lines 35–6) and presenting testing as part
of the pre-surgery process (lines 181–5). The patient then produces a positive
assessment "well that'd be wonderful.=" (line 188). It is unclear exactly which

part of the previous talk this assessment refers to, for example, having a normal blood test, or being able to go ahead with the surgery. After providing further information about the operation and addressing the patient's question about the likelihood of the problem recurring, the surgeon provides an overall assessment: "°↑it's a good operation¿ ↑°" (line 209).

In lines 213 and 215, the patient seeks more information to inform her decision. She asks for the surgeon's *personal* opinion (rather than his objective, professional opinion): "if it were your wife would you be suggesting it for your: [signif(h)ic(h)-ant oth(h)er¿". The surgeon responds positively (line 214). If the patient is looking for a reason not to have surgery, it has not yet been given by the surgeon. However, the surgeon subsequently introduces a condition: "depends_ o'l it depends how much ↑trouble you're having" (lines 217–18). The surgeon starts an "if–then" contrast for when surgery is appropriate, "y'know if your f- if your foot hurts you¿" (line 221); however, the patient heads off the second part by denying that her foot hurts (line 223). The surgeon then provides the contrasting "then": "then I wouldn't ↑do it" (line 224) before formulating it in full: "if your foot isn't painful I wouldn't_ °I wouldn't° °°(have an oper]ation).°°" (lines 233–5). The patient now agrees (lines 237, 239).

The final decision is made when the surgeon proposes "so why don't we leave it and [see what (you like)" (line 241), reversing the polarity of the question in line 160 (i.e., go ahead vs leave it) and the patient agrees by echoing the proposal (line 243). Now, the surgeon readily agrees with the patient: "absolutely" (line 244). The patient returns to her previously mentioned (non-surgical) treatment, orthopaedic shoes, downplaying it as a somewhat secondary and incidental treatment consideration in relation to surgery with "only because" and "knowing I was coming to see you" (lines 245–7).

In this consultation, there is a sustained orientation by both parties to the relevance of surgery and its privileged status as a treatment. The treatment decision that the participants ultimately negotiate is that the patient will not have surgery (now), but will get a prescription for orthopaedic shoes. With the benefit of hindsight, it seems that the patient made this treatment preference available at the beginning of the consultation. However, the preference proffers were ambiguous, sometimes mitigated, and complicated by the cross-cutting nature of surgery as not wholly positive. When the patient stated she was "not anxious to have surgery neces[sar-ily¿" (Extract 6a, line 29), it was treated as prudent cautiousness. Similarly, the patient's questions about the risks of surgery do *question* the surgeon's recommended treatment (and as such, could be taken as resistance); however, they do not *challenge* the recommendation. Instead, the questions are aligned with the project of considering surgery. The patient can be understood to be seeking information for an informed decision.

7.6   Concluding Discussion

This chapter focused in detail on examples from orthopaedic surgery consultations in which patients resisted surgeons' recommendations. When resisting treatment recommendations, patients participated in the negotiation of the decision by invoking aspects of their medical history – including previous investigations, treatments and medical professionals consulted – and their symptoms – including, severity, duration and life impact. They balanced these against the risks and benefits of treatments – that is, the likely success and duration of the intervention; recovery – for example, pain, disability, rehabilitation time and life impact; and risks of complications – for example, infections, side-effects, reactions. Throughout these examples, patients and surgeons can be seen to be oriented to the omni-relevance of surgery as well as the cross-cutting nature of treatments in this context as neither wholly good nor wholly bad. Patients, like surgeons, balanced the risk of surgery and the likely benefit in relation to the magnitude of their problem in the context of their life.

The context of orthopaedic surgery consultations as a secondary care setting is consequential for the organization of treatment recommendations and patients' resistance of them in a number of ways. First, because seeing an orthopaedic surgeon in Canada and in many other countries requires a referral from another medical professional, patients have necessarily consulted with at least one other health professional about their problem. This provides patients with rights to claim a degree of professionally-endorsed legitimacy of their problem (Heritage 2009). Second, alongside having sought prior medical advice, patients have often tried one or more treatments that have been ineffective. Third, either or both the patient and the referring professional saw that the orthopaedic surgeon was the appropriate specialist to potentially manage the patient's problem. As such, patients have an established history of experiential and professionally-informed knowledge about their condition and they can draw on these epistemic resources when resisting surgeons' suggested treatments.

The inherently mixed nature of treatments in orthopaedic surgery adds a complicating lens to how patient preferences for treatment and resistance can be heard and what they can be understood to be doing. Not "being anxious to have surgery" can be general warranted cautiousness towards the risks of surgery, or it can be a genuine preference. Resisting a non-surgical treatment can be resisting the threat to legitimacy that a non-surgical treatment can imply, without necessarily indicating the patient wants to have surgery.

Treatment recommendations in orthopaedic surgery are tied into legitimacy and the seriousness of the patients' problems and as well as the surgeons' professional role. In medical consultations generally, receiving treatment implicitly legitimates the patient's problem as "doctorable" and validates the decision to seek care (Heritage 2009). In orthopaedic surgery consultations, surgery is the treatment that implicitly and wholly legitimates patients' problems as "surgeonable", or "surgeon relevant" (see also Heritage and Robinson 2006 on "doctorable"). Surgery is the treatment that implicitly and wholly utilizes the professional role of the surgeon (i.e., the treatment that the surgeon is uniquely sanctioned to perform). Recommendations *not for* surgery pose a potential threat for the legitimacy of patients' problems and their decision to consult with the surgeon. Recommendations *not for* surgery can also leave the participants with "symptom residue" (Maynard and Frankel 2006). That is, the treatment offered may not resolve the patients' problem, leaving them in a position of living with and managing a condition that may be causing them substantial pain and disability. It may also leave them to consult further with other health professionals.

Patient resistance to a treatment recommendation indicates some misalignment between the surgeon and patient, and can require lengthy negotiation to reach consensus. However, patient resistance is not necessarily negative. Treatment recommendations provide a sequential environment for patients to participate in decisions about their care. The negotiation of treatment decisions through patients' active resistance is shared decision-making and patient participation in action. Current trends in healthcare delivery emphasize greater patient involvement in consultations (Collins et al. 2007). The process of consensus-building is an opportunity for surgeons to explore patients' treatment expectations and reasoning bases, as well as explain their own medical reasoning.

Interactional research can contribute novel understandings about treatment options and decision-making in orthopaedic surgery. Medical research is dominated by quantitative research. Random controlled trials are the gold standard to inform objective and unbiased evidence-based medicine. Determining the efficacy of interventions through clinical trials is, of course, important; however, treatment decisions are not only based on efficacy or objective reasoning. This chapter has demonstrated that treatments have important socio-relational dimensions that factor into the negotiation of treatments in orthopaedic surgery consultations. Explicating how issues of legitimacy, responsibility and patient and surgeon identities are implicated in the design, delivery and uptake of treatment recommendations can inform surgeons' (and medical practitioners' more broadly) understandings about factors that impact on decision-making. Such research can contribute to a new evidence basis. However, the next challenge is to disseminate and translate the research. This volume takes an important step towards that goal. Further work is now needed to translate and adapt interactional research to reach busy practitioners on the ground.

The negotiation of treatments in orthopaedic surgery consultations is complex. Treatment decisions are jointly negotiated to take into account medical criteria, patients' preferences, social situations and life experiences. Understanding the nature of the complex interplay between medical and life-world knowledge and experience, the omni-relevance of surgery, legitimacy and the cross-cutting nature of treatments in this context can benefit surgeons by providing insight into the sensitivity and interactional flexibility that is required in these negotiations.

Acknowledgements

Many thanks to Geoffrey Raymond who contributed to work that this chapter builds on. We are grateful for his insightful analysis which has informed our understanding of the data. Any errors or deficiencies remain our own.

Dr Hudak is a recipient of a Career Scientist Award from the Ontario Ministry of Health and Long-term care. Financial support for this study was provided in part by a grant from the Social Sciences and Humanities Research Council of Canada (# 410-2006-0126). This support is gratefully acknowledged. The results and conclusions are those of the authors and no official endorsement by the above organizations is intended or should be inferred.

References

Clark, Shannon J., and Pamela L. Hudak. 2011. When Surgeons Advise Against Surgery. *Research on Language & Social Interaction* 44: 385–412. doi: 10.1080/08351813.2011.619313

Collins, Sarah, Nicky Britten, Johanna Ruusuvuori and Andrew Thompson. 2007. Understanding the Process of Patient Participation. In *Patient Participation in Health Care Consultations: Qualitative Perspectives*, edited by Sarah Collins, Nicky Britten, Johanna Ruusuvuori and Andrew Thompson, 3–21. Maidenhead, UK: McGraw-Hill International.

Gardner, Rod. 2001. *When Listeners Talk*. Amsterdam: John Benjamins.

Heath, Christian. 1992. The Delivery and Reception of Diagnosis in the General-Practice Consultation. In *Talk at Work: Interaction in Institutional Settings*, edited by Paul Drew and John Heritage. Cambridge: Cambridge University Press.

Heritage, John. 2009. Negotiating the Legitimacy of Medical Problems: A Multiphase Concern for Patients and Physicians. In *Communicating to Manage Health and Illness*, edited by Dale E. Brashers and Daena J. Goldsmith, 161–78. New York: Routledge.

Heritage, John, and Jeffrey D. Robinson. 2006. Accounting for the Visit: Giving Reasons for Seeking Medical Care. In *Communication in Medical Care*, edited by John Heritage and Douglas W. Maynard, 48–85. Cambridge: Cambridge University Press.

Hudak, Pamela L., Shannon J. Clark, and Geoffrey Raymond. 2011. How Surgeons Design Treatment Recommendations in Orthopaedic Surgery. *Social Science & Medicine* 73: 1028–36. doi: 10.1016/j.socscimed.2011.06.061

Hudak, Pamela L., Shannon J. Clark, and Geoffrey Raymond. 2013. The Omni-Relevance of Surgery: How Medical Specialization Shapes Orthopedic Surgeons' Treatment Recommendations. *Health Communication* 28: 533–45. doi: 10.1080/10410236.2012.702642

Hudak, Pamela L., Virginia Teas Gill, Jeffrey P. Aguinaldo, Shannon Clark and Richard Frankel. 2010. "I've Heard Wonderful Things about You": How Patients Compliment Surgeons. *Sociology of Health & Illness* 32 (5): 777–97. doi: 10.1111/j.1467-9566.2010.01248.x

Maynard, Douglas W., and Richard M. Frankel. 2006. On Diagnostic Rationality: Bad News, Good News, and the Symptom Residue. In *Communication in Medical Care*, edited by John Heritage and Douglas W. Maynard, 248–78. Cambridge: Cambridge University Press.

Peräkylä, Anssi. 1998. Authority and Accountability: The Delivery of Diagnosis in Primary Health Care. *Social Psychology Quarterly* 61: 301–20. http://www.jstor.org/stable/2787032

Peräkylä, Anssi. 2002. Agency and Authority: Extended Responses to Diagnostic Statements in Primary Care Encounters. *Research on Language & Social Interaction* 35: 219–47. doi: 10.1207/S15327973RLSI3502_5

Pilnick, Alison, and Robert Dingwall. 2011. On the Remarkable Persistence of Asymmetry in Doctor/Patient Interaction: A Critical Review. *Social Science & Medicine* 72: 1374–82. doi: 10.1016/j.socscimed.2011.02.033

Robinson, Jeffrey D. 2001. Asymmetry in Action: Sequential Resources in the Negotiation of a Prescription Request. *Text – Interdisciplinary Journal for the Study of Discourse* 21: 19–54. doi: 10.1515/text.1.21.1-2.19

Robinson, Jeffrey D. 2003. An Interactional Structure of Medical Activities during Acute Visits and Its Implications for Patients' Participation. *Health Communication* 15: 27–59. doi: 10.1207/S15327027HC1501_2

Schegloff, Emanuel A. 1998. Reflections on Studying Prosody in Talk-in-Interaction. *Language and Speech* 41: 235–63. doi: 10.1177/002383099804100402

Schegloff, Emanuel A. 2007. *Sequence Organization in Interaction: Volume 1*. Cambridge: Cambridge University Press.

Stivers, Tanya. 2002. Participating in Decisions about Treatment: Overt Parent Pressure for Antibiotic Medication in Pediatric Encounters. *Social Science & Medicine* 54: 1111–30. doi: 10.1016/S0277-9536(01)00085-5

Stivers, Tanya. 2005a. Non-Antibiotic Treatment Recommendations: Delivery Formats and Implications for Parent Resistance. *Social Science & Medicine* 60: 949–64. doi: 10.1016/j.socscimed.2004.06.040

Stivers, Tanya. 2005b. Parent Resistance to Physicians' Treatment Recommendations: One Resource for Initiating a Negotiation of the Treatment Decision. *Health Communication* 18: 41–74. doi: 10.1207/s15327027hc1801_3

Stivers, Tanya. 2006. Treatment Decisions: Negotiations between Doctors and Patients in Acute Care Encounters. In *Communication in Medical Care*, edited by John Heritage and Douglas W. Maynard, 279–312. Cambridge: Cambridge University Press.

Stivers, Tanya. 2007. *Prescribing under Pressure: Parent-Physician Conversations and Antibiotics*. Oxford: Oxford University Press.

ten Have, Paul. 1991. Talk and Institution: A Reconsideration of the "Asymmetry" of Doctor-Patient Interaction. In *Talk and Social Structure: Studies in Ethnomethodology and Conversation Analysis*, edited by Deirdre Boden and Don H. Zimmerman, 138–64. Cambridge: Polity Press.

White, Sarah J., Maria H. Stubbe, Lindsay M. Macdonald, Anthony C. Dowell, Kevin P. Dew and Rod Gardner. 2014. Framing the Consultation: The Role of the Referral in Surgeon-Patient Consultations. *Health Communication* 29: 74–80. doi: 10.1080/10410236.2012.718252

Shannon J. Clark is a Research Fellow in the Centre for Research and Action in Public Health at the University of Canberra, Australia. She also holds a visiting fellowship with the School of Literature, Languages and Linguistics at the Australian National University. Shannon's specific research interests are centred on analysing interactions between patients and a range of professionals, including psychotherapists, orthopaedic surgeons, nurse practitioners and midwives. Shannon completed her PhD in Linguistics at the Australian National University and worked as a post-doctoral fellow at the University of Toronto, Canada, with Dr Pamela Hudak.

Pamela L. Hudak trained originally as a physical therapist before completing her PhD in Medical Sciences. She worked for over a decade as a Scientist in Toronto, Canada studying communication between patients and physicians, and patient and physician decision-making. Currently, Pamela is a Qualified Mediator and Principal at The Alternative Dispute Resolution Practice Inc. in Toronto, where she applies her knowledge of communication to workplace mediation and the restoration of relationships at work.

SECTION II
THE OPERATING THEATRE

8 Transactions between Matter and Meaning: Surgical Contexts and Symbolic Action

David G. Butt, Alison Rotha Moore and John A. Cartmill

8.1 Why Model Symbolic Complexity in Surgical Contexts?

Surgery – and all of the levels, phenomena and systems the term encompasses – has evolved into a complex system of high degree. Attempts (however well-meaning) to influence it inevitably underestimate that complexity, with unintended consequences. Evolved systems are typically robust and for the most part adaptive – as demonstrated by their having "evolved" at all. Medical processes are among the strongest anticipatory arrangements in societies; and they involve enormous allocations of expertise and budgets (at least in technologically developed countries). Nevertheless, the very strengths of their developments, regulations and traditions can become obstacles to efficacy when, for instance, contexts of surgery are not seen for what they are – contexts in which our value systems and meanings are contested in the face of the material and social imperatives of illness. In that contest, the regulations and ideologies of governments, the boundaries between specializations, and the insulation between the medical environments and the community, all may need renegotiation. But such renegotiation – such management of change – needs to encompass the methical analysis of the complex, symbolic – that is, semiotic – structure that our predecessors have passed on to us (Halliday 1973, 1976, 1978).

The word "semeion", from which we derive the term "semiotics" – the science of signs in our community living – was first applied by the ancient Greeks to the interpretation of a symptom or the reading of a physical sign. In this context "semeion" meant the manifestation by which a physician interprets the aetiology of illness, what the signal means. The signs of redness and swelling, for example, may signal inflammation. The word for language or for reason or thought was predominantly "logos". In this discussion, we set out reasons for bringing these two concepts together: the broader notion of signs and the idea of a working language around surgery. Our view is that surgery is a highly coded context of extremely diverse signs and the meanings those signs carry, and that this diversity is characteristically brought together by experienced surgeons into an ensemble of interlocking systems, in much the same way that the options in a language can be described in systems for choosing to say things one way, and not a different way. Such an ensemble may encompass idiosyncratic elements (a practical "idiolect", which practitioners sort out over the instances of their individual experience). But more typically the signs (and what we have learned over the millennia as to what those signs *mean*) are an evolved expression of collective wisdom, whether implicit or explicit, in the training and college tradition of mentoring to which practitioners have been exposed.

Our argument here is that there is much to be gained by regarding the spectrum of meanings signalled and interpreted in a Department of Surgery as a complex system of systems (of signs). The first task is to make vivid the ways in which a semiotician will be drawn to the diversity of sign types in what can reasonably be called the *ecology* of surgery. We can then consider the ways in which the diversity can be systematized and sub-categorized. We also carry our analysis into the symbolic complexities which are less likely to have already been noted by the wider community, and even by some professional "insiders". The work overall is the result of an ongoing investigation of "systemic safety in contexts of surgical care", which began as an Australian Research Council Discovery Project: see details below and in Moore (Chapter 11 in this volume).

The motivation for the research was to examine those parameters of surgical contexts which were most likely to produce misadventure through misunderstandings of the semantic and systemic force of signs around surgical processes, along with the corollary: namely, to elucidate those routine arrangements which may lend robustness to surgical team behaviour and the system overall – arrangements from political governance to the contact between surgical instrument and human tissue.

A priority in our thinking was the development of anticipatory structures in the environment of operating theatres (OTs) and in their management. While medical and health contexts are notable for their evolved safety procedures – their explicit regulation of what can take place – we believed that modelling the OT experiences as transactions between matter and meaning, and, moreover, between meaning and meaning (i.e., as contested meanings), would provoke new ways of seeing difficulties in the environment.

The data of the project were drawn from participants' interpretations of the contexts of surgical care, their own roles, and the roles of others. Such interpretations were based on the direct observation and/or videoing of c. 20 lists in the operating theatre. Other levels of surgical and hospital activity were investigated through interviews with key institutional and professional stakeholders.

Interpretations by professionals of their own roles in relation to others can be crucial in the development of an effective team or ensemble of effort. Interpretations can become a source of divergence, with team members pulling in different directions by construing their roles in different ways, or by misconstruing the contribution of others in their team (Lingard 2011). Interpretations can be modelled in a series of levels, these being levels of meanings or values. While actions by others on different levels of a health system may exert semantic "pressure", the actions do not *cause* a reaction in the mechanical or organic sense of *cause*. The meaning-bearing behaviours of others do change our circumstances, however, in that we go on to interpret, or construe, the new state of our context. Let us explore how this can be discussed and rendered diagrammatically.

8.2 What We Mean when We Speak of a "Health System"

It has long been a commonplace to speak of the governance and conduct of medicine as a "health system". At the outset of our collaboration in this project, however, four important themes concerning systems were becoming insistent in the intellectual milieu:

- the notion of system was undergoing conceptual renovation and broader application in thermodynamics – for an overview see Mainzer (1997 [1994]) – and through cybernetics – for instance, see the work by Bertalanffy (1969);
- this change was refined by the graduation of chaos theory into complexity theory, with the understanding that small shifts of initial conditions produced systemic perturbations that were not unequivocally subject to human agency and blame (Cohen and Stewart 1994);
- the public was "talking about" these ideas: even the tabloid press, although always keen to find a villain, showed some accommodation to the idea of system safety, while also still projecting indignation and blame (Moore, Butt and Cartmill 2005);
- the expansion of "information" (the information era) created an awareness of the importance of communication and meaning, not just of energy and matter (Davies and Gregersen 2010; Gleick 2011).

Linguistics was also at its own "tipping point": after years of formalistic proposals about the abstract nature of a genetically determined mental organ for "syntax", many linguists had well and truly moved away from the hegemonic intuitionism and "universalism" of Chomsky, and turned back to the traditions of their subject – namely, to the traditions of observation, of empiricism, and to the gathering of authentic data from direct contact with the variation in communities. Boas and Sapir in the U.S., and Malinowski and Firth in Britain, in the first half of the 20th century, had ensured that linguists engaged in a natural science of meaning. Linguistics had long developed its own methods of what was later brought together and applied in medical and other circles as "grounded theory" (Glaser and Strauss 1967; Strauss 1987; Strauss and Corbin 1998). A form of pragmatics and contextualism had re-emerged. Systemic Functional Linguistics (SFL), as used in our projects, is a contemporary form of a context-based method which has been continuous in social linguistics since the early–mid 1900s (Butt 2006). While American Formalism (especially the work of Chomsky on an innate "syntactic organ") has obscured these continuities in linguistics, the commitment to empirical social research is strong again now in spite of criticisms from "Cartesian linguistics" (as Chomsky chose to characterize his approach in 1966). In fact, functional linguistics, in its various forms, has significant connections (and collaborations) with neuroscience, given the contemporary emphasis on the role of interaction in the evolution and ontogenesis of human brains and our collective "psyche" (Trevarthen and Hubley 1978; Edelman and Tononi 2000; Meares 2012; Arbib 2012; Damasio 2012).

This specific form of functional language theory used in the present project – Systemic Functional Linguistics (SFL) – should be thought of through one central concept, a principle that has prodigious tool power for the mapping of surgical contexts and health services in general. Since 1964, SFL has set out complexity in language as interdependent choices, in a network. The pathway you take through the available choices is your meaning: not just the explicit track of what you did, but what you did in relation to the other choices that you did not take up. The value you invoke is defined, then, by what you set aside as action or meaning.

8.3   Surgical "Ensembles": From Levels of Governance to Teams

It may seem precious to refer to surgical teams as ensembles; nevertheless, we are claiming more. This word incorporates the meaning of those who contribute differently and who must be "in sync" for the fulfilment of a goal – for an important exploration of being "in sync", see the work of systems mathematician Steven Strogatz (2003). Some part of this activity may be scripted and parts improvised on the basis of shared training and experience. The script may be agreed upon in only general terms and even unstated for some group members who will follow a "lead". The first point for the outsider to appreciate is the careful organization of space, set to a purpose, to which the OT team must accommodate. As emphasized in discussions of the present research elsewhere (Moore, this volume), the closeness is like that of wrestlers and lovers – potentially highly charged interpersonal proximity. And it is sustained for hours.

Within that space there are conventional and well recognized allocations of responsibilities. Along with the temporal sequence of responsibilities (viz., from the nursing team setting up the theatre, to the anaesthetist managing patient sedation, to the surgeon initiating the procedure and further phases) there are zones

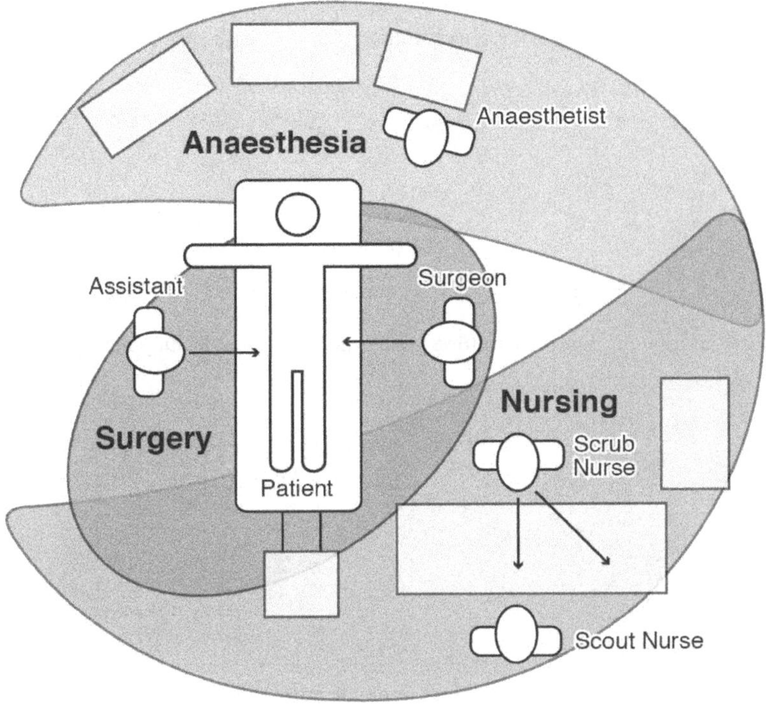

Figure 8.1: Zones of responsibility "in" and around the patient

of responsibility (Figure 8.1), including the "inner sanctum" of contact with the patient.

A much more poorly understood phenomenon, which turns out to index responsibilities in the OT team, is differentiation in communication, and its structure and texture. We foreshadow some of our results at this point in the chapter because they illustrate our argument that understanding surgery involves understanding crucial alignments between the material and symbolic "orders".

Some key relations between communication and team responsibilities can be gauged immediately by Figures 8.2–8.4. These present an iconic representation of the exchanges between certain members during a specific five-minute segment of one apparently routine operation. The thickness and direction of each arrow indicate the amount and the direction of symbolic traffic, or in other words the frequency of messages exchanged between pairs within the team, along with the frequency of messages sent compared with those received by each member. Additionally, the messages are coded by grey tone according to their speech function – whether the message took the form of a command, a question, a statement or an offer. While unbroken lines indicate speech, broken lines represent communication through gesture, gaze or orientation.

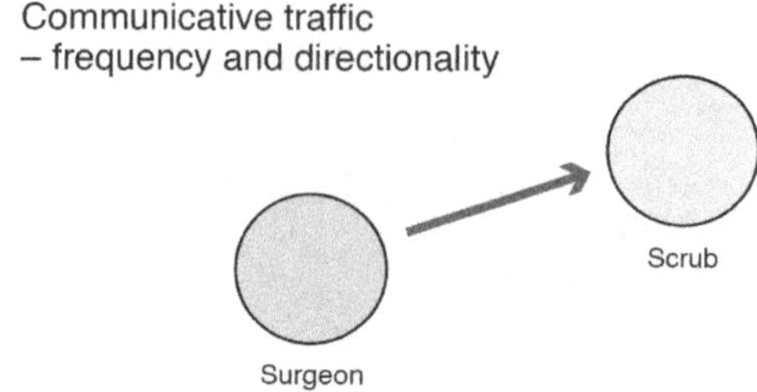

Figure 8.2: Representing symbolic traffic in operating teams – indicating message direction

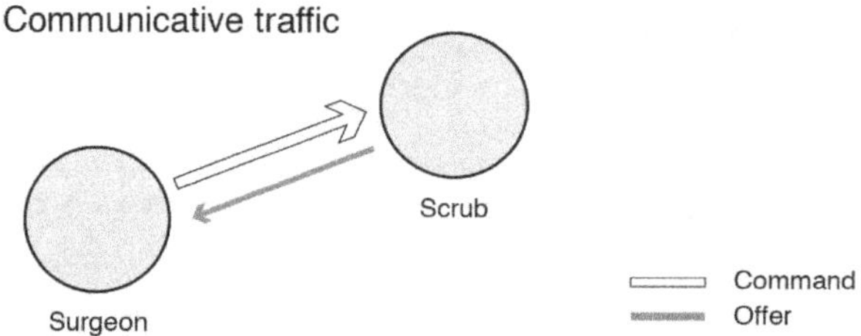

Figure 8.3: Representing symbolic traffic in operating teams – indicating speech function

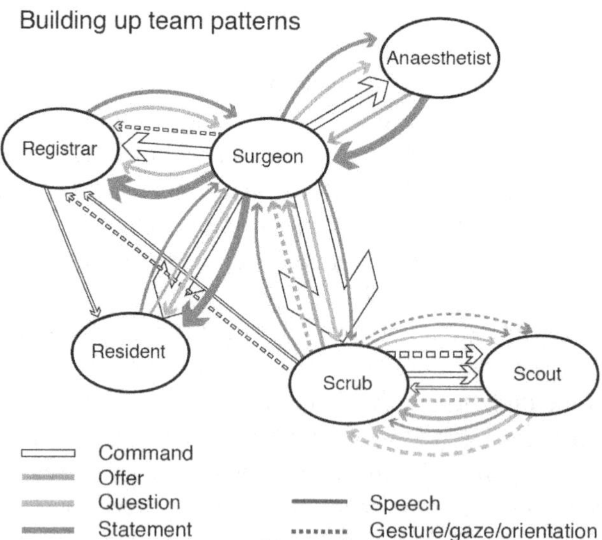

Figure 8.4: Relative frequency, directionality and speech function of messages exchanged between operating theatre team members in a five-minute period

As Figure 8.4 indicates, the most frequent symbolic traffic (thickest arrow) runs from the surgeon to the scrub nurse, and represents commands, although in our study these were generally commands with a diminished imperative style, unlike the more direct imperative forms reported elsewhere (Bezemer et al. 2011). It should be noted that very little detailed research on grammatical and semantic variation in surgical or other medical registers has been published, so it is difficult to ascertain the extent to which the patterns displayed here are a function of the semiotic style of the surgeon, the surgeon-nurse dyad, the local or national surgical culture, the particular phase of the procedure observed or other factors.

Yet this is only a beginning. The surgical environment bristles with signs. There are the overt uses of *conventional wordings* as warnings and regulations; and these extend to detailed information about, for instance, the number of operations performed month by month in the previous year. There is also an enormous variety of *iconic signs* – the technical name for images that supposedly resemble the meaning in their very form, including pictures and schematic versions of equipment or actions or prohibitions. But most of all, surgery depends on *indexical signs*: these are those in which there is a natural connection with the phenomenon they signal – swelling is to inflammation as smoke is to fire, and as a footprint is to the size of the foot.

The refinement of indexical signs in particular through the experience of medical "touch" becomes very elaborate (Bezemer and Kress 2014), perhaps similar to the discrimination of an expert musician to the range of "expression" in performance. Butt and Cartmill have pursued this meaning potential through its "vocabulary" and bodily configurations – its structures (see Cartmill and Butt [2012] and this volume, Chapter 13). It should be noted, in passing, that the whole disposition of space in a hospital is a theory of what can happen and what is expected to happen within the institution: spaces *invite, encourage, inhibit, limit* and *prevent*; they *imply* roles and hierarchies; they make certain social structures more or less likely. An example from another social institution is the movement from the old to the new Parliament House in Canberra, Australia, and the new difficulty of reporters and politicians in meeting casually, thus giving advisors more control over ministerial statements (explained by veteran reporter Laurie Oakes).

The locus and actions of an OT team are made possible only because of a number of layers of culture – in fact many levels of governance, training, management and interactions with other agencies. These levels need to work as an ensemble because that is how they came about – they are an *evolved* arrangement of how society addresses the phenomena of illness and wellbeing. This includes beliefs about sickness, about resources, about expertise, about legal rights and responsibilities, about remuneration and about many other matters besides. It is in teamwork that most people can see the role of cooperative action; but it is in a second notion of ensemble that systemic safety has its most compelling challenge: How might one intervene to improve upon the arrangements that have grown up from the myriad of

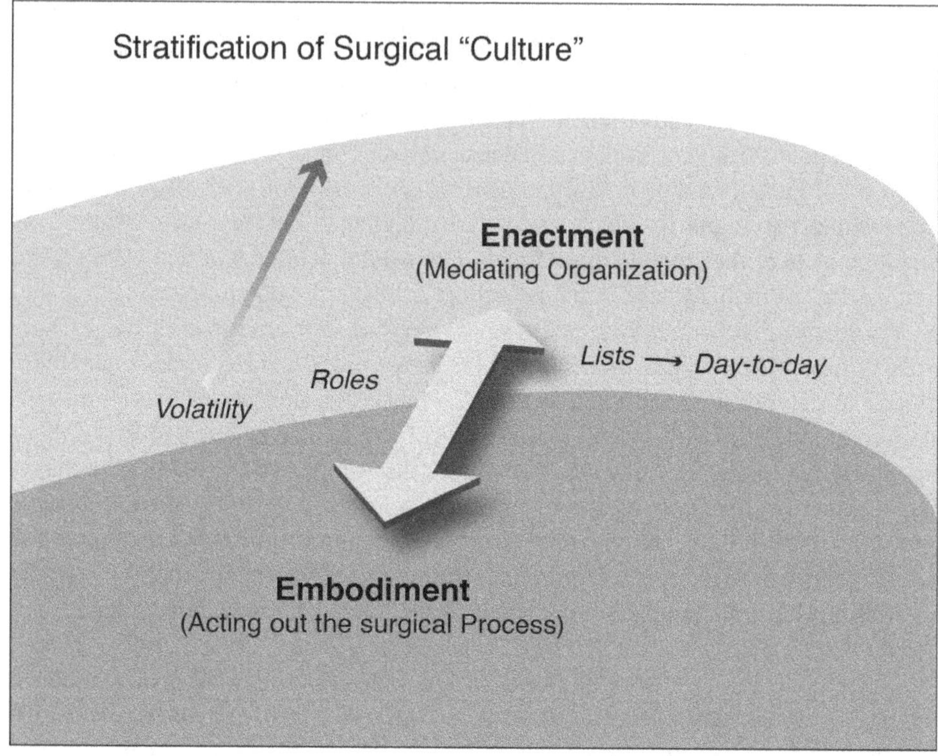

Figure 8.5: Stratification of lower, more concrete levels of surgical "culture"

conscious and unconscious, goal-directed decisions that community members have contributed over generations? Who can see the latent dependencies in a system that has involved collective effort and adaptations to so many past human circumstances? Must not any intervention be considered in "fear and trembling"?

Let us move therefore to explaining this idea of levels through the next set of figures. In the Stratification of Surgical "Culture" (Figure 8.5), we can see the dimensions of the system that we began to incorporate into our initial modelling of contexts of surgical care. There is the embodiment of the operation on the lower level. This is – just as in the previous figures – one material place at one time. But above that concrete level there is the management of the operating theatres as a unified department: the allocation of a theatre, the nomination and rostering of an appropriate team, the coordination of rosters and patient lists, the adjustments according to late changes in staff or suitability of patients, and perhaps the needs of emergency cases that must "trump" all preceding arrangements (e.g., emergency caesarian sections). In addition to the explicit order codified for these two levels, there is also a body of implicit knowledge that shapes the context. An example here is the budget for the department: there are judgements to be made about the amount of service the section can offer – itself dependent on the way the service is supported by ephemeral government and insurance provisions (and such provisions will force us to look beyond these two levels of organization for the dynamics of the overall system – see further below).

A more adequate grasp of systemic dynamics is offered, then, when we view the context of surgery in the four levels, as presented in Figure 8.6, namely, **Environment** (policy and resources); **Enactment** (hospital and department as mediating organization); **Embodiment** (actions of the surgical team); and below those initially considered is the **Substance** (the way technology and tissue are brought together, noting that technology gives form to meaning in "tools" much as social institutions determine the "value" placed upon an action or procedure).

To put the situation pragmatically, for anything to happen at all in healthcare, there must be simultaneous alignments across a number of levels of "order". Everything must line up and happen at once for anything to happen at all. A college of specialists and a whole health system are in many ways like a language – they are the product of an enormous number of social and individual human contingencies. Many levels of human participation have interacted to produce its extant

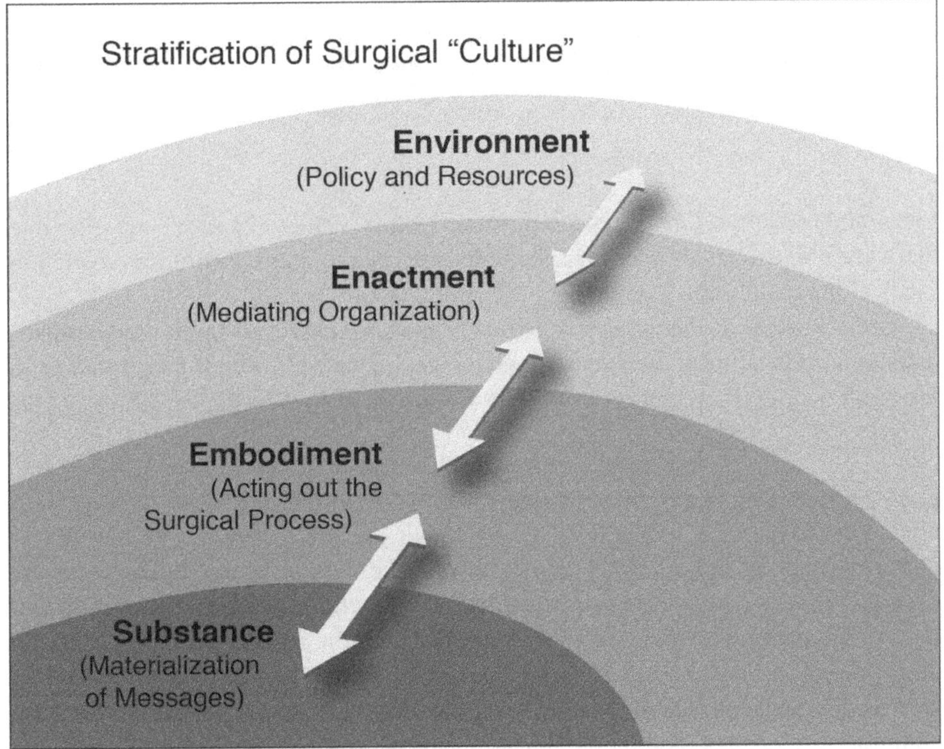

Figure 8.6: Further layers of the surgical "culture"

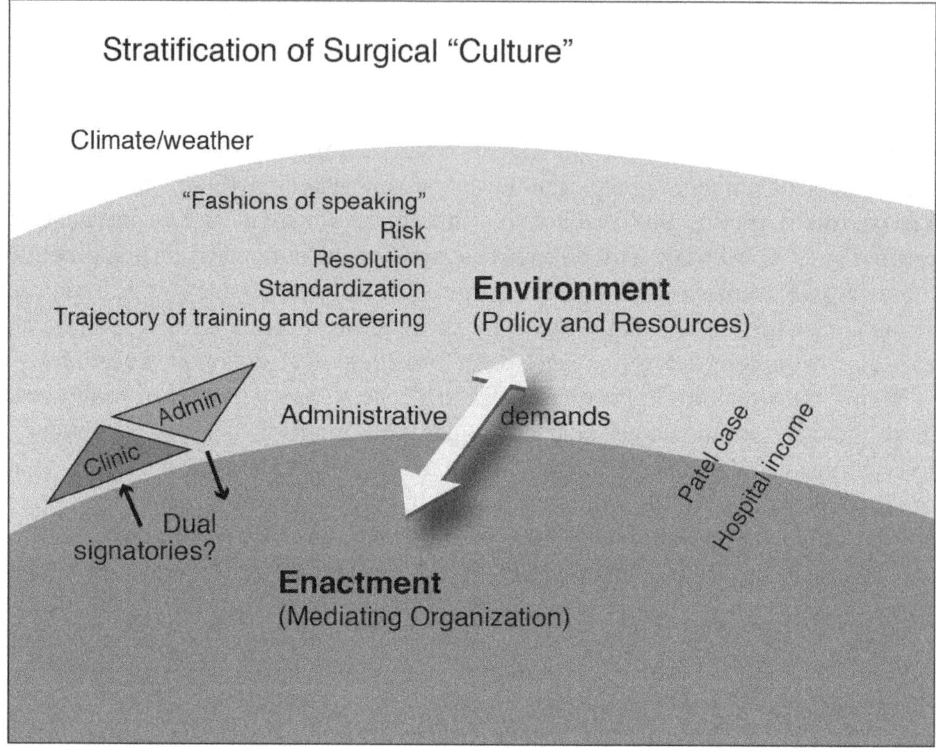

Figure 8.7: The higher and at times less obvious layers of surgical "culture"

forms and functions. Given a heterogeneous history, it should not be surprising that there are idiosyncrasies and unpredictable aspects about any institution – whether medical, financial, religious, military or pedagogical.

A brief review of the upper two levels (Figure 8.7) helps us think more realistically about the cultural dynamics of what takes place "at the coal-face", that is on the two lower levels of action and tissue already described in Figure 8.5.

8.4   Early Observations, Findings and Implications

Our observations and analyses produced what we took to be some local, specific findings, and a number of ideas concerning the general properties of complex systems – the parameters that were likely to increase the robustness of institutional arrangements.

An early, local clarification in our research was the inverse relationship between communicative roles of surgeon and scrub in the theatre: the surgeon can choose to engage and command on any channel to any person in the theatre; similarly, he or she can also choose *not* to engage with any symbolic traffic on any channel. The scrub, inversely, has to stay available on all channels, including dealing with requests for equipment from teams in other theatres, and an initial indication of the intensity of this symbolic traffic for the scrub is seen in Figure 8.4 above, though note that this is from one "channel" only (the surgeon). Furthermore, the scrub has to anticipate the needs of the surgeon in real time, whether or not the stage of the operation has been made explicit to her (or him[1]) or not. Her own work is both interpretive and procedural: her attentiveness to the needs of the surgeon is evaluated (often through micro-behaviours taken as indexical signs of inattention, discussed in Chapter 11 by Moore and Chapter 13 by Butt and Cartmill). So too, there were the explicit regulations – her public counts of swabs and instruments, as well as her broader management of common contingencies (e.g., the desire of the surgeon to change to the other side of the patient), and of unanticipated intrusions (the appearance of pharmaceutical representatives; an electrician; and those requests from other theatres: e.g., sharing equipment).

To this convergence of profound responsibilities and professional scrutiny, we gave the general term "role creep". By this we meant that there had been a drift of multiple tasks to one person and that the tasks went with little discretionary authority – certainly not authority commensurate with the difficulties and responsibilities. The key to this situation was that it went underappreciated "in the system", and often overlooked, we were told, by surgeons who saw themselves as the unequivocal protagonist (viz., actor of first importance) in the drama of this form of "theatre". The comparison of theatres and operating theatres is itself illuminating; and has been elaborated by Butt, Cartmill and Moore (2009) and Riley and Manias (2005).

This low visibility was a particular problem in public hospitals. In private hospitals the surgical list was easier to control for diversity of procedure, timing, consistency of OT team and responsibilities for training new staff. Surgeons could regularize and limit teams and rosters in private hospitals, building up thereby the knowledge of those working together with respect to surgical and interactive styles. In public hospitals, the OT department is much more often contested ground, and teams and priorities are subject to real-time decisions concerning personnel, theatre allocations and even minor equipment (e.g., availability of a particular staple gun). Furthermore, an emergency in one theatre (even the discovery that a patient is allergic to latex) could affect the whole department – for example, by shutting down previously rostered arrangements, with consequences for all staff with reasons to go or arrive at previously established times (for instance, those with responsibilities at home). It needs to be noted that the greater continuity, and predictability,

---

1 We use the female pronoun from here on as this represents the most typical case in our own data.

of arrangements at a private hospital are a function of the narrower range of operations performed, and the different "temporal horizon" in medical action – e.g., non-emergency.

In public institutions, furthermore, the responsibility for training new surgeons and OT staff is a constant and critical role. This is accepted as "going with the territory". But it is not addressed equally by all; and, as a pedagogic role, it challenges the ideology and professional judgements of everyone in the context. Surgeons and OT teams are not specifically trained to train, nor are there regulations as to how authority is to be articulated (whether pedagogical or not). Consequently, a wide spectrum of reactive behaviours can ensue, depending on the assumptions of the senior surgeon. These assumptions may range between egalitarian and positional (authoritarian) modes of "advisory" behaviours. Variations in authoritarian style do not, we were assured by one senior nursing officer, fall out simply along generational lines. As in universities (with which we were most familiar) and other institutions, younger staff can be more categorical and some older staff less likely to adopt a direct (quasi-military) style of "command structure". (See the example of "taking over" in Chapter 11 of this volume, and for a linguistic analysis of the same episode see the detailed example by Moore in Lukin et al. [2011]).

But, as we ought to have expected, professional ideologies are not predictable or homogeneous and are not insulated from other beliefs which a person brings from home and culture. The OT department is a site of semantic variation, of different styles of behaviour or interpretation as to what is appropriate in the ways in which experience and responsibility influence interpersonal meanings. The daunting consequences of error are seen by some as a justification for positional command, and by others as a cause for team-building collegiality (but this is a theme to be elaborated in a future article, and may be explored in the literature on culture and safety: viz., Reason 1997; Helmreich and Merritt 1998).

The immediate relevance of these reports and observations of interpersonal exchanges is how they affect the role of those in a surgical team, firstly with respect to the scrub nurse. The responsibility for teaching changes the layers of meaning in any context of work. While that appears obvious with respect to the surgeon, the most dramatic rise in complexity is for the scrub nurse. The surgeon has to act surgically and offer experience to those who need to be taught that action. But the surgeon is at the apex of immediate authority. The scrub nurse may be the most experienced person in the room (by the criterion of surgical lists completed in her career); yet, with the enactment of teaching, she has the problem of accommodating two or more levels of surgical expertise. Yet her authority to direct (and correct) personnel is equivocal, and hence one more stressful consideration.

As noted above, Figures 8.2–8.4 attempt to show the symbolic traffic around the theatre in the space of five minutes. The arrows for statements, questions, commands and offers are indicative of the amount of discourse directed at a person or role in the theatre. The "hotspot" of the scrub in all this messaging emerges immediately when tracked. But the point is that this potential for "volatility" in the system is underappreciated due to some traditional/historical and some practical characteristics of her mediating role.

But let us return to the logic of the surgical context and its codifications by law and by collegial tradition. A survey of other responsibilities in our culture suggests that there are many day-to-day activities with such potential for disastrous consequences; yet they are not categorized and administered with the same gravitas and "gatekeeping" which set apart the practitioners of medicine. Intercity and urban bus driving, train driving and long-haul trucking are extremely critical responsibilities, for example. This is particularly the case when they have come together in collisions. There is a prodigious literature on community safety – studies of ports, like Hutchin's celebrated *Cognition in the Wild* (1995); of aviation; of engineering; and of institutions, especially hospitals. As seen in the Ashgate library of publications, considerable attention has drifted to cultural effects in contexts of critical care, with the highlighting of the role of beliefs and assumptions about authority (for example, in the operation of hierarchy in air disasters: see the work of Helmreich generally and Helmreich and Merritt [1998]). It is useful to seek the parameters of work and responsibility that define the role of the surgeon uniquely. As in all environments of interpretation, such parameters are not self-evident. There are dimensions of medicine to which our community responds in its demand for specialized training, and for remuneration. We will keep this issue in sight as we elaborate our investigation below. The weight of responsibility and the social position of physicians have not been constant in Western cultures: the role has become less metaphysical and more technical since the inception of early Greek medicine, with an interesting role played by the "forensic" observations of the historian Thucydides. His naturalistic account of the Plague of Athens (c. 402 BCE) – an affliction close to SARS – is a significant step away from attributing disease and its amelioration to "the gods" (see Kappagoda 2004 for a full account of this, and an exploration of the development of medicine through the efficacy of metaphoric thinking, with symbols acting like a "sixth sense").

In Figures 8.5–8.7, we can see more of the phenomena that are focal in the culture of surgical practice – that are the sources of variability and the consistency of change in human institutions. We are trying to understand an ecosocial system, as depicted by Lemke (1995). Such systems are stratified. And we illustrate the meaning of this, and of all the other terms invoked below in this chapter. The ensemble effects can be weird (as widely discussed in complex systems). We list some characteristics of such realizational systems: (1) *Stratified (layered)*, as each part presupposes the whole – all strata or none! (2) *Inter-related by realization*, not causation: levels "express" each other, rather than drive each other sequentially. (3) *Evolved*, not designed: prediction can only be ventured through heuristic modelling and probabilities, not linearly. (4) *Adapted*, creating a weird/ quasi-teleological illusion of progressive adaptation (when viewed historically).

(5) *Stable*, or "metastable": because changes are occurring all over the system all the time, the system sustains itself. (6) *Goal-directed*, since it is responsive to unconscious (habits), subconscious (wishes, drives), and conscious (problem-solving) decisions by human agents. (7) *Describable* through networks of points of "choice" (based on the five primitive terms – *or*; *and*; *both*; *only when/if*; and *choose over again*). (8) *Quantifiable*, when we count typical choices along the lines of the system most relevant to its efficacy (this involves dimensions based on community values, on surgical meanings and on the interpretations of matter: see exemplum in section 8.7 below). (9) *Subject to diverse construals*, that is, it will be viewed differently depending on whether one is responsible for outcomes, or costs, or waiting lists, or training, or if you come to the system as a patient; each observer will foreground the facets of the system from their point of view and from the level through which they enter the domains of systemic experience – consequently, there are also many possible modes of analysis. (10) *Recognizable* as a realizational system: for instance, when problems run across the scale of phenomena from ideological values at the abstract end of the scale all the way to mechanical tools at the material end, it follows that you are dealing with a meaning-expression system of realizations, not just causations.

The point here is that perhaps we do not understand our institutions as well as we assume – why one activity is so highly valued, and another, adjacent role is treated as less specialized and quotidian. By exploring the semiotic complexity of a context, we can better understand how and why we have come to value it. We may also separate the practical necessity and adaptive character of an institutional tradition from any accretions of humbug. In fact, the benefits of such analysis of complexity may be both general and local. They are general in that the interdependencies of a health system are further illuminated and decisions and interventions may be framed with improved anticipation of problems and potential cascades across the layering of the system overall. This general benefit is a form of cultural cartography. The benefits are local when the needs of particular environments and even of individual participants (including stakeholders/patients) are more clearly defined. It also becomes more plausible to characterize often-invoked notions like "patient-centred care" relative to the particulars of specific surgical procedures and conditions (for instance, is patient-centred care the "same" through surgery conducted on unconscious patients as it is for those who, as in eye surgery, will be fully aware of each step of the surgery?).

As indicated at the outset of this chapter, our research and our review of the systemic environment of surgery suggest that the perception of surgery as a confrontation between the uncompromising character of sick tissue (living matter) and the techniques of the surgeon is misleading. The surgical environment appears to us to be characterized chiefly by nodes of interpretation and choice. Interpretation and choice are processes with which a surgeon must be engaged on many levels. It is for these acts of construal and decision that a surgeon is most valued since such decisions have to encompass domains as diverse as the materiality and extent of a tumour, on the one hand, and the often highly politicized issues of resources and expenditure, on the other. Alongside these are the deep issues of ethical behaviour and "fairness".

8.5   The Aims and Methods at Inception

This project was supported by an Australian Research Council grant: "Systemic safety in contexts of surgical care". The central aim of the project was to adopt a systemic perspective on safety and error in the day-to-day actions of Operating Theatres and their hospital Departments. The researchers began by introducing themselves to all members of a colorectal surgical team at Nepean Public Hospital in the (at that time) Wentworth Area Health Service; surgeons and their junior medical officers, scrub nurses, scouts, anaesthetists and their trainees, and anaesthetic nurses. This resulted in a list of volunteers from which staff could be drawn as an operational unit or "team" on any operating day when the researchers were present. However, any subject could withdraw at any time and have destroyed any recordings with which they were unhappy. On several occasions surgeons working on challenging cases asked for recording to stop to reduce any chance of distraction.

Consent was also required from each patient for the researchers to sit in on and record the operation. Ethics committee approval was granted by the Area Health Service and Macquarie University.

The researchers combined the ethnomethodological strategies of grounded theory (Strauss and Corbin 1998) with the longer established but similar approaches of anthropologists and field linguists, namely: *observe*; *note*; *include* all relevant texts and phenomena; *interview*; *check* the professional and legal frameworks within which a procedure can take place; *consider* the point of view and "interests" of those who are acted upon as well as those who are agentive; *examine* how decisions are made pertaining to the "locus" as a work space; *review* the history of authority within the institution (e.g., as senior nurses become department managers); try to *limit* one's intrusion on customary practices; *include* meanings at the margins (what were the concerns that preoccupied those in informal exchanges – e.g., in the tea room: see Long, Iedema and Lee [2007]); *evaluate*, where appropriate, any accounts of the context made by the participants themselves; *attend* to the issues raised in post hoc discussions of the OT team members; *look for* the origin of any outsider impression of the "strangeness" of arrangements, especially those that are taken for granted and are considered "natural" to the insider.

Our experience suggested that nonverbal communication in the operating room is part of a generalizable system of communication, one that may function well or poorly under different conditions and one that, like any language, may be taught. It should not be regarded merely or passively as a function of the individual personality of the surgeon about which nothing can be done. However, before this can happen, there needs to be a systematic account of how nonverbal skills are "articulated" in different surgical contexts. Hall and, more recently, Martinec are two researchers who have looked at the meaning expressed by proximity, that is, what is conveyed by how close people stand to each other and how they align their bodies. The concepts of Hall (1959) and Martinec (2001) were used in this study to examine how members of the surgical team communicate nonverbally (Chapter 11, this volume; Moore et al. 2010).

At first the researchers merely sat in on procedures, quietly taking notes and making sketches; next, after a consensus of all participants, a relatively non-intrusive hand-held camera was introduced. Finally, full video and wireless sound recorders were agreed to, and these became just one more aspect of the organization of the OT over approximately 12 months in which we awaited suitable rosters and the other conditions.

Over 50 hours of videotapes were obtained. Sections of video were analysed frame by frame using a functional linguistic framework for all messages, including a framework for nonverbal signalling based on Hall and Martinec: that is, interpreting orientation, visual target and vertical alignment. With respect to the latter nonverbal semiotics, the analysts examined single frames of videotape looking at the body position of each team member, where their eyes were looking, what their hands were doing, how high they held their heads, nods and glances, as well as what tone of voice was used, what was being said, what was meant and what was actually happening during the procedure.

The data were charted onto ELAN spreadsheets, which line up each dimension being analysed. Next, the information was mapped onto diagrams (with, for example, unbroken and dotted lines for spoken and unspoken, respectively) to generate "maps of symbolic traffic".

8.6   Results and Discussion

A telling finding regarding the importance of the gestural/proxemic mode was that even with the sound turned off it was possible to follow the "rhythm" of the interactions, to identify who was operating and who assisting, whether things were going well or whether the case was difficult, and even very specific information such as whether an assistant was helping as much as he or she could.

For instance, a surgeon who is engrossed in work might have made a nonverbal request for an instrument by holding out a hand; the experienced scrub nurses tell from the shape of the hand which instrument is required. This may happen when surgeons find themselves lost for words because the task that requires their full attention is so "spatial" or topological in nature. Another example is of a scout subtly alerting a surgeon to the position of a foot pedal under the drapes with just a nudge. We found that the scrub nurses in particular had to master two systems of communication for two different physical zones, the operative field and the wider context (including beyond the room for purposes of instrument swapping).

The diagrams produced from this analysis illustrate the density of the overlay of verbal and nonverbal exchanges. The operating theatre was certainly a stage for intense symbolic exchange, much of which – whether verbal or nonverbal – tended to implicitness. The expectation of being understood turned out to be high. By this we mean that minimal signs functioned to carry highly specific meanings, much of which depended on knowing the logical next step in the operation and construing the surgeon's needs. Such semiotic minimalism is characteristic of expert exchanges, even across putative language boundaries (see Nguyen 2002, in which cardiac surgeons from Vietnam and China evaluated patients on the basis of the iconicity provided by x-rays and the common experience expressed in a "patch-work" of code switching across Vietnamese, Chinese and English).

Given that expert team members know "how to proceed" from this or another point in the context of culture, an elaborate code could be an obstruction to goal-directed action. Such a minimalist approach to explicit instruction is foregrounded in other domains of performance too – for instance, in martial arts training. One might say that learning by repetition is favoured over reiteration: the task is to be emulated and "handed on" through the mastery of the teacher. Certain traditions ("tradire": Latin for "to pass on") never move far from reminding practitioners that they are embodied knowledge. While there is skill and a "wisdom of the hands" to be achieved in surgery, there are at least **five significant dangers** in the implicitness of pedagogy that coexist with intense symbolic exchange.

The **first problem** is that experts may not notice how they achieved aspects of their expertise and may assume that novices have just either got "the right stuff" or they are not "cut out" to be surgeons. As with the nature of institutions mentioned above, we can find individuals who operate well within the system but who have a poor sense of the structure and roles which sustain that institution. Rather than appreciate the way they themselves were socialized over time into an operational skill *and* a value system, some practitioners appear insensitive to the process that brought about their current level of achievement when this process is not "spelt out", that is, when it is not made explicit. This "blindsight" to experience can be met with in any activity that is intricate and that therefore takes time to learn.

The **second problem** emerges from the first, namely that the gatekeeping for new practitioners may be biased by a value system irrelevant to the skills and judgements realistically involved in medical outcomes. The novice who does not speak or reflect the social style of the college may be subtly excluded. This kind of bias was obviously used against women in the past; but in a highly implicit code of learning, there is always opportunity to "find" shortcomings in any individual's performance, that is, when the steps for contributing in a surgical team are not brought out clearly by observation and explanation (especially when unrealistic notions are held by those who believe they exemplify such contributions).

The **third problem** is with the patterns of socialization into a profession with complex forms of decision-making, with profound responsibilities and with challenging ethical dilemmas. When the roles of different practitioners are not appreciated – as in a system with high levels of implicit action and/or of implicit positional authority – the chances of quarrels and bullying behaviours are increased. Some practitioners may carry over an authoritarian, hierarchical framework from their own training. These may be intensified by more general values which they carry from family and culture. An assumption of positional authority may manifest itself in confrontation instead of cooperation. In fact, the combination of problems 2 and 3 can be seen in cases reported to us of devaluing the complex role of the scrub nurse (explained above) and other surgical roles. There is a strong likelihood that a "command structure" will emerge when the difficulties others face are underappreciated. Such styles of imperative-based interaction run counter to the consultative styles which are endorsed explicitly by most public institutions today.

The **fourth problem** derives from the underestimation of the work of others. For instance, should a surgeon be passed an instrument in an irregular way, or in a way not favoured by the surgeon, then it is easy for anyone unaware of the strain of the scrub nurse's divided attentions to assume that she is "having a bad day" or is not really "on the mark". With the intensity of meaningful signals around the deep responsibilities of patient care, every action is interpreted. From interpretation follows evaluation. In a context in which much is left implicit, any one-to-one correspondence between a posture or action and a meaning is hard to ascertain. The message conveyed by physical methods of communication depends on the context over time. For example, a scrub nurse who used a posture appropriate for laparoscopic surgery inadvertently conveyed a message of lack of interest in the proceedings by using that posture during open surgery (Chapter 11, this volume). So, evaluation needs to be realistic about the difficulties that a person is managing. The symbolic traffic is one way of measuring such difficulties. In terms of symbolic traffic, the scrub nurse may be the most challenging role in the operating theatre.

A **fifth issue** concerns management at different levels in a hospital. The Operating Theatres usually constitute a distinct department within a hospital. The OT manager allocates authority over rosters and the use of resources, among many other matters. The manager may well be a senior nurse whose previous roles included working with surgeons in those theatres. Now the surgeons must come to petition for changes or special conditions from the manager. This is one only of a number of potential areas of conflict between perceptions of medical authority and actual institutional power. The senior nurse manager may have vastly more experience than the surgeon; but further up the levels of governance there is more chance of there being a divide between clinical judgement and financial priorities (van der Weyden 2005), with the possibility (which appears to have been one factor in the

Patel Case) that a financial officer signs off on clinicians' employment contracts without the oversight of a clinical supervisor.

8.7 Exemplum: Risks and Opportunities within Realizational Systems

Decision-making in complex institutions is difficult; we all appreciate this as fact. But what is the basis of the difficulty? "Misadventures", as the etymology of the word suggests, are often attributed to "human error" (including due to overwork, lack of appropriate training etc.). Other attributions are "equipment failure" (including insufficient maintenance, outmoded instruments, budget stringencies etc.) and canonical "accidents" (improbabilities, "acts of god", alignments of invidious conditions – now referred to as "perfect storms", without any need to be connected to weather). A crucial dimension of talk around "misadventure" is whether or not the event was foreseeable, whether it was predicted by modelling, by certain individuals, or whether or not it was implicit in available data, but unread. Reflect on how this applies to Hurricane Katrina in New Orleans; the multiple construals of the Liverpool football disaster; the U.S. attempt to fly helicopters to Tehran during the "hostage crisis"; Fukushima and earlier atomic power disasters.

"Error" is the classification for what humans could have foreseen, anticipated and addressed, but did not. It also is applied to the decisions made after some terrible event is in train, when those decisions fail to ameliorate the situation.

Difficulties in complex systems are often latent – unseen because they are not directly in touch in time and space with the consequences which express the new state of the system. But this does not mean that they cannot be anticipated. Some general principles around anticipations and interventions did arise from reflecting on this project.

It is precipitous to modify any aspect of a working system without revisiting all major variables that determine outcomes. One example brought to our attention was the intervention of government lawyers in relation to perceived legal exposure of the hospital: that the pneumatic anti-thrombosis stockings for patients during operations, which were regularly reused, might become (according to the legal advice) the basis of a suit by a patient. Consequently, the government stopped the double use of the stockings. At over $50 per pair, the additional budget over a year, for c. 10,000 operations, amounted to more than 250,000 dollars for the Department at the hospital. This had implications for rosters and other ways of cost-cutting. These cuts then become part of the conditions of work, thinning out the resources across the system, as may be happening with other pieces of "silent legislation". The factor is covert, as any individual failure in the system is not traceable back to this action specifically. It is likely that such symbolic/material alignments around cost-containment are responsible for many potential and actual medical "errors" and even population health disasters. A recent example may be the proposed link between IMF cuts, clinician shortages, and the spread of ebola within and beyond Guinea, Liberia and Sierra Leone (Kentikelenis et al. 2014).

Authorities and experts need to make decisions together, not individually; and, in the "core business" of an institution, changes need to be subject to veto (or to being held over for adjudication) by the personnel trained first and foremost for that core expertise. In hospitals, for instance, this means that administrators cannot introduce change without the assent of representatives of clinicians. Whatever the facts of the Patel Case in Queensland, a systemic problem existed in that an administrative head signed off on contracts on the basis of short-term financial perceptions – i.e., without clinical expertise providing the complementarity of judgement (the way dual Consuls and a Tribune could veto decisions in Republican Rome). In universities, autocratic executive powers, lines of "report" and short contracts have been introduced along corporation lines with little community knowledge of how such instruments of control change the nature of the institution: command structures do not equal transparency or responsibility, and certainly these elements combined change the perception of time for innovation. Institutions can change, for better and for worse, by semantic increments. Consider the semantic pressure of "clients" instead of "patients" or "students". In fact, as in any culture, whether of hospitals, universities or governments, emphasizing pyramids of command can make less likely any admission or discussion of problems and errors.

Even with the best-planned systems, some mundane decisions made "on the run" can have considerable consequences. As staff call in "unavailable", the roster has to be reworked in minutes, modifying surgical teams and times. Furthermore, operations "running late" on a shift mean that staff are then late to other obligations; yet this additional effect is not registered in the workload. Unexpected changes to teams and unrecognized sacrifices create resentment that often gets expressed in the tearooms. Along with "role creep" – the increasing number of roles that a person may be assigned – there is a syndrome around the "weight of exposure" (rather than of "responsibility"). Feeling the stress of unrealistic exposure leads to lower satisfaction with the conditions of work. We suggest that this probably leads to higher rates of unproductive exchange amongst hospital personnel, as well as adding to the degree of interpersonal volatility in the teamwork. But let us change focus: to exemplification of successful decisions around a complex system.

Surgical emergencies presenting to public hospitals in Australia have traditionally been admitted under the care of an individual surgeon, rostered on-call for a specific period. The on-call period is typically 24 hours, or a full weekend in larger city hospitals, but could be a full week in a smaller country hospital. All patients admitted under the surgeon would typically remain that surgeon's responsibility for all investigations, decision-making, surgery and post-operative care for the duration of their stay; be it days or months. This responsibility, impossible to predict in advance, could be considered the "tail" of the on-call period and it must be managed and integrated across all of the surgeon's subsequent "on-call" periods as well as their pre-arranged elective work of consulting, operating and teaching across a number of unrelated hospitals and institutions. The ideal of "patient-centred care" is impossible to achieve under such conditions. The central concept of the realizational system, that everything must coincide for anything to happen at all, helps us to understand how a single patient's priorities cannot come first in a system with such profound and inevitable conflicts of availability. A surgeon can only be in one place at a time. Such a system could be described instead (without prejudice) as surgeon-centred.

It is easy to see how such a system evolved from the British heritage of charity hospitals for the poor. This was a simpler system, where surgical expertise was not only in short supply but, in relative terms, a much greater component of the whole of the determinants of a patient's outcome. In this traditional system surgeons essentially "owned" their patients; and with that benign paternalism came accountability, continuity of care, patient advocacy and other priceless values. This surgical legacy is worthy of respect not least because it has "endured"; however, its evolved state does not mean that it cannot be subjected to rational critique and interventions.

In 2005 and 2006 the Prince of Wales and Nepean Public Hospitals changed this long-standing model of patient care (Cox et al. 2010) by forming a specialized acute surgical unit to which all emergency surgical patients would be admitted. Surgeons continue to serve the unit on a regular roster; however their commitment is a dedicated, but finite, 24 hours at a time: 12 hours of which are spent by the surgeon in the hospital, while for the other 12 hours they are immediately and unequivocally available to the hospital. From the surgeon's perspective, there is no "tail", and life and work are simpler. For the patient the optimum resources are more likely to be available more efficiently. With a surgeon always available there is one less factor that has to "line up" for the decision to be made, for the surgery to be booked, for the care to progress. Priorities for individual patients can be determined within the local setting of the hospital and its resources. The acute surgical unit is not truly patient-centred, but it is much closer to that ideal; no patient can be the centre of a realizational system all of the time. The patient will be the centre of the realizational system (will **be** the "realization" in fact) as circumstances and resources allow and these "start to line up" more readily with a surgeon immediately on hand.

Particular expertise accrues to this (busy) unit with its staff of trainee surgeons and experienced clinical nurse specialists, with a rotating roster of senior surgeons. The success of the intervention is demonstrated in patient outcomes and efficient use of the operating theatres (Parasyn et al. 2009; Pepingco et al. 2012).

8.8 Modelling Symbolic Complexity in Contexts of Surgical Care

It seems self-evident that surgical procedures are the central figure of the surgical process. Our purpose in this discussion has not been to deny the obvious. What has been obscured in considering surgical practice, however, has been another order of fact: namely, that the surgical procedures only take place because our community has, through time, come to various agreements – some legally explicit, some tacit, and many latent or even covert – as to how we will allocate resources to maintaining the organic wellbeing of our community members. These social facts have become slowly shifting layers of laws; of research evaluations; of modes of training and professional "gatekeeping"; of institutional management and delegation of responsibility; of ethical accountability (of practice, and of expenditure); of formal and informal associations into teams; of quasi-proprietorship ("Whose patient is...?": as in the example of the "tail", discussed above); and even of our perceptions with respect to duty and self-sacrifice, for example in the extended training and "availability" of Operating Theatre professionals.

Consequently, we suggest that a "figure–ground" reversal may be, at this moment, a highly practical way of evaluating safety in contexts of surgical care: rather than just seek a culprit within any instance of surgical misadventure, the vast background of contested meanings around surgery needs a different kind of systemic analysis. With the complexity of such community arrangements, linear thinking is limiting. The notion of a realizational system is one step in the direction of conceptualizing and managing the non-linear complexity of institutions with deep historical roots. It also is more representative of the efforts of all levels of medical professionals in that it assists us to attend to the "energy" involved in the systems of symbolic traffic in medicine: the persuasion on behalf of a patient; the consultations with patients; the maintenance of "esprit de corps" in a team; the mentoring; the bidding for, and the sharing of, resources; the representations to governments, whether on budgets or as to who can offer medical advice to the public; the adjudication as to what constitutes a new specialist area (viz., emergency; palliative care); and so on... Consider for instance the time spent by emergency doctors on the rhetorical challenge of having a patient accepted into an already busy ward or the emergency caesarean section trumping the operation for the perforated appendix.

When decisions have such consequence for human lives, it should not surprise us that the whole domain of surgery is turbulent with the meanings and values of the wider community, and its history. We need to do a better job of bringing this background of contested meanings into the picture when we are evaluating the day-to-day actions we take.

References

Arbib, Michael. 2012. *How the Brain Got Language: The Mirror System Hypothesis.* Oxford, New York: Oxford University Press.

Bezemer, Jeff, and Gunther Kress. 2014. Touch: A Resource for Making Meaning. *Australian Journal of Language and Literacy* 37: 77–85.

Bezemer, Jeff, Ged Murtagh, Alexandra Cope, Gunther Kress and Roger Kneebone. 2011. "Scissors, Please": The Practical Accomplishment of Surgical Work in the Operating Theatre. *Symbolic Interaction* 34: 398–414.

Bertalanffy, Karl Ludwig von. 1969. *General System Theory: Foundations, Development, Applications.* New York: George Braziller.

Butt, David G. 2006. Firth, Halliday and the Development of Systemic Functional Theory. In *History of the Language Sciences,* edited by Sylvain Auroux, E.F.K. Koerner, Hans-Josef Niederehe and Kees Versteegh, Volume 2. Berlin and New York: Walter de Gruyter.

Butt, David G., John C. Cartmill and Alison Rotha Moore. 2009. Space, Light and Shadow in Theatres of Critical Care. The Surgeon as Protagonist and as Mentor. Plenary presentation at Brawijaya University, East Java.

Cartmill, John C., and David G. Butt. 2012. Engineering the Surgical Imagination. *The Medical Journal of Australia* 196: 497.

Cohen, Jack, and Ian Stewart 1994. *The Collapse of Chaos: Discovering Simplicity in a Complex World.* London: Penguin.

Cox, Michael R., Linley Cook, Jennifer Dobson, Paul Lambrakis, Shanthen Ganesh and Patrick Cregan. 2010. Acute Surgical Unit: A New Model of Care. *ANZ Journal of Surgery* 80: 419–24.

Damasio, Antonio. 2012. *Self Comes to Mind: Constructing the Conscious Brain.* London: Vintage.

Davies, Paul, and Niels Henrik Gregersen (eds.). 2010. *Information and the Nature of Reality.* Cambridge: Cambridge University Press.

Edelman, Gerard, and Giulio Tononi. 2000. *A Universe of Consciousness: How Matter Becomes Imagination.* New York: Basic Books.

Glaser, Barney G., and Anselm Strauss. 1967. *Discovery of Grounded Theory: Strategies for Qualitative Research.* Mill Valley, CA: Sociology Press.

Gleick, James. 2011. *The Information: A History, a Theory, a Flood.* London: Fourth Estate.

Hall, Edward. 1959. *The Silent Language.* New York: Doubleday.

Halliday, Michael A.K. 1973. *Towards a Sociological Semantics: Explorations in the Functions of Language.* London: Edward Arnold.

Halliday, Michael A.K. 1976. *System and Function in Language.* London: Oxford University Press. Edited by Gunther R. Kress.

Halliday, Michael A.K. 1978. *Language as Social Semiotic: The Social Interpretation of Language and Meaning.* London: Edward Arnold.

Helmreich, Robert L., and Ashleigh C. Merritt. 1998. *Culture at Work in Aviation and Medicine: National, Organisational, and Professional Influences.* Aldershot, UK: Ashgate.

Hutchins, Edwin. 1995. *Cognition in the Wild.* Cambridge, Massachusetts: MIT Press.

Kappagoda, Astika. 2004. Semiosis as the Sixth Sense: Theorising the Unperceived in Ancient Greek. Unpublished PhD thesis, Macquarie University.

Kentikelenis, Alexander, Lawrence King, Martin McKee and David Stuckler. 2014. The International Monetary Fund and the Ebola Outbreak. *The Lancet,* December 22. http://dx.doi.org/10.1016/S2214-109X(14)70377-8, last accessed December 30, 2014.

Lemke, Jay 1995. *Textual Politics: Discourse and Social Dynamics.* London: Taylor & Francis.

Lingard, Lorelai. 2011. Beyond "Communication Skills": Research in Team Communication and Implications for Surgical Education. In *Surgical Education: Theorising an Emerging Domain,* edited by Heather Fry and Roger Kneebone, 199–211. London: Springer.

Long, Debbi, Rick Iedema and Bonsan Bonne Lee. 2007. Corridor Conversations: Clinical Communication in Casual Spaces. In *The Discourse of Hospital Communication: Tracing Complexities in Contemporary Health Organizations,* edited by Rick Iedema. London: Palgrave.

Lukin, Annabelle, Alison Moore, Maria Herke, Rebekah Wegener and Canzhong Wu. 2011. Halliday's Model of Register Revisited and Explored. *Linguistics and the Human Sciences* 4(2): 187–243.

Mainzer, Klaus. 1997 [1994]. *Thinking in Complexity: The Complex Dynamics of Matter, Mind and Mankind,* 3rd edition. Berlin: Springer.

Martinec, Radan 2001. Interpersonal Resources in Action. *Semiotica* 135: 117–45.

Meares, Russell. 2012. *A Dissociation Model of Borderline Personality Disorder.* New York: Norton & Company.

Moore, Alison Rotha, David G. Butt and John Cartmill. 2005. Systemic Safety in Surgery: Risk, Responsibility, System. Paper presented to COMET-VELIM 05 – 3rd Interdisciplinary Conference on Communication, Medicine and Ethics. University of Sydney and Macquarie University, June 30–July 2, 2005.

Moore, Alison Rotha, David G. Butt, Jodie Ellis-Clarke and John Cartmill. 2010. Linguistic Analysis of Verbal and Non-Verbal Communication in the Operating Room. *ANZ Journal of Surgery* 80: 925–9.

Nguyen, Huy Quang. 2002. Anticipating Miscommunications amongst Health Specialists: Field, Tenor and Mode in the Vietnamese Health System. Unpublished PhD thesis, Department of Linguistics, Macquarie University.

Parasyn, Andrew, Philip Truskett, John M. Bennett, Sharon Lum, Jennie Barry, Kourosh Haghighi and Philip Crowe. 2009. Acute-Care Surgical Service: A Change in Culture. *ANZ Journal of Surgery* 79: 12–18.

Pepingco, Lester, Guy Eslick and Michael Cox. 2012. The Acute Surgical Unit as a Novel Model of Care for Patients Presenting with Acute Cholecystitis. *Medical Journal of Australia* 196: 509–10.

Reason, James. 1997. *Managing the Risks of Organisational Accidents.* Aldershot, UK: Ashgate.

Riley, Robin, and Elizabeth Manias. 2005. Rethinking Theatre in Modern Operating Rooms. *Nursing Inquiry* 12(1): 2–9.

Strauss, Anselm L. 1987. *Qualitative Analysis for Social Scientists.* Cambridge: Cambridge University Press.

Strauss, Anselm L., and Juliet M. Corbin. 1998. *Basics of Qualitative Research: Grounded Theory Procedures and Techniques.* 2nd edition. New York: Sage Publications.

Strogatz, Steven. 2003. *Sync: The Emerging Science of Spontaneous Order.* London: Hyperion.

Trevarthen, Colwyn, and Penelope Hubley. 1978. Secondary Intersubjectivity: Confidence, Confiding and Acts of Meaning in the First Year. In *Action, Gesture and Symbol*, edited by Andrew Lock. London: Academic Press.

van der Weyden, Martin. 2005. The Bundaberg Hospital Scandal: The Need for Reform in Queensland and Beyond. *Medical Journal of Australia* 184(6): 284–5.

David G. Butt, PhD, is an Associate Professor of Linguistics at Macquarie University, Sydney. He has published widely on systemic functional linguistic theory and applications including literary stylistics, educational linguistics and health discourses – in particular surgery, oncology and psychotherapy. He began discussions with John Cartmill at the recommendation of Professor Miles Little; and this connection led to their focus on the semantic complexity of institutional systems.

Alison Rotha Moore, PhD, is a Senior Lecturer in English Language and Linguistics at the University of Wollongong and an Honorary Research Associate with the Language in Social Life Research Network at Macquarie University, Sydney, where she held an ARC Project on interaction within surgical teams, with John Cartmill and David Butt, among other joint endeavours. She currently publishes on medical discourse, animal studies and functional linguistics, in particular register theory.

John A. Cartmill is a senior consultant surgeon at Nepean Public and Macquarie University Private Hospitals and a founding Professor in the Faculty of Medicine and Health Sciences at Macquarie University, Sydney. Professor Cartmill has played a leading role in developing the emerging area of postgraduate surgical education in Australia. A fortunate introduction to David Butt and Alison Moore has led to a fascination with the power of linguistics to unlock many of the (hitherto) intangibles of the specialty he enjoys so much.

Drawings by **Marcus Cremonese**, biomedical illustrator.

9 Operating Together: The Collective Achievement of Surgical Action

Lorenza Mondada

9.1 Introduction

The study of social interactions in medical work has primarily dealt with doctor-patient consultations in which the body is often talked about rather than actually manipulated. Another field in which medical work directly deals with the body, radically transforming it during a procedure, is surgery. In this practice, we can say that the anatomy is situated and collectively achieved during a surgical operation, both through the way in which it is locally seen and interpreted for the practical purposes of surgical action, and through the way the anatomy is actually cut, dissected, cauterized and repaired. Moreover, surgery is typically a collective activity, performed by a team, requiring timely, detailed and precise forms of coordination.

This chapter deals with surgical practice as it is locally shaped within the course of an operation; it focuses on the way in which surgical action shaping the body for the local purposes of an operation is timely, situational and interactively organized. In order to do this, I offer a systematic analysis of the instructions given by a chief surgeon to his or her assistant in the operating room during a surgical operation, and of the instructed actions of the assistant following the directives of the surgeon. In this way, the chapter aims to show how surgery is a methodic collaborative achievement, relying on finely tuned coordination between staff members. More generally, it aims at presenting a systematic and detailed analysis of instructions as situated accomplishments in time, and of instructed action as resulting from an embodied and indexical understanding of directives and requests as they are produced in time and in context.

Thus, adopting an ethnomethodological and conversation analytic perspective, the chapter deals with instructions in the operating room as a pervasive feature of operating as collective and collaboratively distributed work. Within surgical team coordination, instructions in the form of directives and requests are a frequent type of action, crucial for the achievement and progression of ongoing surgical work. Although the work of a team can be tacitly performed without saying a word, instructions are often produced by a surgeon to his or her assistants – for example in order to direct their action or to request various instruments. Instructions in the form of directives and requests are mostly performed in a routine way, but they can also acquire an urgent character, responding to possible contingencies, unforeseen events and the emergence of risks. Instructions reveal the orderly character of the situated action of a surgical team. They also reveal how this action is achieved within the surgical field and within the praxeological context of surgery. Instructions are intelligible and observable only for a "professional vision" (Goodwin 1994), able to see them as part of an ongoing procedure and as orienting to the relevant anatomical landmarks.

After sketching current studies of surgical practice and the type of actions – instructions, requests, directives – that are crucial for the collaborative achievement of surgery, and after having described my data, I offer an analysis of instruction in three contexts of team collaboration in surgery: manipulation of the endoscopic camera, activation of the coagulating hook and the position of an assistant's hands. In all the cases, the sequential environment of these collaborative actions is organized first by an instruction followed by the instructed action. This analysis is further developed by describing how a team treats the indexical features of action, coordination and instruction by using its underlying knowledge, experience, expertise and skill.

9.2   Surgery as a Situated Collaborative Action: Video Studies

Although surgery is one of the most spectacular and prestigious forms of medicine, studies focusing on the detailed ordinary work of surgeons in the operating room remain scarce.

Some important ethnographic studies have outlined the actual work of the surgeon – for instance, Hirschauer (1991) on the transformation of the patient in an operable body, Katz (1999) on the ritual aspects of surgery, Pettinari (1988) on the various types of discourse in the operating room and Prentice (2012) on surgical training.

Video recordings of naturally occurring surgical operations have offered a new way of not only observing surgery but also analysing it in detail as it unfolds in real time in actual work environments (Heath, Hindmarsh and Luff 2010; Mondada 2003a, b, 2006a). This has made it possible for ethnomethodological and conversation analytic studies to unpack the complexities of what happens in the operating room. This line of research has described both the ordinary work of surgeons and the work of training surgeons in the operating room, showing how they notice, gaze, scrutinize, categorize and discover the details of the anatomy while they operate (Koschmann et al. 2007, 2011; Koschmann and Zemel 2011; Mondada 2003a, forthcoming a), how they collaborate (Hindmarsh and Pilnick 2002, 2007; Mondada 2007a; Sanchez Svensson 2005) and how training and demonstration are embedded in the work of operating (Koschmann et al. 2011; Mondada 2006a, 2007c, 2011, forthcoming b; Sanchez Svensson, Heath and Luff 2009).

These analyses of surgical work show the importance of coordination in the operating room and, thus, the crucial role of instructions, requests, directives and orders in the conduct of a surgical procedure. For instance, Sanchez Svensson, Heath and Luff (2007) and Bezemer et al. (2011) show how instruments are exchanged in the surgical theatre; while Mondada shows the systematic way in which the coagulating hook manoeuvred by the surgeon is activated by the assistant (2011), studies the way in which the endoscopic camera is directed by the surgeon, making the very action of operating possible (2003a, forthcoming a) and analyses how the surgeon directs the assistant's hands in open surgery (forthcoming c).

This chapter elaborates on these studies by focusing on various contexts in which a surgeon requests an action from an assistant, instructing him or her how to do the action, and the assistant responds by complying with the request, performing the instructed action. This focus of analysis contributes to our understanding of how coordination in teams works in real time and how trajectories of action constitutive of the surgical procedure are both methodically and situatedly organized, taking into account the local ecology of action.

9.3   Instructions, Instructed Actions, Directives and Requests

Although there is a long-standing interest in pragmatics and linguistics in the study of how speakers order and request something of other people, the study of the way in which participants get someone to do something in naturally occurring social activities – and even more so in actual specific social contexts such as the workplace – is still scarcely developed. In this chapter, I rely on two complementary traditions, one coming from ethnomethodology and dealing with instructions/ instructed actions, and the other one coming from conversation analysis that studies requests and directives.

First, this study is inspired by the ethnomethodological insights of Garfinkel (2002) about instructions and instructed action. Garfinkel (2002: ch. 6) is interested in the way in which members follow instructions – for example when they read a manual or look at a map or when they build a piece of furniture or search for a location. Garfinkel shows that instruction does not unilaterally determine instructed action. Rather, it acquires its meaning through being followed. His way of describing the following of instructions recalls Wittgenstein's (1953) view about following a rule. An instruction is achieved as such only by and through the action of interpreting the instruction and following it. Instructions are essentially incomplete (Garfinkel 1967: 29), since they cannot provide the detailed account of an embodied action's practical aspects that is required to realize them (Suchman 1987). This indeterminacy builds the efficiency of instructions, a matter that crucially relies on the situated interpretation of participants. The way in which an instruction is implemented in a responsive action – the instructed action – relies on the skilled interpretation of the recipient, his or her competent grasp of what is going on and the relevant features of the local ecology. The situated sense of directives is irredeemably tied to the particular activities and context in and through which a particular action required by the directives is produced (Amerine and Bilmes 1988).

Second, this study refers to a long-standing tradition in linguistics and conversation analysis dealing with the way in which action is formatted. Historically, the conditions of interpretation of direct and, mostly, indirect acts have been widely discussed within the speech acts tradition (Searle 1975). Within sociolinguistics and discourse analysis, the social relationships indexed by directives have been privileged. Most of the literature considers that directive formulations are determined by social aspects such as politeness, power, hierarchy and status (Ervin-Tripp 1976). Aggravated forms of directives, such as orders and demands in the imperative form, imply that a speaker can legitimately impose on another by stating his or her requirements boldly. By contrast, the use of mitigated forms expresses these acts in downgraded ways and allows a speaker to avoid offending another (Labov and Fanshel 1977: 63, 84–6).

Within the conversation analysis tradition, requests and directives initiate a sequence where complying constitutes the preferred response and rejection of the non-preferred one. Participants design requests so as to prevent non-preferred responses and this accounts for the use of pre-requests and other pre-sequences (Davidson 1984; Schegloff 1980), as well as other formats that are sensitive to different forms of entitlement (Craven and Potter 2010; Curl and Drew 2008; Heinemann 2006; Lindström 2005; Wootton 2005).

Within this literature, most of the directing and requesting actions studied concern future actions that are solicited, often in phone conversations, and granted within a verbal agreement. By contrast, directives and requests concerning actions that are to be performed immediately within the same setting and in an embodied way have been much less studied. Exceptions are studies by Cekaite (2010) and Goodwin and Cekaite (2012) of directives addressed by parents to children concerning tasks to be carried out in an immediate context, a study by De Stefani and Gazin (2014) of directives during driving lessons and a study by Lindwall and Ekström (2012) of instructions teaching how to do crochet. Other studies by Mondada (2013, 2014) of home activities, like playing video-games or cooking, show how time crucially matters for the embodied production and response to directives and requests that rely on the moment-by-moment, exactly synchronized coordination of the participants collectively engaged in an activity. This chapter elaborates on these previous studies by showing how a surgeon directing the action of his or her team organizes their collective action here and now in a situated, embodied and timely way (cf. also Mondada 2011, forthcoming a).

9.4 Data and Methodology

Between 1996 and 1998, I conducted extensive fieldwork in the surgical department of a large university hospital in France. The data collected during this fieldwork concerned both surgical operations – 25 hours of video recordings of laparoscopic and open surgeries – and video conferences in which surgical staff discussed diagnoses and clinical decisions with other colleagues in Europe, the U.S. and Japan – constituting 30 hours of audio/video recordings.

On the basis of this large corpus, I have been interested in the way in which instructions are produced in various operations and surgical procedures: instructions concerning the manipulation of the endoscopic camera in laparoscopic surgery (Mondada 2003a, forthcoming a), instructions concerning the activation of the cautery while the surgeon is both operating and demonstrating an operation (Mondada 2011), and instructions embedded in demonstrations (Mondada 2007b).

Data have been collected and transcribed according to the principles of conversation analysis. This means an emphasis on naturally occurring activities, which are recorded either by a researcher or by participants themselves – as is the case here – documented as they happen ordinarily; this also means in-depth transcription of the relevant actions and the resources they mobilize. In the cases analysed in this chapter, multimodal transcription integrates the talk of the participants, their surgical gestures, the movements of the instruments and the movements of the endoscopic camera. These details are temporally arranged within the relation of both successivity and simultaneity. The actions of the participants are finely timed, and this aspect is crucial for the understanding of their coordination. Therefore, these temporal features are precisely annotated in the transcripts and exploited in the analysis of the sequential organization of patterns of actions.

In this chapter, I rely on video recordings of both open and laparoscopic operations.

Open operations – for instance, the operation for an inguinal hernia – are achieved by a surgeon operating with one assistant. The former uses coagulating forceps or scissors with his or her right hand while the left hand and the hands of the assistant are busy with forceps, retractors, graspers and other instruments holding the tissues and making the surgical field visible and accessible for dissecting. Most of the instructions produced by a surgeon to an assistant concern the position of his or her hands and of the instruments for the progression of the ongoing procedure. This responds to a practical problem the surgeon faces while operating: surgery is a complex activity that mobilizes a number of instruments, which require more than just two hands; consequently, teamwork is required, and, more precisely, the coordination of one's own and others' hands.

Laparoscopic surgery, also called minimally invasive surgery, is performed with surgical tools and an endoscopic camera inserted in the body of a patient through small holes, called trocars. The endoscopic image is projected on monitors in the operating room that are used by the surgical team. In the case studied here, the image is also projected to a remote amphitheatre where the audience and experts watch the operation live; all participants have access to the same endoscopic image, constituting the visual evidence on which the operation is based. The operations studied here were held within an international course for advanced trainees. Each surgeon and their team did not only operate but also explained the operation (here I do not focus on this latter aspect, but see Mondada 2006b, 2007c, 2011 about demonstrations during live surgery).

The following analyses aim at describing the way in which instructions are organized in the operating room – concerning the passing of instruments, actions to be done and the manipulations of the camera. First, I analyse the way in which basic and more complex forms of instructions and instructed actions occur in these three domains, showing the similarities that they permit us to observe. Second, I focus on two issues that are central for teamwork organization: the way in which participants go beyond the indexicality of instructions and achieve a common vision and interpretation of the ongoing surgical action and the way in which skill and experience are manifested through the organization of both instructions and instructed actions.

9.5   The Organization of Collaborative Action: Instructions/ Instructed Actions as Paired Actions

In this section, I focus on requests and directives through which a surgeon instructs the action of an assistant in three praxeological contexts. First, I describe how the endoscopic camera is directed by the surgeon instructing the assistant holding it (9.5.1); second, I show how the surgeon asks the assistant to activate the coagulating hook he or she is manipulating (9.5.2); third, I analyse how, in open surgery, the surgeon directs the assistant's hands (9.5.3). These three types of instructions/ instructed actions constitute instances of collaboration and coordination crucial for the achievement of surgery.

9.5.1   Directing the Endoscopic View

In laparoscopic operations, the endoscopic camera is generally manipulated by an assistant under the supervision of a surgeon who instructs him or her. This is a key aspect for the achievement of the activities carried out – both of operating and demonstrating. In the operation, the camera is indispensible for making the next surgical step, under the control of vision – such as cutting, dissecting, coagulating, clipping, cleaning etc. In demonstrations, the camera is crucial for making visible anatomical landmarks and relevant peculiarities, the shapes, forms and colours characterizing the anatomy. These aspects, which are to be seen by an audience, are not only focused on by the camera assistant but also indicated by the surgeon in different ways. So, the relevant and efficient manoeuvring of the camera is mandatory for the activity at hand and for the production of the *visibility* of the operating field.

The endoscopic camera held by an assistant constantly adjusts in a tacit way to the surgical action it makes possible, both following and anticipating the actions of the chief surgeon. However, in some circumstances, for instance when the surgeon initiates a new step in a procedure, changes the surgical orientation or spots a new problem, the position and zoom of the camera is specifically instructed by him or her. In this case, the surgeon initiates a sequence constituted by a directive followed by a complying action by the camera assistant.

Some occurrences are illustrated in Excerpts 1–5:

Excerpt 1 (1106k1d2-11.31)

```
1   SUR       %zoom arrière.
              zoom back
              %im.1
2             (0.2) + (0.3)+ %
    cam               +zooms back+
    im                        %im.2
```

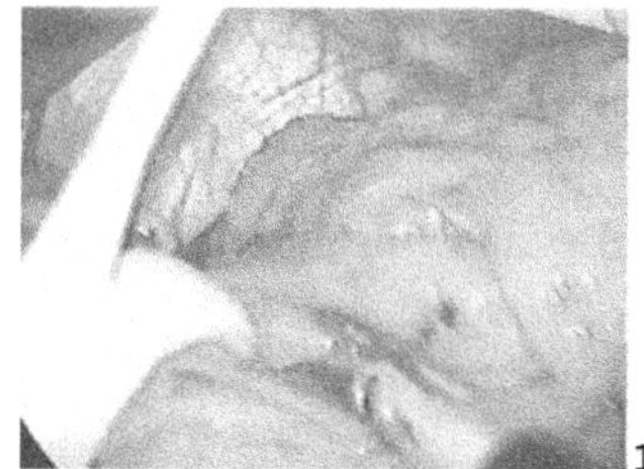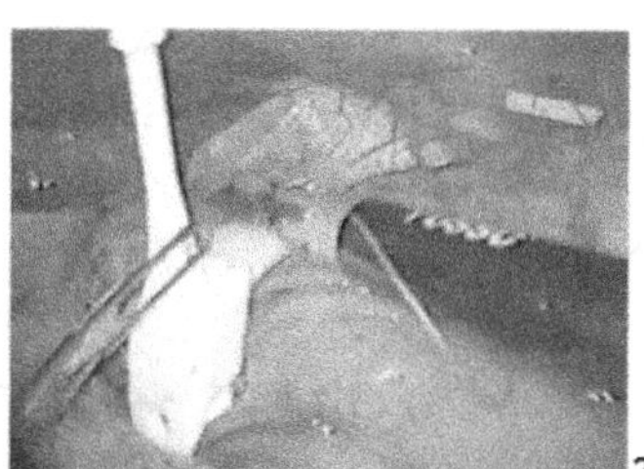

Excerpt 2 (2702k1d1-8.17)

```
1   SUR       %au: milieu s'il vous pla+ît,
              in the middle please
    cam                           +recenters-->
    im        %im.3
2             (3.+3)%
    cam         ->+  %
    im              %im.4
```

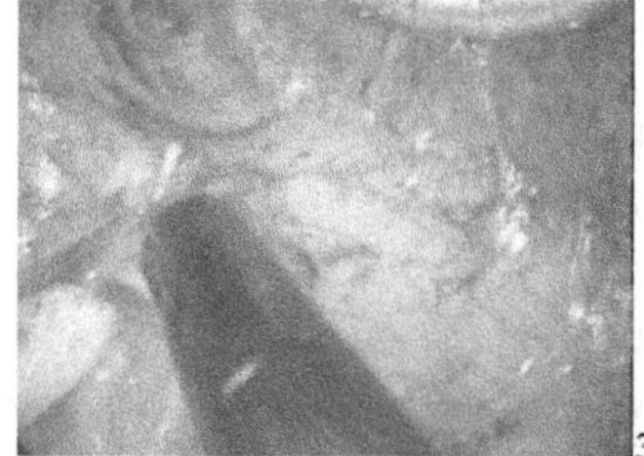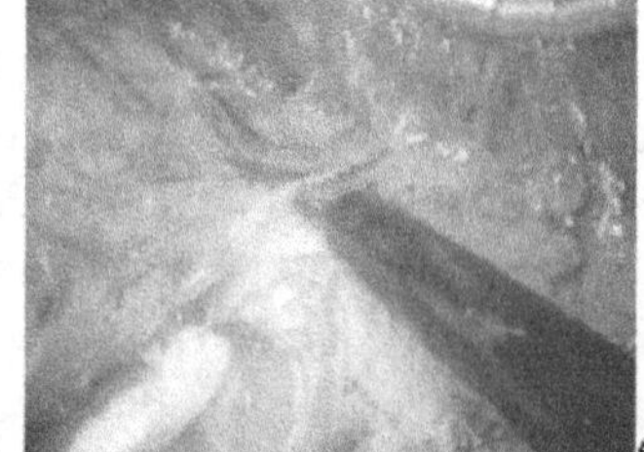

Excerpt 3 (2702k1d1-27.16)

```
1   SUR       %°okay. get close°
    im        %im. 5
2             +(0.9)
    cam       +zoom in-->
3   SUR       °okay°.+%
                  ->+
    im             %im.6
```

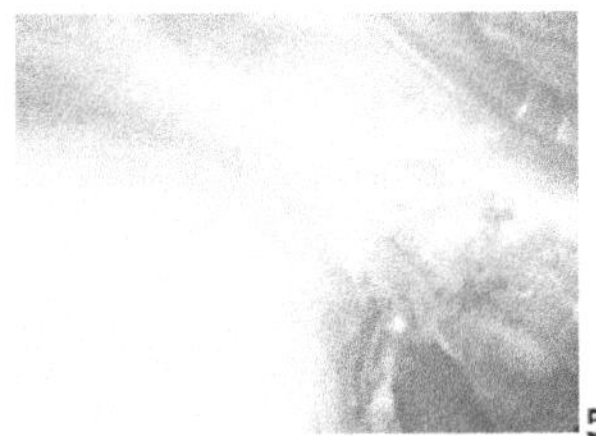 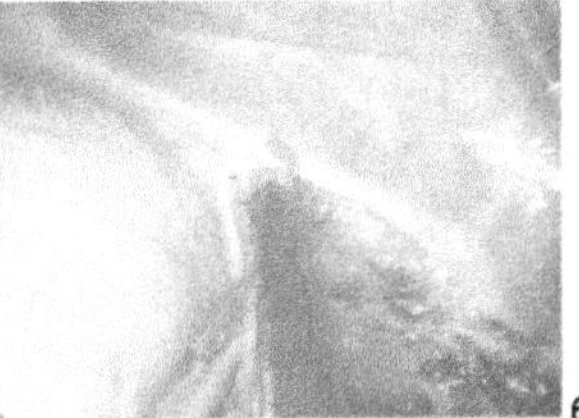

Excerpt 4 (2702_k1d1- 43.24)

```
1   SUR       center +here, that little+ vein
    cam             +goes below and centres+
```

Excerpt 5 (2702_k1d2-50.23)

```
1   SUR       get close to the spleen now
2             +(0.8)+
    cam       +zooms in+
```

In all cases, an instruction is produced, followed by a movement of the camera operated by a (silent) assistant. The instructions are implemented in directives, which can take different forms. They are generally brief, essentially formulated by a verb of action, often in the imperative form but also in the present progressive ("get close" 3, 5; "zoom arrière" 1; "center here" 4), and accomplished through spatial indication ("close" 3, 5; "au: milieu" 2; "arrière" 1; "here" 4), which is most frequently expressed by a deictic expression. Less frequently, a more precise landmark is formulated ("that little vein" 4; "to the spleen" 5). Often, the instruction is produced by code-switching into French, the language of the operating team (Mondada 2007b).

These paired actions raise several questions. The main analytical issue here concerns how the assistant is able to move the instructed camera in a way that successfully complies with the directive – given that the directive is produced in a very indexical way. This adequate response of the camera assistant is precisely what practically achieves the visual arrangement for the ongoing surgery (see below).

9.5.2 Requests to Activate Coagulation

Another collaborative action recurrent in my data is the cauterization of tissue during dissection. Although it is common for surgeons to activate their own cautery, in the cases observed this action is performed in a distributed manner by the team. A chief surgeon dissects with a coagulating hook, an electrocautery device, which uses heat from an electric current to perform division and haemostasis of tissues. The hook is manipulated by the surgeon, but its coagulation is activated by his or her assistant: their coordination is achieved by the surgeon giving a verbal instruction to the assistant, uttering "coag" or "coagulation", and the assistant activating, by dint of a pedal, the current that allows the surgeon to cauterize the tissue. This simple action, coagulating, although possibly realized by the surgeon alone, is, therefore, organized as a collective action.

This collective action is constituted by two paired actions: the directive and the granting of the directive.

Excerpt 6 (coag 2.35)

```
1   SUR       coag
2             (2+.6)
    ast          +activates coagulation
```

Excerpt 7 (coag 14.30)

```
1   SUR       coag
2             (0.5) +(1.7)
    ass             +activates coagulation
```

In order to better understand the complex coordination going on here beneath the apparent simplicity of these expressions, a more appropriate transcription is needed in order to capture the time of the actions and the interplay of coordinated gestures between the participants. The following transcript has been realized with the ELAN alignment tool:[1]

---

1 ELAN is an alignment software developed at the Max Planck Institute of Nijmegen; it is available for the research community on the website www.lat-mpi.eu/tools/elan/. It permits synchronization of a transcript with a video or audio signal.

Excerpt 8 "coagulation"

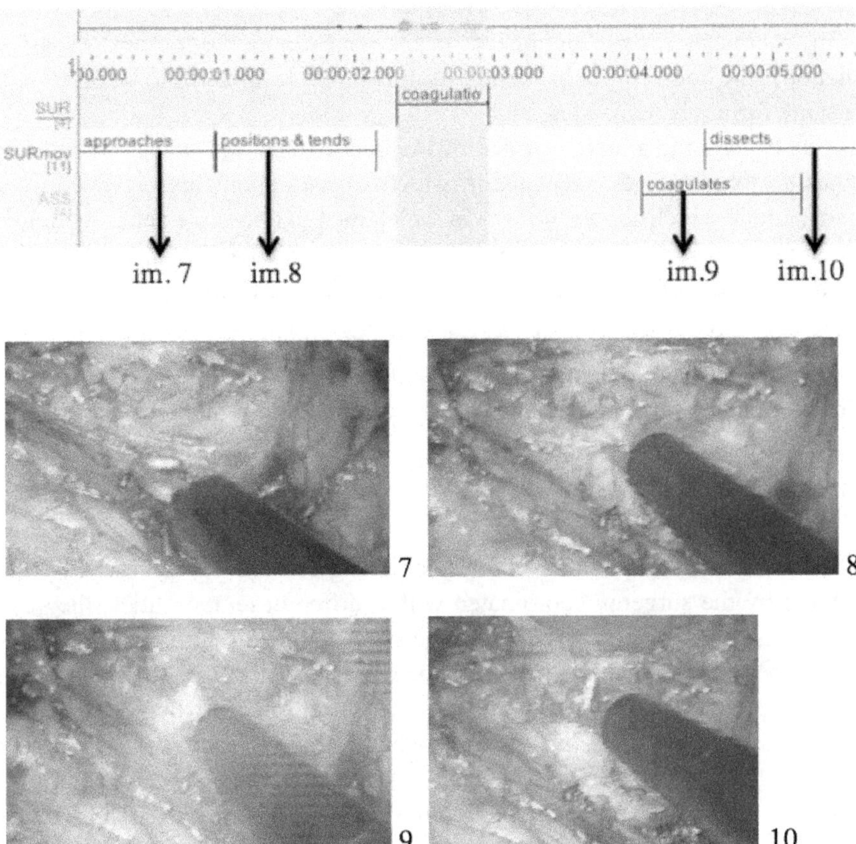

This transcript describes an action that takes less than five seconds. The sequence organization (Schegloff 2007) can be detailed in the following way:

- The surgeon approaches the point that has to be dissected with his hook (image 7);
- He positions the hook in an adequate way, beneath the fatty tissue to be dissected (image 8);
- He utters the instruction ("coagulation");
- The assistant responds by activating the cautery (image 9); coagulation is performed by using a current that produces a rapid rise in temperature in the cell, which makes it explode. This process is visible since it produces vaporization.

In our transcripts, the multimodal description of the assistant's action ("+activ. coag") is annotated as soon as this vaporization is visible.

- The hook is further tensed and performs the dissection (image 10);
- Once the point has been dissected, the hook moves away.

This instruction is serially organized; in the next round, for the next "coag" / "coagulation", the hook comes back, approaching the relevant area to be dissected, and the same format is realized again.

Thus, far from being a matter of just two paired actions, the "coag" instruction constitutes a more complex sequence in which paired actions are preceded by a preparatory move which shows the area in which the next possible action will take place, thus permitting the assistant to project the requested action and to respond to it in a relevant and efficient way. The complex sequence format is the following:

- Preparation (hook's approach and adequate positioning);
- First pair part: verbal instruction ("coagulation");
- Second pair part (a): achievement of the instruction by the assistant (activation of the cauterization);
- Second pair part (b): achievement of the dissection by the surgeon (manipulation of the hook).

The second pair part has the specificity of being collectively achieved by the assistant and by the surgeon, coordinated within different temporalities; they can either operate simultaneously or be slightly dissociated. More importantly, "coagulation" can be uttered when the hook is already positioned (when the preparation has been completed) or while it is still moving. Often this instruction is uttered within a series, and this repetitive format enhances the possibility of anticipating the next step. Indeed, in a series, whereas the first occurrence of "coagulation" is produced in a manner timed at the end of the preparatory move, the subsequent occurrences are produced in an anticipated way, well before the hook is in place. This shows that the response of the assistant is not a mechanical reaction to a command; the assistant follows the movements of the hook and displays his or her own interpretation of the adequate place and moment where the cauterization has to be done. This makes possible both anticipations of the cauterization before the instruction and coagulations without any instruction.

9.5.3   Directing the Assistant's Hands

In open surgery, the work of the surgeon and his or her assistant is organized in a complementary way; the assistant's hands and the left hand of the surgeon hold the tissue in a way that produces tension, making dissection or cauterization possible. The right hand of the surgeon operates, dissects or coagulates, by means of scissors or cauterizing forceps. Maintaining the relevant tension along with the progression of the dissection is the condition of possibility of the operating surgeon's action. Thus, tension and dissecting represent the core actions constituting the surgeon and assistant's joint activity – changes in the tension of the tissues are managed through directives by which the surgeon asks the assistant to modify the orientation of the tissue forceps.

This directive takes the form of a simple paired action as we see in Excerpts 9 and 10.

Excerpt 9 (PEL 5.10)

```
1   SUR   °prends là°
          °grasp there°
2   ASS   ((changes position of his forceps))
```

Excerpt 10 (PEL 3.42)

```
1   SUR   vas-y tends
          come on tend
2   ASS   ((tends with pliers))
```

If we look closer at what happens in open surgery when a surgeon utters his or her directives, we find the complex praxeological configuration illustrated in Excerpt 11.

Excerpt 11 "reprends plus près" / "take it closer again" (2.15)

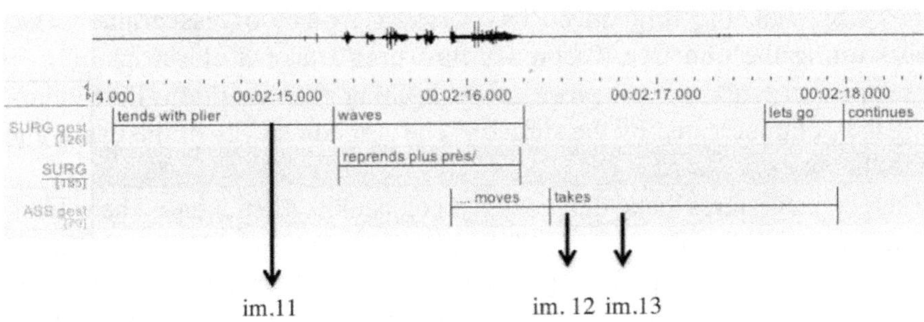

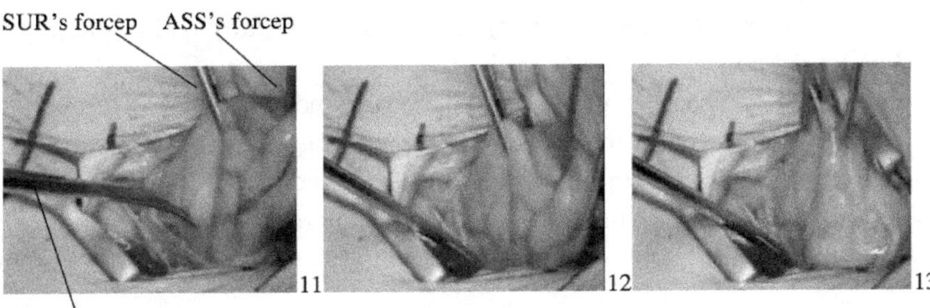

The surgeon is grasping a piece of tissue with forceps while he dissects with scissors at the base of the tissue (image 11). As he goes on, the space he dissects is transformed and the tension on the tissue is not sufficient any more. This makes the point of retraction maintained by the assistant not useful any more. Consequently, the directive asks the assistant to change the position of his forceps.

When the surgeon utters his directive ("reprends plus près"/"take it closer again"), he waves the tissue to be grasped. Thus, the directive is not just produced by means of verbal resources, but also gesturally – the waving of the item – constituting a form of pointing and highlighting of the relevant object. Consequently, the assistant drops the tissue he was holding with his forceps (image 12) and grasps the indicated item, closer to the surgeon's forceps. As soon as the assistant grasps the piece in this new position (image 13), the surgeon continues his dissection.

Excerpt 12 presents another similar example.

Excerpt 12 "reprends plus près" / "take it closer again" (3.19)

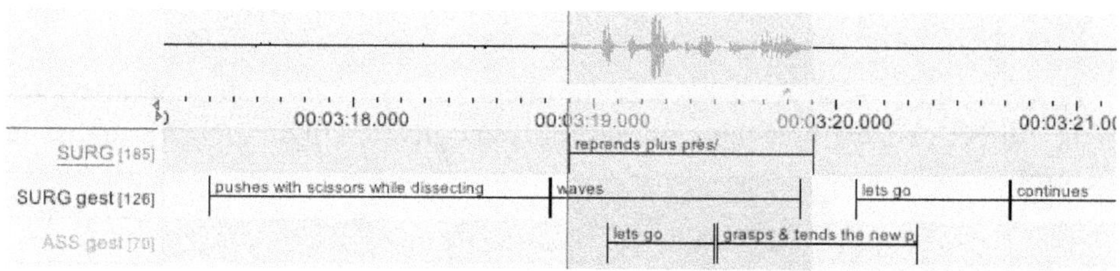

In this fragment, the surgeon pushes forward a piece of tissue and waves it when uttering the directive ("reprends plus près"/"take it closer again"). In response, the assistant drops the piece he was holding and repositions his forceps, grasping the point indicated by the surgeon. The surgeon lets go of the tissue and continues his work.

The surgeon's gestures make the process recognizable. First, the way he is tending the tissue is functional to the dissection; it also prepares and projects further steps in the dissecting action. These gestures indicate the trajectory of the ongoing operation; they permit the assistant to anticipate the next step. Thus, the instruction is precisely positioned and embedded in the surgical procedure and is made relevant and meaningful thanks to its position in this temporally and sequentially organized course of action.

Second, when the surgeon waves the tissue, he suspends the ongoing dissection in order to communicate with the assistant. The waving is not in service of the action of dissecting but is a communicative movement addressed to the assistant, both giving him the tissue to hold and highlighting the relevant point to be held. In this sense, waving the tissue works like a pointing gesture – even an insistent pointing gesture.

So, as for the previous actions, the sequence organization of these directives takes the form of a paired action, which is constituted by a series of actions by the surgeon, producing intelligibility and the conditions for a response from the assistant following the action. The sequential format is, therefore, constituted by a *complex multimodal gestalt* temporally arranged in a finely tuned way.

In this case, the sequential format is the following:

- *Preparation:* the surgeon is dissecting along a line and places the tissue in tension;
- *First action:* a verbal directive or request instructing the assistant and a visible gesture;
- *Second action:* instructed action of the assistant responding.

The *first action* of the sequence is formatted through a variety of multimodal resources. One is verbally, where instructions often take the form of imperative verbs, deictics (either the pronoun "ça", or locations like "là", "plus près") and more minimal forms (like "mhm"). Another is through gesture where instructions are generally preceded by a series of embodied actions that initiate the sequence, either in the form of pointing gestures done with scissors or haemostatic forceps or in the form of the surgeon's grasping of a relevant point/piece of tissue, which is visibly waved. These gestures accomplish various tasks: they highlight the visibility of a point, thus focusing the attention of the assistant (and of the audience); they display a detail within an action that is not one of dissection but makes available a further step in the dissection. The repeated way in which these gestures are done both highlights the visibility of the target, securing the identification of the relevant object/point to be grasped, and possibly expresses some "insistence" in a gesture that is repeated until the action of following the gesture is achieved or at least initiated.

The *second action* of the sequence completes the indexicality of the instruction by offering a situated interpretation incorporated in the response (Garfinkel 1967: ch. 1; Wieder 1974; Zimmerman 1971). Instructions are inescapably indexical, incomplete and illusive, and their intelligibility relies on the understanding of the procedure, which unfolds in a series of orderly moves recognizable within locally projectable trajectories as well as within the global surgical procedure. Their intelligibility also depends on the skills and competences of the assistant, his professional vision (Goodwin 1994) allowing him to see the relevant details within the ecology of the current activity, and the changing relevance of details as the dissection and the operation progress. Instructions and instructed actions mutually shape one another since a complying action anticipates the outcome of the sequence and prefigures it, and the outcome retrospectively confirms what the expected and adequate action was. Both the intelligibility of the first action and the understanding exhibited by the second one shape the variable temporality of the sequence and the way in which multimodal resources are distributed within it.

This section has shown how instructions are interactively achieved and rely on a finely tuned coordinated collaboration between a team's members. Moreover, instructions are not formulated in a vacuum. They are produced in relevant contexts of action, which reflexively give instructions their intelligible and even their evident character. In the next section, I deal with the way in which the participants deal with the indexicality of instructions by focusing on two recurrent praxeological environments that reflexively make instructions to the camera accountable.

9.6   The Indexicality of Instructions

As we have seen, instructions are inescapably indexical. The camera operator does not merely respond to what is said in the instruction but does much more than that. How does he or she know what exact camera movement and view are requested at which precise moment? How is the response to instructions formatted in a relevant way?

In order to grant a directive, an assistant mobilizes other multimodal, embodied and material resources, interprets the praxeological context and the ecology of the ongoing action, and displays his or her professional vision (Goodwin 1994). In the following, I develop the analyses of section 9.5.1 and investigate two praxeological contexts in which the work of making accountable and of interpreting indexical instructions concerning the endoscopic camera is observable.

9.6.1   When the Camera Follows Pointing Gestures

In the first type of environment, verbal instructions, often containing a deictic term, co-occur with "pointing gestures" made by the surgeon with the hook; he suspends the dissection and literally points towards the relevant space to cover with the endoscopic camera.

Excerpt 13 (= Excerpt 2) (2702k1d1-8.17)

```
1   SUR       au*: mili*eu s'il vous pla+%ît,*
              in the middle please
                 *hook back and forth*          *positions hook-->
    cam                                       +recenters-->
    im                                          %im.14
2             (3.+%3)
    cam       ->+
    im          %im.15
```

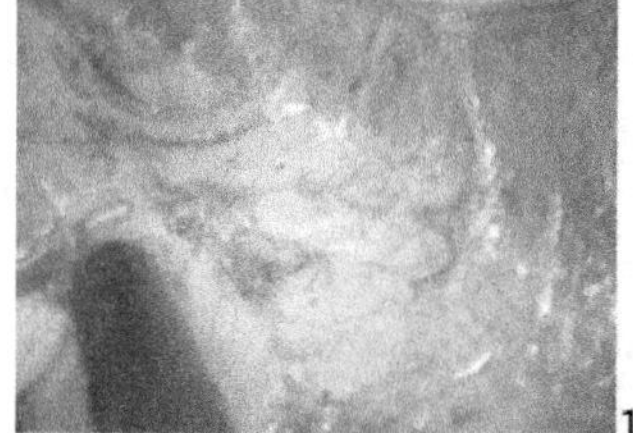

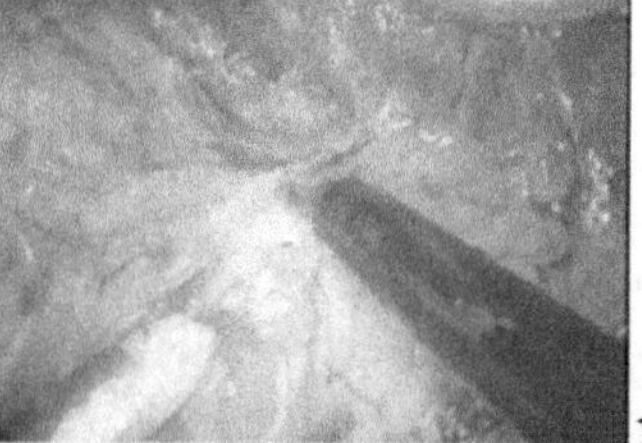

In this fragment, which reproduces Excerpt 2 with a detailed multimodal tran-scription, the surgeon stops using the hook to dissect and moves it back and forth, indicating the place that is supposed to be visualized in the middle of the screen. This zone was originally visible on the left side of the picture (image 14); after the instruction, it ends up being in the centre (image 15). In this case, operating constraints merge with more aesthetic criteria, relative to the presentation of the operating field for an audience.

In Excerpt 14, the instruction is uttered in French, code-switching in the middle of an ongoing explanation, and contains a deictic term ("à gauche"):

Excerpt 14 (2702k1d1-35.59)

```
1   SUR      after that we know *that montre à gauche (.)
                                         show on the left
             >>hook gest above last clip*shows on the left->
2            *on +the RIGHT si:de,+ we have no problem,
             *hook covers a yellow surface various times->
    cam          +moves to the left+moves below following hook->
3            and the dissection* will be very+ very easy, .h
                        -->*hook goes down----------->>
    cam                      -->+cam goes down-->>
```

The instruction "montre à gauche" co-occurs with the hook showing something on the left of the screen; at that point, the camera begins to move to the left too (line 2). The next camera movements literally follow the hook. Interestingly, the use of French for the instruction and English for the comment refer to two different spaces that are oriented in opposite ways. The former ("à gauche") refers to what is visible on the screen, while the latter ("on the RIGHT side") refers to the body of the patient. This shows that the relevant space of action for the camera operator is not the body itself, but the visible field – both being seen within two different praxeological perspectives.

In Excerpt 15, the relation between the camera work and the work of showing to the audience – in order to make them see the relevant aspects of the operating theatre – is particularly clear.

Excerpt 15 (1106k1d1-50.24)

```
1   SUR      you see* here, (.) eh:: eh eh zoom arrière jean,
                                            zoom back
             >>.....*points w hook-->>
2            +(0.5)+
    cam      +zoom out+
```

The operating surgeon first addresses an instruction to the audience ("you see"), accompanied by pointing with the hook; then he produces a directive addressed to the assistant. Here, the directive achieves the instructed vision of both the audience about what has to be seen and the camera operator about what has to be relevantly shown.

9.6.2   When the Camera Orients to the Ongoing Trajectory of Dissection

There is a second type of environment for instructions directing the endoscopic camera. In it, there is no pointing, neither addressed to the audience nor to the camera operator; instead, the operating surgeon is fully engaged in the surgical procedure. The sequential organization of the surgical action projects the next step to come and reflexively instructs the camera operator. The next two fragments document this coordination between the surgeon's hook and the assistant's camera.

Excerpt 16 (= Excerpt 3) (2702k1d1-27.16)

```
1   SUR       °okay. get close°
              >>dissecting-->>
2             +(0.9)+
    cam       +zooms in--->
3   SUR       °okay°.+
                 --->+
```

The operating surgeon is working with the hook at a particular point visible on the screen; his action constitutes the focus of his indexical instruction ("get close", line 1). Indeed, the camera assistant immediately operates a zoom in focusing on that particular place. The camera movement and its completion are further directed by the terminal "°okay°" in third position (line 3).

In a similar way, in Excerpt 17, the instruction is formulated first with a deictic ("here", line 2); the camera next moves as soon as the verb is uttered and continues to move as this spatial description is completed, with a demonstrative ("that little vein", line 2).

Excerpt 17 (= Excerpt 4) (2702_k1d1- 43.24)

```
1             *(1.5)                          *(0.5)*
    sur       *approches a bleeding spot w hook*cauterizes it*
2   SUR       center +here, that little+ vein
    cam              +goes below and centres+
3             *(2)
    sur       *continues cauterization->
```

The operating surgeon is cauterizing a bleeding spot apparent from blood pooling and from the surgical action that treats the spot. The camera assistant grants the instruction even *before* the demonstrative description is completed. So, here we have an *early response* by the camera assistant, who orients to the projections made possible by the operating actions of the surgeon and anticipates them in his response.

Interestingly, this early response is also observable in some cases in which the verbal spatial description of the surgeon is particularly explicit, as in Excerpt 18.

Excerpt 18 (2702k1d1-28.18)

```
1  SUR      *okay. .hh +°show me this+ ligament°
           *moves the scissor tow the ligamt+dissects->
   cam                +moves in dir of the scissor->
```

The surgeon moves his scissors towards the ligament before naming it, and the camera operator orients immediately to his action, following the movement of the scissors before the verbal instructions. Moreover, the surgeon begins immediately to dissect – an action that relies on the relevant visualization of the operative field – before the anatomical landmark has been uttered. So, although the instruction is particularly explicit, the instructed action is achieved *before* it. In this context, the explicit character of the description seems to orient to the fact that the surgeon is not just operating but also demonstrating the operation – it is addressed more to the audience of trainees than to the assistant.

In sum, these *early movements* show that, although instructions are always indexical, their indexicality is often not a problem since they are accountably formulated within a *praxeological context* that reflexively achieves their intelligibility. This context is configured by trajectories of the surgical action that highlight and project the relevant landmarks for the next surgical step. In these early camera movements, the assistant controlling the camera and the surgeon directing it display their common orientation to the ongoing surgical action. The assistant exhibits through these anticipating moves, his skilled participation in the operation (see Sanchez Svensson, Heath and Luff [2007] about a team's anticipation of the next move while passing instruments).

The camera response can be produced relatively early or late, depending on the way in which this praxeological context evolves dynamically within the temporal and sequential unfolding of the surgery. Responses tend to be fast in the course of a projectable trajectory of action (see also Mondada 2011); they tend to be delayed when a new surgical step is initiated or when the movement of the hook initiates a new trajectory – i.e., in cases in which the incipient praxeological context is not yet intelligible enough to permit a recognition of the relevant operating space to be focused on by the camera.

After the early occurrences analysed above, in the next two fragments I give instances in which the camera response occurs quite late after the instruction, being granted only once the position referred to has been clearly indicated by the placement of the hook.

Excerpt 19 (2702k1d1-6.04)

```
1  SUR      on+ va là+ he*in
            we go there okay
            >>moves hook-*turns the hook---->
   cam        +moves slightly+
2             (1.2)
3           on se rapproche enco*+re,+
            we go closer again
                              ---->*positions hook for dissection->
   cam                            +zoom+
```

When the surgeon says "on va là" (line 1), the camera moves slightly, responding to the directive but without clearly moving to a specific target. A pause follows (line 2) in which the surgeon rotates the hook without orienting or using it in a precise direction. The second directive (line 3) is completed as the hook is finally positioned for the dissection. At that precise moment, the camera operator immediately zooms in to the relevant point. We can clearly see here that although the movement of the camera displays an immediate response to the verbal directive, it actually grants it only once the emergent spatial configuration indicated by the hook has been made recognizable.

Difficulties in recognizing this configuration can delay the camera response, as in Excerpt 20.

At line 1, the surgeon's instruction is *not* followed by a camera movement. At that point, the context is still evolving; a new spatial configuration is defined first by the movement of the hook (images 16–17), which was almost out of the screen at the beginning of the "°oké°" (line 1), and then by the "peanut" (the nickname for a special grasper having a piece of mesh gauze rolled and fixed on its tip), an instrument manoeuvred by another assistant, which becomes visible in image 18. Both the hook and the peanut enter the visual field of the camera and position themselves progressively in the middle (image 19). This positioning is completed when the surgeon announces the new step in the procedure (line 3) and shows the adrenal vein with his hook positioned just under it (at the end of "now", line 3, see image 19). At that point, the camera assistant responds to the instruction and does a fast zoom in towards the adrenal vein (image 20) just before the surgeon describes his action and space of action (line 5). Again, what seems to be crucial for the assistant to be able to grant the directive is the recognizable emergence of a visual field graspable in terms of the surgical action the camera will make possible.

In sum, the analysis of the instructed action of the camera assistant cannot rely only on the description of the paired action directive/compliance but has also to include the progressive establishment of a relevant praxeological context that makes the instruction intelligible and accountable. The temporality of the instructed action depends on the emergent character of this context, and is further characterized by early versus late responses, displaying the possibility of anticipating versus

Excerpt 20 (2701 k1d1-13.55)

```
1   SUR     %oké* on va se rapprocher enco*re%
            okay we get closer again
                *hook advances-->
    im      %im.16                              %im.17
2           (0.2! %0.8* 1.5)
    pea      !peanut enters the field, advances till is positioned->
    sur          ->*hook is positioned-->
    im           %im.18
3           so we begin no%w!*
                        -->*hook under adrenal vein back and forth->
    pea                 --->!
    im                    %im.19
```

```
4           (1.0) + (0.5)
    cam           +zooms in quickly->
5   SUR     to pass% under+ the (1.0) the adrenal vein
    cam              ->+
    im           %im.20
```

following the requested action. These responses, then, adjust to the different trajectories of either a continuous (thus projectable) or a new course of action.

Moreover, these responses exhibit the competent action of the assistant, to which we now turn.

9.7   Skilled Collaboration in the Operating Room

The very possibility that the requested action can be made by a skilled assistant even without instructions raises the question of the intelligibility of instructions (cf. section 9.5) and also that of the skilled character of instructed action. The latter point is discussed here on the basis of the paired action "coag"/activation of cautery, developing the analyses of section 9.5.2 above.

This analysis is based on two operations using the same approach to the same pathology and performed by the same chief surgeon. The modes of coordination within the team are different in these two cases – and this casts light on the mechanisms of collaboration as well as on the experience and skills required to perform the instructed action.

During the first operation, recorded in 1998, from which are extracted the data analysed so far (see section 9.5.2), the mode of coordination with the assistant is very stable. The surgeon systematically says no more than "coag" or "coagulation". This is systematic, although the precise sequential moment at which the directive is produced may vary, as well as may the time of the response. However, in another video recording of the very same operation, performed by the surgeon seven years later (in 2005) with another assistant, Anna, the paired action is realized in two different coordination modes, showing different degrees of explicitness of the instructions. The next excerpts focus on the latter case.

While in the other operation the action of coagulating is never topicalized or negotiated, in this operation, it is striking that the paired actions – "coag" and the response, cauterizing the tissue – are explicitly formulated. In the first part of the procedure, the surgeon indicates that the verbalization of the instruction can be omitted, but announces that, in the second part, this will not be the case.

In this excerpt, the surgeon formulates the mode of coordination between his action and the assistant. It is not necessary to verbalize the instruction since the assistant "knows" (lines 1–2). Interestingly, the very next activation of the coagulation is, nevertheless, done by means of an instruction in the form of "oui, h" (line 4), which appears to be responsive to the assistant tacitly asking for it, and which is followed by the activation of the coagulation. This is the case of the next one (line 8) too (see the single and double arrows). On the contrary, the subsequent case (the assistant activates the coagulating hook, line 11, when the surgeon utters "follows") is realized without any instruction, as is the next one (line 13, see the thick arrow). At line 16, the surgeon gives the instruction again ("oui h") but does not do so for the following one (line 18). So, immediately after the formulation of the instruction's rule, we observe a mixed mode of coordination, alternating between tacit and explicit instructions. This "mixed" regime is adjusted to the embeddedness of the operation and the demonstration that constitutes the multi-activity. The instruction "oui" is uttered between one

Excerpt 21 (2005/"Vous y allez sans que j' vous l' dise")

```
 1  SUR        très bien vous y allez sans que j'vous l'di:se
               very well you go on without me telling you anything
 2             puisque vous savez anna hein?
               since you know Anna don't you?
 3             (0.6)
 4  SUR  →     oui, h (.) +pour la veine cave on fera autrement
               yes          for the vena cava we'll proceed differently
    ass  ⇉           +activ. coag
 5             (0.5)
 6  SUR        okay so:, (.) we c- we can use the scissors or the hook,
 7             (.)
 8  SUR  →     oui:
               yes:
 9             (+3.1)
    ass  ⇉      +activ. coag
10  SUR        and you see that the retractor, (0.3) of the first
11             assistant, (0.6) +follows+ the: hoo:k,
    ass  ➡          +activ. coag+
12             (0.3)
13  SUR        and so we have a very good +traction,+ (0.6)
    ass  ➡                                +activ. coag+
14             during all the dissection.
15             (1.3)
16  SUR→       oui h,
               yes h,
17             (+2.4)
    ass  ⇉      +activ. coag
18  SUR        very important to go on the right +si:de,+ (0.5) even
    ass  ➡                                       +activ. coag+
19             if we know that the gland is:, on thee (.) internal
20             part of the (0.5) of the monitor,
```

completed unit and another (lines 8, 16), i.e., when the temporality of the operation fits with the temporality of the talked demonstration; on the contrary, when the relevant moment for coagulating is situated in the middle of a syntactic unit, the instruction is omitted and the activation of the coagulation is achieved tacitly by the assistant following the operating action of the chief surgeon (see section 9.5 for evidences of participants' orientations to linguistic units and for a detailed description of this alternating organization of the multi-activity).

The instruction concerning the management of the coagulating hook, lines 1–2, is promptly restricted to a particular phase of the operation. In line 4, the surgeon announces that the rule will be different when they come nearer the vena cava. In this way, he differentiates two moments in the operation and displays that the second needs a revision of the collaboration mode established in the first.

Indeed, later on, when they come closer to the dissection of the vena cava, we can observe a new formulation of the rule (Excerpt 22).

Excerpt 22 (2005/"maintenant c'est moi qui dis")

```
 1  SUR        we have also the good plan because we need to have (0.4)
 2              a posterior good plan. (0.2) and to take off all the:
 3              fat, (0.5) around the: h (1.4) thee adrenal gland. h
 4              (0.3)
 5  SUR        coag
 6              (1.0 + (0.5)
    ass              +activ. coag
 7  SUR        uh (.) là maintenant c'est moi qui l'di:s,
               eh (.) right now it's up to me to tell you,
 8              (1.0)
 9  SUR        coag,
10              + (4.8)
    ass        +activ. coag
11  SUR        ouais h
               yeah h
12              (0.8) + (0.8)
    ass              +activ. coag
13  SUR        so we need to extend a little bit the: (0.2) dissection
14              because we want now, coag
15              + (2.3)
    ass        +activ. coag
16  SUR        to see the vena cava.
```

In line 7, the surgeon highlights the "here" and "now" as being the starting point of a new rule ("c'est moi qui l'di:s"), which contrasts explicitly with the first formulation ("vous y allez sans que j'vous l'di:se", line 1 – Excerpt 21). In the remaining part of the operation, he systematically produces the instruction before the assistant activates the coagulation. This modification of the rule happens when they come closer to the adrenal gland and the vena cava, as announced, i.e., when they arrive in an area presenting more risks.

In this same operation, "coag" can be integrated in a variety of expressions, elaborating the instruction and showing the variety of features the coagulation has to take into consideration, as in Excerpt 23.

Excerpt 23 (2005/"pas d'coag")

```
 1  SUR        and so: it will be: (0.2) easier to mobilize a
 2              little more the: (0.8) coag, (2.1) the liver,
 3              (0.6)
 4  SUR  →     pas d'coag s'il vous plaît,
               no coag please,
 5              (8.0)
 6  SUR        coag
 7              (2.1)
 8  SUR  →     stop eh,
 9              (1.6)
10  SUR        coag h,
11              (2.8)
```

Here we have two instances of specific instructions modifying the simple "coag" form. In the first, the surgeon initiates a movement of the hook around a vein which is not designed to dissect it but is done in order to make the contour of the vein visible; in this case, the surgeon makes explicitly clear that this is *not* an environment where the coagulation is expected or adequate, by using a *negative* instruction. Immediately after this, the next "coag" is also modified, showing another feature of this instructed action, its length, modulated through the added instruction "stop".

In the operation I recorded in 1998, this latter feature is never made explicit by the surgeon ("coag" is used in a very homogeneous and invariant way through the whole operation). This – *ex negativo* – shows the skilled adjustments constantly performed by the assistant, who adequately achieves the instruction by identifying not only the "here" and the "now" but also the "how" of the relevant action to be performed.

So, we can distinguish between procedures in which the surgeon uses a unique form of directive – "coag" – and procedures in which he uses a variety of instructions – "coag", "no coag", "stop coag". The former orients to the expertise of the assistant within an acquainted team and displays skilled tacit interpretation of the instructed action. The latter shows how the details of the instruction are produced moment by moment accompanying the ongoing closely monitored instructed action. So, expertise, skills and professional competencies are accountably embodied in the organization of action and in its detailed recipient-designed formatting.

9.8 Conclusion

Surgery is a highly collaborative practice, performed by well-coordinated teams. This collaboration can be described at various levels, taking into consideration a diversified set of participants – ranging from anaesthetists to scrub nurses, from the operating surgeon to his or her assistants. This collaboration can also take different forms and be achieved either within multimodal exchanges during a procedure or in a silent and tacit way. In this chapter, I chose to focus on instructions given by the surgeon to one of his assistants, formatted both in a verbal and in an embodied way. These explicit requests and directives display a specific form of complementarity and asymmetry that is related to issues of responsibility and authority.

This chapter has analysed three key actions in which these requests and directives can be observed: instructing the manoeuvring of the endoscopic camera, directing the assistant's hand positioning and requesting the assistant to activate the coagulating hook. These actions are central for achieving the visual access and visual intelligibility of the procedure, for securing the coordination of the surgeons' gestures and for achieving dissection. Various formats of instructions have been described through which the surgeon directs the action of his assistant, and the assistant responds by complying with the instructions, within a particular format of collaborative achievement. These instructions can be described as sequences constituted by a first action projecting and making expectable the second. Moreover, the first action is prepared in a way that makes the second intelligible.

Instructions are a significant example of collaboration. The response to a directive is not a mere reaction to what the directive tells one to do but is an active engagement in a specific form of action assembled as an adequate response under specific circumstances, a specific ecology and a specific course of action. In this sense, if instructions are necessarily indexical, the praxeological environment in which they are initiated and prepared makes them accountable and understandable. Their accountability also depends on the professional vision and the surgical skills of the assistant. In turn, their formatting is recipient-designed in a way that orients towards the supposed competence of the collaborator.

The detailed analysis of instructions shows how this form of coordination is achieved by the participants orienting to and actively considering a range of complex auditive and visual features in the environment of the operating room. This shows, in turn, how actions such as directives or requests instructing an action to be done here and now are profoundly embedded in the local ecology and rely on complex multimodal resources.

The detailed analysis of instructions reveals how coordination and collaboration in the operating room are achieved in a finely tuned way, by the participants both mobilizing a range of auditive and visual resources to communicate together and considering the local ecology of the surgical action and the dynamic anatomic environment in which the surgeon's actions are embedded. More generally, this kind of analysis sheds light on the fine-grained organization of teamwork, which is so crucial for managing surgery in an adequate, efficient and safe way.

Transcription Conventions

The excerpts have been transcribed according to conventions developed by Gail Jefferson and commonly used in conversation analysis (see Chapter 2).

Translation from French is given in italics in the line following the original.

For the conventions according to which descriptions of gestures and actions are transcribed, see below (cf. Mondada [2003a] and a detailed presentation online: https://franz.unibas.ch/fileadmin/franz/user_upload/redaktion/Mondada_conv_multimodality.pdf).

* *	a gesture is delimited between two symbols and synchronized with corresponding stretches of talk
cam	the participant making the movement is identified in the margin if (s)he is not the same person as the actual speaker
-----	the gesture is held until the next closing boundary symbol
---->	the gesture is held until the next symbol, situated on the following line
. . . .	gesture preparation
, , , ,	gesture retraction

References

Amerine, Ronald, and Jack Bilmes. 1988. Following Instructions. *Human Studies* 11: 327–39.

Bezemer, Jeff, Ged Murtagh, Alexandra Cope, Gunther Kress and Roger Kneebone. 2011. "Scissors, Please": The Practical Accomplishment of Surgical Work in the Operating Theater. *Symbolic Interaction* 34(3): 398–414.

Cekaite, Asta. 2010. Shepherding the Child: Embodied Directive Sequences in Parent-Child Interactions. *Text & Talk* 30(1): 1–25.

Craven, Alexandra, and Jonathan Potter. 2010. Directives: Entitlement and Contingency in Action. *Discourse Processes* 12(4): 419–42.

Curl, Traci S., and Paul Drew. 2008. Contingency and Action: A Comparison of Two Forms of Requesting. *Research on Language and Social Interaction* 41(2): 129–53.

Davidson, Judy. 1984. Subsequent Versions of Invitations, Offers, Requests, and Proposals Dealing with Potential or Actual Rejection. In *Structures of Social Action*, edited by J. Maxwell Atkinson and John Heritage, 102–28. Cambridge: Cambridge University Press.

De Stefani, Elwys and Marie-Danielle Gazin. 2014. Learning to Drive: Timing and the Spatial Embeddedness of Instructional Sequences in a Mobile Setting of Interaction. *Journal of Pragmatics* 65: 63–79.

Ervin-Tripp, Susan. 1976. "Is Sybil There?": The Structure of Some American English Directives. *Language in Society* 5: 25–66.

Garfinkel, Harold. 1967. *Studies in Ethnomethodology*. Englewood Cliffs, NJ: Prentice-Hall.

Garfinkel, Harold. 2002. *Ethnomethodology's Program*. New York: Rowman and Littlefield.

Goodwin Charles. 1994. Professional Vision. *American Anthropologist* 96(3): 606–33.

Goodwin, Marjorie H., and Asta Cekaite. 2012. Calibration in Directive/Response Sequences in Family Interaction. *Journal of Pragmatics* 46: 122–38.

Heath, Christian, Jon Hindmarsh and Paul Luff. 2010. *Video in Qualitative Research*. London: Sage.

Heinemann, Trine. 2006. "Will You or Can't You?" Displaying Entitlement in Interrogative Requests. *Journal of Pragmatics* 38: 1081–104.

Hindmarsh, Jon, and Alison Pilnick. 2002. The Tacit Order of Teamwork: Collaboration and Embodied Conduct in Anaesthesia. *Sociological Quarterly* 43: 139–64.

Hindmarsh, Jon, and Alison Pilnick. 2007. Knowing Bodies at Work: Embodiment and Ephemeral Teamwork in Anaesthesia. *Organization Studies* 28(9): 1395–416.

Hirschauer, Stefan. 1991. The Manufacture of Bodies in Surgery. *Social Studies of Science* 21(2): 279–319.

Katz, Pearl. 1999. *The Scalpel's Edge: The Culture of Surgeons*. Boston: Allyn and Bacon.

Koschmann, Tim, Curtis LeBaron, Charles Goodwin and Paul Feltovich. 2011. "Can You See the Cystic Artery Yet?" A Simple Matter of Trust. *Journal of Pragmatics* 43(2): 521–41.

Koschmann, Tim, Curtis LeBaron, Charles Goodwin, Alan Zemel and Gary Dunnington. 2007. Formulating the Triangle of Doom. *Gesture* 7(1): 97–118.

Koschmann, Tim, and Alan Zemel. 2011. "So That's the Ureter": The Informal Logic of Discovering Work. *Ethnographic Studies* 12: 31–46.

Labov, William, and Dan Fanshel. 1977. *Therapeutic Discourse: Psychotherapy as Conversation*. New York: Academic Press.

Lindström, Anna. 2005. Language as Social Action: A Study of How Senior Citizens Request Assistance with Practical Tasks in the Swedish Home Help Service. In *Syntax and Lexis in Conversation*, edited by Auli Hakulinen and Margret Selting, 209–30. Amsterdam: Benjamins.

Lindwall, Oskar, and Ekström Anna. 2012. Instructions-in-Interaction: The Teaching and Learning of a Manual Skill. *Human Studies* 35: 27–49.

Mondada, Lorenza. 2003a. Describing Surgical Gestures: The View from Researchers' and Surgeons' Video Recordings. In *Proceedings of the First International Gesture Conference, Austin, July 2002*. http://gesturestudies.com/files/isgsconferences/Contributions/Mondada/Austin-Mondada-txt_new.htm (accessed July 10, 2013).

Mondada, Lorenza. 2003b. Working with Video: How Surgeons Produce Video Records of Their Actions. *Visual Studies* 18(1): 58–72.

Mondada, Lorenza. 2006a. La compétence comme dimension située et contingente, localement évaluée par les participants [Competence as a situated and contingent dimension, locally evaluated by the participants]. *Bulletin VALS-ASLA* 84: 83–119.

Mondada, Lorenza. 2006b. Video Recording as the Reflexive Preservation of Fundamental Features for Analysis. In *Video Analysis*, edited by H. Knoblauch, J. Raab, H.G. Soeffner and B. Schnettler, 51–68. Bern: Lang.

Mondada, Lorenza. 2007a. Bilingualism and the Analysis of Talk at Work: Code-Switching as a Resource for the Organization of Action and Interaction. In *Bilingualism: A Social Approach*, edited by M. Heller, 297–318. New York: Palgrave.

Mondada, Lorenza. 2007b. Operating Together through Videoconference: Members' Procedures for Accomplishing a Common Space of Action. In *Orders of Ordinary Action*, edited by S. Hester and D. Francis, 51–67. Aldershot: Ashgate.

Mondada, Lorenza. 2007c. Turn taking in multimodalen und multiaktionalen Kontexten [Turn-taking in multimodal and multiactivity contexts]. In *Gesprächals Prozess: Linguistische Aspekte der Zeitlichkeitverbaler Interaktion [Talk as Process: Linguistic Dimensions of Temporality of Verbal Interaction]*, edited by Heiko Hausendorf, 237–76. Tübingen: Narr.

Mondada, Lorenza. 2011. The Organization of Concurrent Courses of Action in Surgical Demonstrations. In *Embodied Interaction, Language and Body in the Material World*, edited by Jürgen Streeck, Charles Goodwin and Curtis LeBaron, 207–26. Cambridge: Cambridge University Press.

Mondada, Lorenza. 2013. Coordinating Mobile Action in Real Time: The Timed Organization of Directives in Video Games. In *Mobility and Interaction*, edited by Pentti Haddington, Lorenza Mondada and Maurice Nevile, 300–41. Berlin: De Gruyter.

Mondada, Lorenza. 2014. Instructions in the Operating Room: How Surgeons Direct Their Assistant's Hands. *Discourse Studies* 16(2): 131–61.

Mondada, Lorenza. forthcoming a. Cooking Instructions and the Shaping of Things in the Kitchen. In *Interacting with Things*, edited by Maurice Nevile, Pentti Haddington, Trine Heinemann and Mirka Rauniomaa. Amsterdam: Benjamins.

Mondada, Lorenza. forthcoming b. The Temporal Orders of Multiactivity: Operating and Demonstrating in the Surgical Theatre. In *Multiactivity in Interaction*, edited by Pentti Haddington, Tiina Keisanen, Lorenza Mondada and Maurice Nevile. Amsterdam: Benjamins.

Mondada, Lorenza. forthcoming c. "Zoom Avant": Directing the Endoscopic Camera during Surgical Operations. In *Video at Work*, edited by Mathias Broth, Eric Laurier and Lorenza Mondada. London: Routledge.

Pettinari, Catherine. 1988. *Tasks Talk and Text in the Operating Room: A Study in Medical Discourse*. Norwood: Ablex.

Prentice, Rachel. 2012. *Bodies in Formation: Remaking Anatomy and Surgery Education*. Durham: Duke University Press.

Sanchez Svensson, Markus. 2005. *Configuring Awareness: Work, Interaction and Collaboration in Operating Theatres*. PhD thesis, University of London England.

Sanchez Svensson, Markus, Christian Heath and Paul Luff. 2007. Instrumental Action: The Timely Exchange of Implements during Surgical Operations. In *ECSCW '07: Proceedings of the Tenth European Conference on Computer Supported Cooperative Work*, edited by Liam Bannon et al., vol. ii, 41–60. Berlin: Springer.

Sanchez Svensson, Markus, Paul Luff and Christian Heath. 2009. Embedding Instructions in Practice: Contingency and Collaboration during Surgical Training. *Social Health & Illness* 31(6): 889–906.

Schegloff, Emanuel A. 1980. Preliminaries to Preliminaries: "Can I Ask You a Question?" *Sociological Inquiry* 50: 104–52.

Schegloff, Emanuel A. 2007. *Sequence Organization in Interaction: A Primer in Conversation Analysis*, vol. 1. Cambridge: Cambridge University Press.

Searle, John R. 1975. Indirect Speech Acts. In *Syntax and Semantics*, vol. 3, *Speech Acts*, edited by Peter Cole and Jerry L. Morgan, 261–86. New York: Academic Press.

Suchman, Lucy. 1987. *Plans and Situated Actions: The Problem of Human Machine Communication*. Cambridge: Cambridge University Press.

Wieder, Lawrence. 1974. Telling the Code. In *Ethnomethodology*, edited by Roy Turner, 144–72. Harmondsworth: Penguin.

Wittgenstein, Ludwig. 1953. *Philosophical Investigations*. London: Blackwell.

Wootton, Antony. 2005. Interactional and Sequential Features Informing Request Format Selection in Children's Speech. In *Syntax and Lexis in Conversation*, edited by Auli Hakulinen and Margret Selting, 185–207. Amsterdam: Benjamins.

Zimmerman, Don. 1971. The Practicalities of Rule Use. In *Understanding Everyday Life*, edited by Jack R. Douglas, 221–38. London: Routledge.

Lorenza Mondada, PhD, is professor of linguistics at the University of Basel. Her research deals with social interaction in ordinary, professional and institutional settings, within an ethnomethodological and conversation analytic perspective. She has published extensively in *Journal of Pragmatics*, *Discourse Studies*, *Language in Society* and *Research on Language and Social Interaction*, and co-edited several collective books on multimodality, mobility, multiactivity and knowledge in interaction.

10 "Coming Up!": Why Verbal Acknowledgement Matters in the Operating Theatre

Terhi Korkiakangas, Sharon-Marie Weldon, Jeff Bezemer and Roger Kneebone

10.1 Introduction

All too often, patient safety is compromised in the operating theatre. It is suggested that communication breakdowns account for the majority of inadvertent harm, patient morbidity and mortality in surgery (Lingard et al. 2006; Makary et al. 2007). Such problems are often implicated in routine practices, for example, the ways in which clinicians transfer information to one another (Lingard et al. 2004). Yet, exactly *how* these failures emerge in daily interactions has remained somewhat opaque. Detailed knowledge should be gained of such routines in order to improve communication and, as Lord Darzi (2008) stresses, the quality of healthcare.

In the UK, the Department of Health (DH) has repeatedly called for attention to learning from other industries in order to improve safety in clinical practice (Department of Health 2006). The implementation of the World Health Organization (WHO) surgical safety checklist (World Health Organization 2008) is a key example of this. Checklists were first introduced in aviation to address human error and to reduce reliance on memory. This approach was modelled to fit with the operating theatre so as to avoid fatal risks, such as wrong-site, wrong-procedure and wrong-patient surgeries, which are more common than thought (Seiden and Barach 2006). While the checklist has reduced surgical morbidity and patient mortality significantly (Haynes et al. 2009), its use is often inconsistent. Inadequacies have been found in team communication whilst using the checklist: the validation of items has been low and team members do not respond to the announcements from the list, sometimes substituting a clear verbal response with a silent nod (Cullati et al. 2013). For some, the WHO checklist has become a "tick-box" exercise that is hurried or not completed at all (Vats et al. 2010) and, as such, can do little for effective communication and patient safety.

In many industries outside healthcare, communication practices that involve speech have been standardized. Consider, for instance, police radio dispatchers, who communicate with field officers through code-language, which enables a fast exchange of information. In restaurant kitchens, teams communicate by *"speaking kitchen"* (in acclaimed pastry chef Shuna Lydon's terms). This means that requests and orders are promptly responded to ("Yes, chef!"), which in turn informs the head chef that their request was heard. Responding clearly to the talk of others serves an important function and can sustain situational awareness – that is, knowledge about "what is going on", what others are doing and what action one should take in a given situation (Endsley 1995; Hazelhurst et al. 2007). Lessons from aviation have taught us that talk which is misheard, or not heard at all, represents the most frequent cause of errors and accidents (Isaac 2007).

Acknowledging or checking what a colleague has said can be crucial even in routine communication, as mistakes happen. Many patient fatalities have been linked to inter-collegial communication. In 2005, a high-profile case in the UK drew attention to *human factors*, showing that errors and accidents happen in much the same way in the clinical context and aviation. In this case, Elaine Bromiley, a patient, lost her life due to an emergency intubation failure during induction of anaesthesia for a routine operation. Elaine's difficulty with breathing quickly escalated into a state of emergency, and retrospective accounts have highlighted how communication broke down between the professionals involved: the consultants, who were "fixated" on their efforts to keep Elaine alive, did not respond to nurses who were speaking to them, and some of the nurses refrained from speaking up to the consultants, even when they knew how to potentially save Elaine's life (Bromiley 2008).

Talk can serve as an important communicative resource, specifically in high-risk environments such as the operating theatre. Indeed, Goffman (1983: 3) has noted that talk, in general, has a specific importance "when something doesn't go as indicated and expected". Spoken practices have been addressed in clinical settings to some extent. For instance, the SBAR (situation, background, assessment, recommendation) briefing model, originally developed in the U.S. Navy, provides a frame and a predictable structure for articulating a message that can facilitate information transfer, such as when a nurse calls a doctor for assistance (Haig et al. 2006). *Check-back* exchange is central: if the doctor orders medication, say, the nurse *repeats* the medication requested, and the doctor *confirms* this. There is some evidence to suggest that the SBAR, like the WHO checklist, has increased patient safety (Haig et al. 2006; Leonard et al. 2004; McFerran et al. 2005); yet breakdowns of communication still occur. It is thus important to more carefully examine communication on the "shop floor" of the operating theatre.

When a surgical operation is in progress, communication between surgeons and nurses is largely organized around requests and responses to these. That is, surgeons ask for something – be it a material *object* (e.g., a surgical instrument) or an *action* (e.g., green lights to be turned on) – and nurses respond to surgeons. These seemingly unremarkable exchanges are fundamental for getting the business done in the operating theatre. Consider how a surgeon needs different instruments for different procedures and issues requests to a *scrub nurse*, who is in charge of instrument exchanges with the surgeon. The scrub nurse should be available to pass the requested instruments in a timely manner, ideally at the precise time of need. Likewise, when the surgeon needs gas, suction or lights to be turned on or off, it is the task of the *circulating nurses* (or circulators) to assist so that the surgical work can continue.

Video-ethnographic methods provide insight into these interactions and how they unfold in real time. Importantly, video can be used to identify issues that often go unnoticed by the professionals who are immersed in their work. To date, a handful of video studies have examined communication between surgeons (e.g., Koschmann et al. 2011; Mondada 2011, 2014a, b; Moore et al. 2010), surgeons and scrub nurses (Bezemer et al. 2011a, b, 2015; Korkiakangas et al. 2014; Sanchez Svensson et al. 2007), and surgeons and anaesthetists (Hindmarsh and Pilnick 2002, 2007). These studies have elaborated on the use of speech and bodily resources, such as gaze, gesture and movements, in understanding what colleagues are doing and gauging the implications for the task at hand. For example, a scrub nurse can anticipate an instrument request from a surgeon's arm movement alone, and the instrument can change hands without either party uttering a word (Bezemer et al. 2011b). Such exchanges can give an air of seamlessness in communication between surgeons and nurses. Yet, as noted, not all communication can happen without speech; one question we explore is: When and how do surgeons and nurses use talk to achieve tasks necessary for the progression of an operation, including the passing of instruments and fixing of equipment?

New social scientific approaches could make an important contribution to patient safety (Iedema 2009; Iedema et al. 2009; Vincent 2009) and surgical practice by studying communication at a more detailed level than is usually done. In this chapter, we offer an examination of a unique corpus of video recordings made at the operating theatre suites of a UK hospital, collected as part of a video-ethnographic project on team communication. The study zooms in on the practice of *responsiveness*: how requests and questions are responded to and how they impact on communication during surgical operations. We will consider different ways in which nurses respond to surgeons: some involve speech and some do not. Surgeons and nurses might not always be aware of how these exchanges impact the "flow" of an operation. Sometimes, things are being done while nothing is being said, and all works well in the theatre. Yet, at other times, when nothing is being said, it can have particular implications even if things are being *done*.

So, what are these moments that do not involve talk? Previous literature has paid some attention to "silences" in clinical communication from different angles.

Some suggest that nurses' silence can relate to many issues, such as power dynamics with surgeons, and that nurses do not often voice their concerns in the operating theatre (Gardezi et al. 2009; Newton et al. 2012). Others suggest that silences indicate "undiscussables": when nurses witness shortcuts, rule-breaking and poor teamwork from clinical colleagues, only one in ten nurses speaks up (Maxfield et al. 2005). However, silences can also emerge in undramatic cases, such as when colleagues request assistance from one another; in this chapter, we will consider such instances. Since emergency situations magnify the need of effective communication, it is important to examine speaking, responding and silences also as part of the mundane so as to understand their mechanisms and impact on safety. Communication involving circulators in the theatre has been rarely studied in detail. Yet, circulators are central for the running of operations, increasingly so of laparoscopic operations that involve frequent fixing of cameras, monitors and the like. Equipment repairs, in particular, require rapid action from circulators, as technical failures are a major contributor to delayed operating times (Gupta et al. 2011). Thus, when requesting assistance, surgeons also talk to circulators. It is of interest how communication is managed when surgeons relay requests to different nurses, and how nurses in different roles respond to surgeons.

10.2 Method

10.2.1 Research Site and Data Collection

This exploratory video-ethnographic study draws on video analysis to examine communication in the operating theatre. Ethical approval was obtained from the NHS Research Ethics Committee for video-based fieldwork in a major teaching hospital in London. The data collection was conducted between August 2012 and January 2013. Two researchers from the team spent a month observing operations, during which time they familiarized themselves with the theatre sites and staff. The surgeons, nurses, operating theatre practitioners and anaesthetists were individually consented to being filmed as the researchers had gradually introduced their wish to collect video data of teamwork during operations. The participants were recruited through convenience sampling, and informed consent often had to be sought continually throughout a day due to a frequent rotation of staff and visitors in the theatres.

During data collection, a total of 29 operations were observed, 20 of which were recorded using two tripod-mounted HD video cameras, producing over 68 hours of film. The filmed operations feature four different consultant surgeons, five registrars, five operating theatre practitioners, four consultant anaesthetists, and 10 nurses involved in general surgical, upper gastrointestinal and bariatric laparoscopic procedures. For the current purposes, a subsample of nine operations has been examined in detail. The cases involve six laparoscopic operations (total duration 480 minutes) and three open operations (total duration 324 minutes), creating a total of 13 hours and 24 minutes of footage that has been analysed.

10.2.2 Data Analysis

All video data were reviewed by two authors (TK & SMW), who created a detailed log of communication events in a subsample of the entire data corpus (see Table 10.1 for an example). This involved a careful reviewing of the operations from start to finish and logging every form of interactional event (e.g., request, question, repetition, response; whether response was produced verbally or nonverbally; associated bodily conduct/position from each team member; and whether any music was played during an operation). The logged events were time-coded, producing a transcript of each operation. The authors logged the first operation together, and random subsamples were taken from following cases to check for the consistency of the logs.

These logs were discussed with the entire team and selected case examples were replayed and analysed. This chapter focuses on one phenomenon identified in the logs: how nurses responded to requests (for objects or actions) from surgeons in the course of an operation. It was noted that sometimes nurses responded to the surgeon *verbally* and sometimes *actionally*. For example, in Table 10.1, at [00:33:41.12] a scrub nurse produces an actional response to a surgeon's request for a Langenbeck (she "moves back to trolley and picks up several instruments"). However, at [00:34:49.00] the same nurse responds differently to a request for

Table 10.1: Example fragment from a coding log

Time	Participant	Action	Verbal description	Nonverbal description	Music
[00:31:42.14]	Consultant	REQUEST		Takes scalpel from trolley.	NONE
[00:33:39.03]	Consultant	REQUEST	"Langenbeck please"	Focuses on operative field.	NONE
[00:33:41.12]	Scrub nurse	RESPONSE		Moves back to trolley and picks up several instruments.	NONE
[00:34:45.15]	Consultant	REQUEST	"Can I have an Alexis please?"	Focuses on operative field.	NONE
[00:34:49.00]	Scrub nurse	RESPONSE	"Yep"	Tilts head to hear consultant, and quickly retrieves object	NONE

an Alexis (instrument): she produces a verbal response ("yep") and an actional response ("tilts head to hear consultant and quickly retrieves object"). Although surgeons can also produce requests in different ways (verbally and/or through action), here we are centrally concerned with spoken requests, which are sometimes addressed to scrub nurses and sometimes to circulators. In this chapter, the actions that might be characterized as directives have been subsumed under the term *request*, for the sake of simplicity.

The chosen methodology responds to a recent call for new approaches in patient safety research. We are drawing on video-ethnography and interactional analysis of fragments of communication as identified in the film. These are critical examples of events that illustrate broader themes in our data set and thus warrant an in-depth analysis of them. In line with this essentially qualitative approach, we first present a quantitative analysis of the distribution of response practices. After this, we subject the selected examples to a detailed interactional video analysis, drawing on the framework of *conversation analysis* (CA) (Schegloff 2007) and multimodal (e.g., body movement) considerations.

The analysis involves a transcription of strips of interaction from the video: making visible how spoken interactions map onto the bodily conduct of nurses and surgeons on a second-by-second basis (see Chapter 2 and Appendix for transcription conventions). Still images have been used to illustrate the key moments transcribed. S*equence organization*, which is the key principle of CA, was used to inform the observations represented in the transcripts. This refers to the ways in which social interactions are organized through recognizable beginnings and ends, such as asking a question and producing an answer. For example, a *request* from a surgeon initiates an interactional sequence, which places constraints on what a nurse should do next: *respond*. That is, when a request or a question (*a sequence initiating action*) is issued, a response (*a responsive action*) is expected to follow (for a more detailed analysis of requests and directives during surgical operations, see Mondada 2014a, b). However, it is not only important that a nurse should respond, but also *when* they should respond: in the sequential space following the request. Although at first glance this might seem trivial, the following analyses show that the type and timing of a response can be consequential to the operation at hand.

10.3 Findings

10.3.1 Distributional Analysis of Different Response Practices

Nurses responded to surgeons' requests either actionally, or verbally *and* actionally (see Table 10.2 for an illustration).

Table 10.2: Request and response formats

SURGEON	REQUEST* Example: • "Scissors please."
NURSE	ACTIONAL RESPONSE Example: • [passes scissors to surgeon] VERBAL RESPONSE** Example: • "Just a moment."

* Requests or directives.
** Verbal responses were followed by actional responses
(approximately within a minimum of 2 seconds).

To consider the distribution of these response practices, the observed request-response exchanges were quantified in a subsample of nine surgical operations (Table 10.3). The frequencies were measured according to the *relevance* of a request for an (implied) addressee. For example, if a request was made for surgical items on the instrument trolley, the implied addressee was the scrub nurse who should respond. If a request was made for action (e.g., gas off, lights on) or for an item beyond the instrument trolley (the sterile field), the implied addressee was (mostly) a circulator. However, sometimes the implied nurse did *not* respond to the request, and these were recorded as "no-responses".

In these nine operations, a total of 831 requests were documented from surgeons; 284 verbal + actional responses, 505 actional responses and 42 no-responses were documented to these requests. Scrub nurses did not respond to initial requests or questions on 12 occasions (2 per cent); and circulators did not respond to initial requests or questions on 30 occasions (12.7 per cent). The no-responses resulted in surgeons repeating their original request or question. A chi-squared test was performed for the overall difference in scrub nurses' and circulators' responses. This was highly significant (X^2=102.3031571 with a p-value of <0.000). A further Z test was performed to see if the differences in distribution were statistically significant (Table 10.3).

Table 10.3: Different response types exhibited by scrub nurses and circulators in nine operations

Response type	Scrub Nurse observed (%)	Scrub Nurse CIs	Circulator observed (%)	Circulator CIs	Total	2-sided p-value
Actional	421 (70.8%)	67.1%, 74.4%	84 (35.6%)	29.5%, 41.7%	505	p<0.00000
Verbal + Actional	162 (27.2%)	23.6%, 30.8%	122 (51.7%)	45.3%, 58.1%	284	p<0.00000
No-response	12 (2%)	0.9%, 3.1%	30 (12.7%)	8.5%, 17%	42	p<0.0001
Total	595 (100%)		236 (100%)		831	

A breakdown of the response types and their p-values using a Z test revealed that scrub nurses used significantly more actional responses (70.8 per cent; Confidence Interval 67.1, 74.4) than circulators (35.6 per cent; CI 29.5, 41.7), and that circulators had significantly more no-responses (12.7 per cent; CI 8.5, 17) compared to scrub nurses (2 per cent; CI 0.9, 3.1). Although circulators exhibited more verbal + actional responses (51.7 per cent; CI 45.3, 58.1) than scrub nurses (27.2 per cent; CI 23.6, 30.8), they still showed significantly more no-responses to the requests. This implies that there is an increased chance for inadequate surgeon-circulator communication, which warrants further examination in the following section.

10.3.2 Interactional Video Analysis

We use qualitative video analysis to consider each of these responses (actional, verbal + actional, and no-response) and their implications for communication.

Actional response: Responding through physical action

Nurses often produced *actional* responses to surgeons' requests (see Transcript 10.1). These responses did not involve talk, but some sort of physical activity. For example, a nurse handed out a requested item to the surgeon.

Transcript 10.1: Actional response [Examples 1, 2, 3]

```
Example 1
[00:27:50.20] Surgeon: Local please
[00:27:52.12] [Scrub nurse passes dish with syringe to surgeon]

Example 2
[00:29:50.29] Surgeon: Scissors.
[00:29:52.21] [Scrub nurse hands scissors to surgeon]

Example 3
[00:09:29.11] Surgeon: Clip
[00:09:30.20] [Scrub nurse passes clip to surgeon]
```

The requests were fulfilled almost immediately through action. In Transcript 10.2, the scrub nurse passed a requested local anaesthetic syringe to the surgeon within approximately one and a half seconds.

Transcript 10.2: Actional response [Example 1]

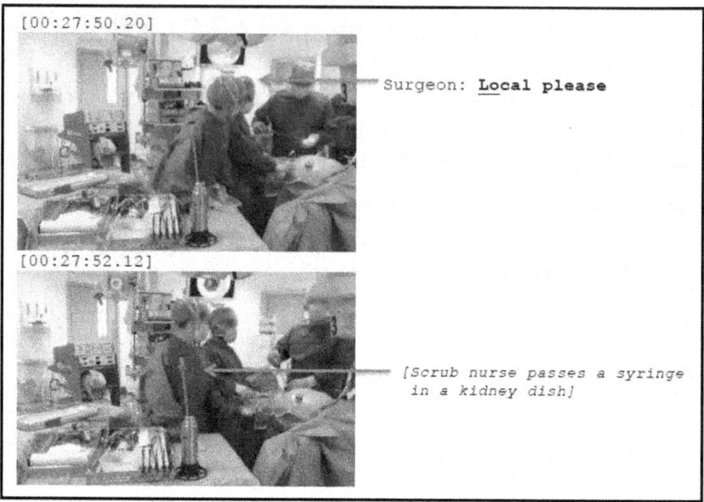

The lapse between a surgeon's request and a nurse's passing gesture was generally approximately 1–2 seconds. This is the time it takes to pick up the item (usually from the instrument trolley) and safely hand it over to the surgeon. When the scrub nurse was already holding the item and had their body aligned with the surgeon, the passings were often swift, with the onset of passing within a second or so from the request. The interactional features of nurse-surgeon object passings have been considered elsewhere (Korkiakangas et al. 2014).

On other occasions, it was the circulator who responded to the surgeon's requests, such as for lights to be turned on or off, a laparoscopic monitor to be moved, or an equipment failure to be fixed. As these requests involve touching of non-sterile objects, they are not the responsibility of the scrub nurse, but rather of the unscrubbed circulator (see Transcript 10.3).

Transcript 10.3: Actional response [Examples 4, 5, 6]

```
Example 4
[00:10:58.06] Surgeon: Gas on please
[00:11:00.28] [Circulator turns gas on]

Example 5
[00:28:17.13] Surgeon: Gas off.
[00:38:23.21] [Circulator turns gas off]

Example 6
[00:43:13.25] Surgeon: Turn the light up to 107 please.
[00:43:17.10] [Circulator adjusts light]
```

Here too the circulator responded through action and no talk was involved. On examining the proximity and visual orientation of the participants, it became evident that in all of these cases (Examples 1–6), the surgeon, scrub nurse and circulator had visual access to each other. So, as the surgeon had uttered his request, he could see (albeit sometimes peripherally) that the scrub nurse, who was positioned near him, was picking up the item and passing it over. Or, the surgeon could see that the circulator was about to turn the gas on and was thereby acting upon the request. Talk might not be needed when a request can be fulfilled more or less immediately and when the actional fulfilment is noticeable.

Verbal + actional response: Responding through talk and action

Not all responses were produced without talk. Occasionally, when a surgeon asked for something, the actional response was preceded by a verbal acknowledgement of the request. In Transcript 10.4, the examples involve requests addressed by the surgeon to different professionals in the theatre team.

Transcript 10.4: Verbal response [Examples 7, 8, 9]

```
Example 7
[00:13:23.24] Surgeon: Can I have a little more head up please Joan.
[00:13:26.00] Anaesthetist: You can

Example 8
[00:16:40.22] Surgeon: Can I have a tonsil swab Mona please.
[00:16:42.22] Scrub nurse: Tonsil swab,

Example 9
[01:22:03.28] Surgeon: Gas on please,
[01:22:05.15]Circulator: Ye:s coming
```

In the above exchanges, each request was first followed by a verbal response. These were used to confirm the receipt of a request. Therefore, these were *different* from the examples where only an actional response was produced. So, why were verbal responses produced here but not in the earlier cases? It is necessary to take closer look at these fragments and to examine what else is happening. Consider again our earlier Example 4 – a request for gas – but now with video stills (in Transcript 10.5). Here the circulator produced an actional response almost immediately by walking over to the gas machine. The gas was turned on in two seconds or so from the request.

However, a similar request for gas received a different response in Example 9 (Transcript 10.6).

Transcript 10.5: Actional response [Example 4]

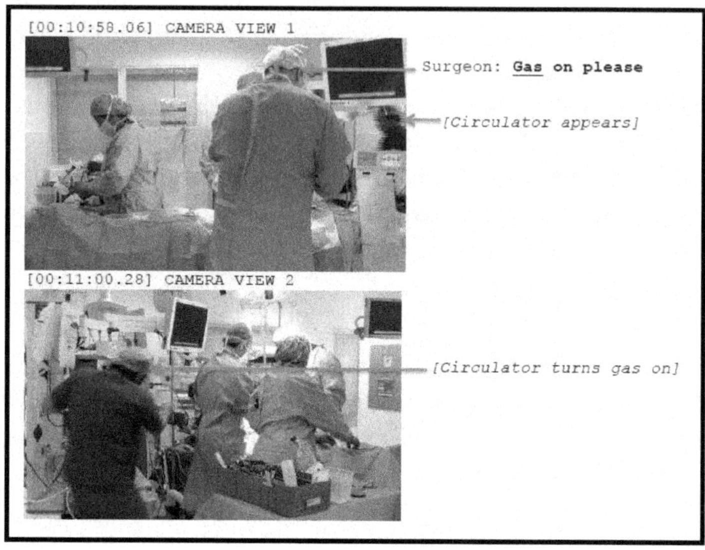

Transcript 10.6: Verbal + Actional response [Example 9]

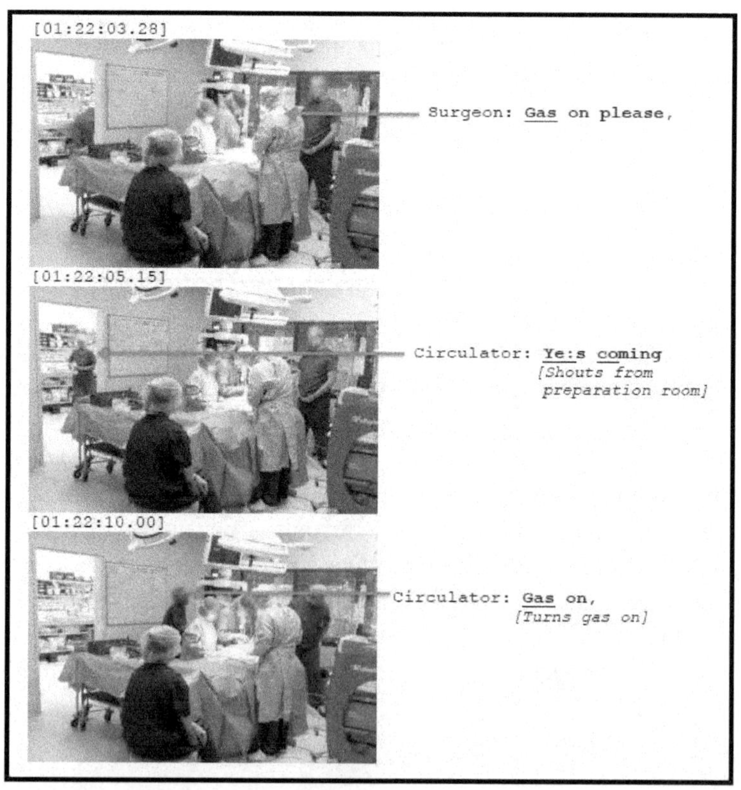

Note again, how in each of the examples, the surgeon asked a colleague to *do* something: to *turn* a switch, to *lower* the table, to *pass* an item. Thus, an action response is required. However, theatre professionals are routinely engaged in *multiactivity* (see Haddington et al. 2014) and orienting to many concerns at once. Therefore they might not be able to change the course of action immediately. As in Example 9, the circulator was momentarily out of the theatre site, in the adjacent preparation room. So when she was called to turn on the gas, she was not readily available to do so. This was accounted for by her verbal acknowledgement ("Yes coming"), which she produced in response to the request. This verbal response oriented to the time it would take her to reach the switch (here approximately 6.5 seconds) and informed the surgeon that the request, nevertheless, had been heard. Also in Example 7 (Transcript 10.7), there was a slight delay before the anaesthetist could act upon the request.

Transcript 10.7: Verbal + Actional response [Example 7]

```
Example 7
[00:13:23.24] Surgeon: Can I have a little more head up please Joan.
[00:13:26.00] Anaesthetist: You can
[00:13:32.00] [Anaesthetist adjusts table]
```

The surgeon asked the anaesthetist to level the patient's head higher: "Can I have a little more head up please, Joan." To do this, the anaesthetist had to first locate a remote control so that the table could be adjusted. Therefore, as the anaesthetist responded, "You can", she acknowledged the request *before* physically adjusting the operating table (approximately 9 seconds after the request).

In Example 8 (Transcript 10.8), the surgeon requested a tonsil swab from the scrub nurse. While the scrub nurse was present by the instrument trolley, she was simultaneously responsible for guarding and preparing the instruments, and for keeping a track of where they were. Sometimes this might impact on her ability to be immediately ready to exchange objects; sometimes locating a requested item might take a while, and therefore a verbal response became relevant. Thus here, as the nurse momentarily turned away from the surgeon, she acknowledged the request ("Tonsil swab") before passing the item over (approximately 6 seconds after the request).

Transcript 10.8: Verbal + Actional response [Example 8]

```
Example 8
[00:16:40.22] Surgeon: Can I have a tonsil swab Mona please.
[00:16:42.22] Scrub nurse: Tonsil swab,
[00:16:46.00] [Scrub nurse passes a swab to surgeon]
```

Delayed actional response: When a verbal acknowledgement is missing

So far we have considered two ways of responding, which orient to the immediacy or delay with which a colleague can do what was requested. The analysis suggests that a delay in an actional response relates to the production of a verbal acknowledgement. However, these acknowledgements were not consistently produced. There was yet a third way in which the professionals dealt with requests: acting upon the request while remaining *silent*. In the following, we consider the implications of this, starting with Example 10 (Transcript 10.9).

Transcript 10.9: Absent verbal response [Example 10]

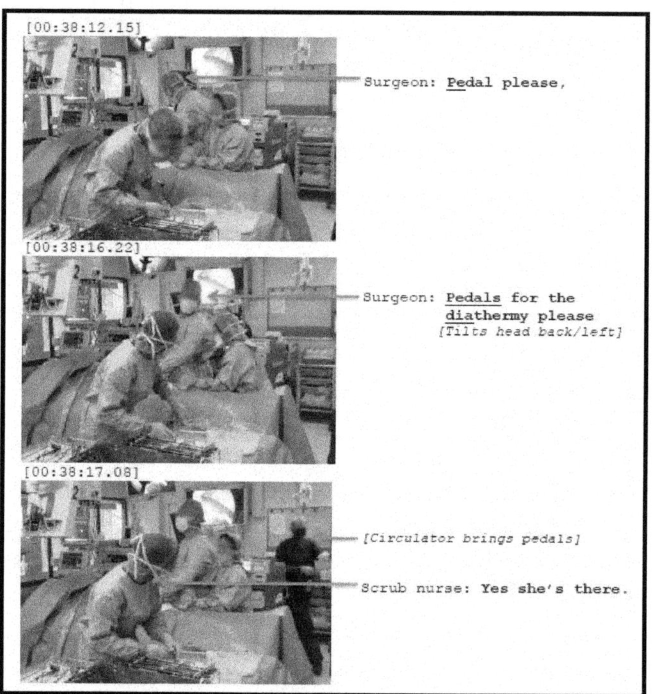

The surgeon asked for pedals for a diathermy machine in order to dissect a piece of tissue. He did not immediately receive a response to this first request. However, from the video we could see that a circulator was busy locating the item behind the theatre equipment (in the background), as there were no pedals immediately at hand. A four-second silent interval passed, after which the surgeon *repeated* his request louder, "Pedals for the diathermy please." While doing so, he turned to look over his left shoulder (apparently in search of a circulator) thereby taking his eyes off the monitor, while holding a surgical instrument inside the patient's body. It was only *after* this repeated request that the scrub nurse quietly responded to him, "Yes she's [the circulator's] there." Shortly after this the circulator appeared carrying the foot pedals.

In this fragment, both of the nurses had apparently heard the surgeon's initial request, however neither of them had acknowledged it verbally. The fact that the pedals were not immediately available, but had to be searched out, would have made an acknowledgement relevant. Secondly, the circulator was not in the visual field of the surgeon, but rather *behind his back*. The lack of visual access and absence of acknowledgement resulted in the surgeon having to repeat himself and reconfigure his body so as to search the room for a response.

If a request is met with silence, a surgeon is likely to believe that no one has heard him or her. These can create momentary interruptions as the surgeon disengages from the operating field and looks around the theatre for a response. In Example 11 (Transcript 10.10), we show a parallel example where no verbal response was produced. The example involves a different surgeon and a different operation, but the same operating theatre. The diathermy pedals were at issue in this example, too. The surgeon made a request for the pedals as he was preparing the patient's skin to be operated on.

Transcript 10.10: Absent verbal response [Example 11]

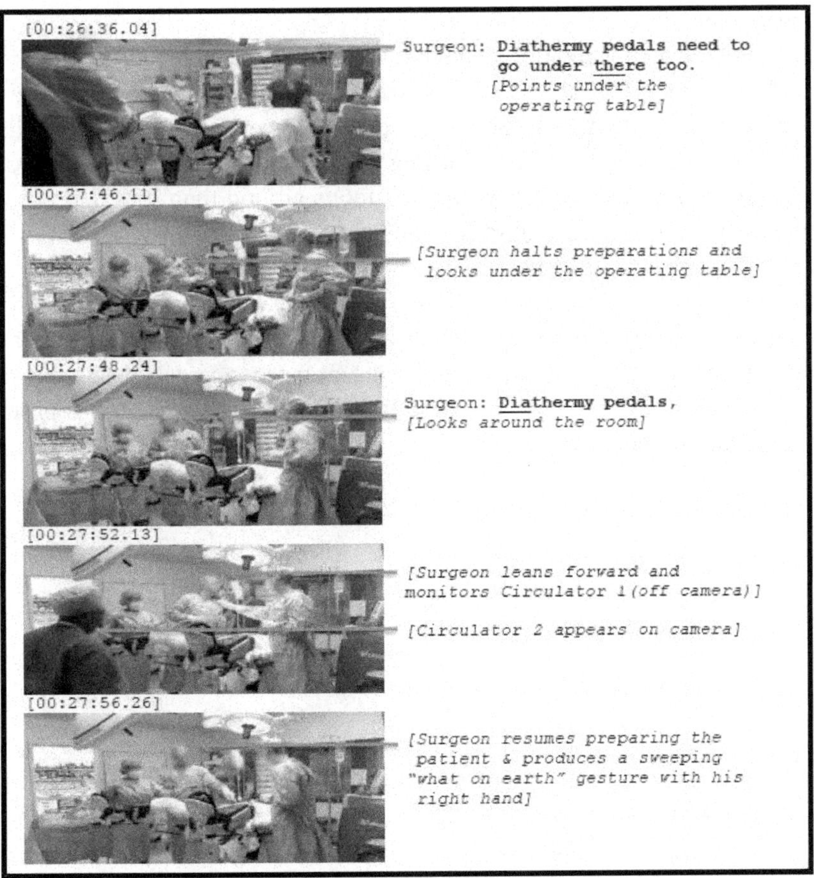

As the surgeon first walked into the theatre, he glanced under the operating table and saw the diathermy pedals missing. He gestured under the table and stated, "Diathermy pedals need to go under there too", addressing one of the two circulators in the theatre (presumably the one who was fastening the sterile gown for him). The surgeon then moved over to the operating table and began to apply antiseptic solution on the patient's skin with a scrub nurse's assistance. A minute or so into these preparations, the surgeon glanced under the table and saw that the pedals were still missing. He looked up and repeated "Diathermy pedals", in a tone of mock-surprise, looking around to see if anyone had heard him. As he shifted his gaze across the theatre, he saw the second circulator behind a stack presumably looking for the pedals. The surgeon leaned over the operating table to catch a glimpse of what was happening, yet probably could not completely see the nurse who was partially behind the theatre equipment. Shortly after, another circulator appeared, attending to the issue. She first glanced under the operating table and then joined the other nurse in her search. Yet even at this stage, there was no verbal update from either of the nurses. As the surgeon resumed preparing the patient, he embodied his thoughts about the silence in a sweeping gesture as if to ask, "what on earth is happening".

The emergent silence did not mean that the nurses were disregarding the request for pedals. Rather, a verbal update was overlooked in the middle of searching for the item, that is, in the middle of taking action. However, when silences like this occur, they prevent surgeons from learning what is happening. During this episode, the surgeon produced seven "questioning" looks around the room. He eventually received the pedals, but seemed to be irritated by this delay.

Our final Example 12 (Transcript 10.11) is drawn from the same theatre site, but involves a different surgeon and different operation. Here, a piece of equipment failed to work properly. The surgeon was about to use a suction machine when he noticed that the machine was not functioning properly and asked, "Is the suction working." Rather than merely requesting information, the surgeon was prompting nurses to attend to the issue.

Transcript 10.11: Absent verbal response [Example 12]

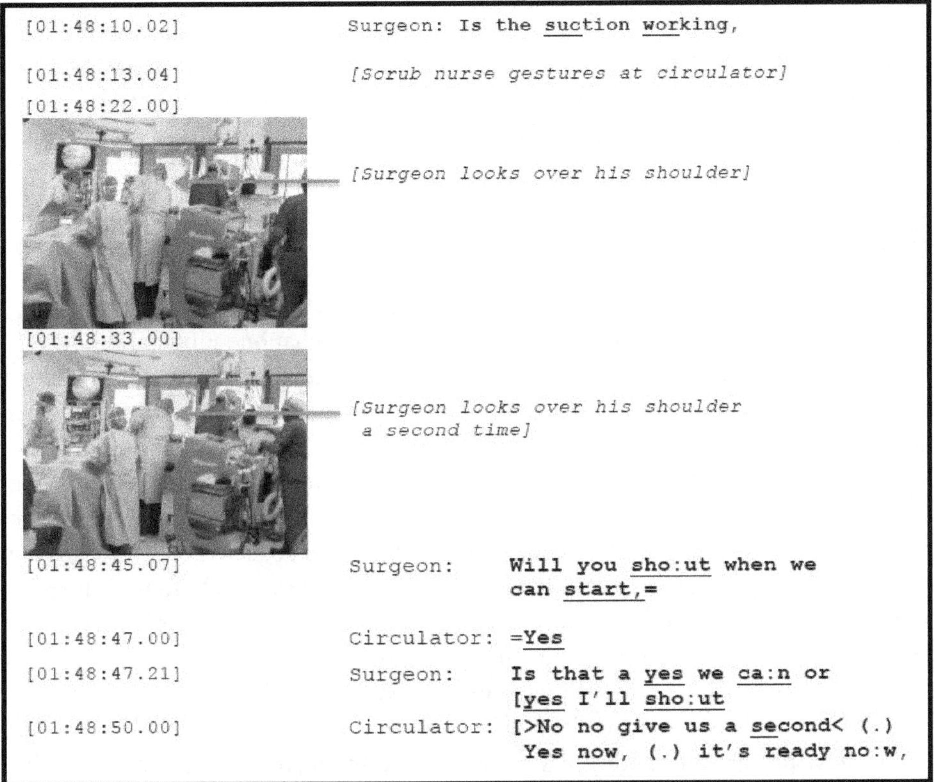

Here the surgeon could see that the scrub nurse in front of him attempted to communicate (mainly by gesturing) with two circulators gathered around the suction machine, but he could not see what was happening behind his back where the machine was located. A substantial 12 seconds later the surgeon turned to look over his shoulder but then returned his gaze to the laparoscopic monitor. After a further 11 seconds he turned again to look over his shoulder, and another 12 seconds later he called a little louder, "Will you shout when we can start." His utterance displayed overt reference to the lack of responsiveness to his initial query about suction: first, in asking the nurses to verbally update him (literally to "shout") when the problem was fixed; and second, in underscoring his apparent confusion about the situation in that he could not see what was happening, did not know how long it might take to fix the problem, and had been left waiting for a response. After this, the circulator's response "Yes" created a further difficulty in that, while she had now verbally responded to his request ("Will you shout when we can start"), it was unclear to the surgeon as to whether the "Yes" meant that the nurses would *update* him or whether they could now *proceed* to use suction.

A silent lapse can create an interval where *ambiguity* develops and, consequently, repeated prompts and interruptions occur. The above cases suggest that when a verbal response is missing, a situation becomes problematic when delays occur and clinicians have no visual access to each other. Timing is also critical: an acknowledgement or other verbal update should be voiced directly after the first request so as to keep colleagues aware of what is happening.

10.4 Discussion

Communication can pose a potential risk to patient safety, while it can also be a key to successful teamwork. The analysis illustrates that what one clinician knows, or does *not* know – their situational awareness – can depend on physical positioning in the theatre and thus visual access to what a colleague is doing. When a request is issued to a nurse, seeing what they are up to can help a surgeon judge whether the nurse has heard the request. Talk becomes relevant when there is a delay in carrying out what has been requested. In our study we sometimes found that verbal acknowledgements, such as "Yes coming!" were voiced so as to notify the surgeon what was "going on". These responses showed nurses' orientation to the surgeon's separate and often limited perspective by the operating table and established mutual awareness of the situation at hand. In these cases, the ongoing operation usually proceeded smoothly with little interruptions. Even if faced with slight delays, the surgeon *knew* that in a short while a nurse was going to carry out what was needed.

So, how do talk and bodily action serve communication? Some video studies have talked about *intercorporeal knowing* between clinicians. As Hindmarsh and Pilnick (2007: 1413) have put it, collaborative work is organized by responding to the "sounds, sights and feel of colleagues", and communication does not always involve talk. We also found that scrub nurses responded to surgeons more often through their bodies rather than through speech. However, these nurses were usually positioned in close proximity to the surgeons, working within their visual field. As such, "silent" communication is not *always* effective; the key is in the noticeability of actions to a colleague. This has specific implications for circulators, who are often *outside* the visual field of other colleagues. When something has been requested of them, a verbal acknowledgement is crucial, as the absence of such acknowledgement can be consequential: the surgeon halts the procedure and looks around for a response, waiting.

The present analysis has shown that professionals do not always respond clearly to one another when mundane issues are in question. Why might this be the case? Some suggest that silences can reflect power dynamics and the hierarchical order of surgeons and nurses in the operating theatre (Gardezi et al. 2009); some have proposed that they represent a more general "silencing" of nurses in the healthcare system (Newton et al. 2012). Care should be taken not to interpret the present findings directly in the light of such power relations. Rather, we are proposing that when nurses do not respond verbally in operations, this may indicate these nurses' immersion in their work, but perhaps also a lack of awareness of how their actions can have a direct impact on others. Mundane exchanges, like those considered in this chapter, can often "fly under the radar" when professionals are going about their business in the operating theatre. Indeed, perhaps paradoxically, nurses sometimes describe communication as being unnecessary during familiar routine tasks.[1]

10.4.1 Implications of Findings

Inadequate communication can potentially lead to harmful incidents and should not be underestimated. Yet, what is *inadequate* has been rarely delineated in detail. Safe communication should not rely on judgements about *seeing* that a colleague has heard you; often, safe communication requires both talk and action. Whether it is responsiveness to checklist items (Cullati et al. 2013), voicing concerns about errors and patient care (Bromiley 2008; Maxfield et al. 2005) or, as here, updating about instrument retrievals or equipment failures, speaking up is important and it should not be taken for granted that it just happens.

Thus, the study has implications both for training and development of systematic communication practices. As in other industries outside healthcare, clear communication should become a standard practice in the operating theatre – a part of the job. We should consider a verbal response neither as an "option" nor as something that only assertive nurses voice in the operating theatre, but rather as something that ought to be done always. New communication strategies can be simple. We recommend that on hearing a request or a question, a prompt verbal acknowledgement (e.g., "Coming up!", "I'm on it!") should be produced, following suit from the field of aviation or professional kitchens. A revision of safety guidelines should include clear instructions as to how and when to respond to requests and questions when an operation is in progress. These could be discussed in team briefings and training courses.

As Leonard et al. (2004) note, introducing practices that make the routine *easier* is a catalyst for a cultural change. Leadership is also crucial, and this is where training is important. Simulation provides a good environment for practising new communication strategies (Husebø et al. 2011), such as verbal acknowledgements and speaking up. Consequently, nurses furnished with standard ways of communicating

---

1 In our own research, some of the theatre nurses mentioned "not needing communication" during routine tasks. On the one hand, this echoes the notion that some communication, at least among experienced theatre nurses, can go on silently without talking. On the other hand, this speaks to the fact of just how easily communication issues, which are hidden in the routine, can be overlooked as unimportant.

can gradually lead others by example: local champions could encourage other team members to follow suit. Our team has run simulation trials with student nurses, operating department practitioners, and in-service operating theatre professionals, and these have looked promising (Korkiakangas et al. 2015, ViSIOT™ training). New awareness of communication could be facilitated combining simulation with video-based training: using different camera angles, participants can explore from video exactly *how* different response practices impact colleagues from the perspectives of surgeons and nurses. Video also helps participants reflect on selected incidents at a broader systemic level and *reinvent* how to conduct their work more efficiently (Iedema et al. 2009).

10.4.2 Areas for Further Investigation

The limitations of the present study should be acknowledged and further lines of inquiry developed. The operating theatre professionals were aware of the presence of two external observers and the video recording equipment, which could have impacted on their communication. However, we are confident that our observation had a minimal impact on the professionals' naturalistic conduct, as the surgeons and nurses were familiar with us prior to the commencement of any filming, and many observers, such as medical students and clinical educators, regularly visit these operating theatres. Overall, our cameras did not draw much attention as the professionals were immersed in their work. We propose that video recording is an important method that could be utilized more fully in future research in the operating theatre.

The present study made use of a convenience sampling of elective routine operations. However, future studies could examine communication during emergency operations. It might be that a state of emergency impacts teamwork and communication differently. Perhaps during relatively uneventful operations, teams might overlook the importance of prompt verbal communication precisely because of no pressing urgency to organize their own behaviour.

Finally, in order for research to achieve "real impact" in clinical practice, we share Vincent's (2009: 1777) view on active engagement between social scientists and clinicians. This involves addressing some of the complexities embedded in daily routines that are hidden, overlooked or dismissed as too mundane to be of actual importance. In the UK Department of Health report, Lord Darzi (2008: 11) reminds us that to improve the quality of healthcare, we should aim for "getting the basics right first time, every time". Thus, by taking seriously also those moments where ambiguities develop during surgical operations – say, when clinicians do not speak when they should do – we could move towards more consistent communication practices. These could keep patients safe with or without emergencies.

Acknowledgements

We are grateful to the patients who gave their consent for their operations to be filmed for research purposes, and to the operating theatre professionals of the participating NHS Trust in the UK for allowing us to video-record and analyse their interactions. We thank Kathy Nicholson for her contribution to the overall research project.

Funding

We thank the Economic and Social Research Council (ESRC) for supporting this research (RES-062-23-3219).

Appendix: Additional Transcription Convention

In addition to the conventions in Chapter 2, the following convention is used in this chapter.

`[Italicized text in square brackets]`   transcription of non-vocal action

References

Atkinson, J. Maxwell, and John Heritage. 1984. Transcript Notation. In *Structures of Social Action: Studies in Conversation Analysis*, edited by J. Maxwell Atkinson and John Heritage, ix – xvi. Cambridge: Cambridge University Press.

Bezemer, Jeff, Alexandra Cope, Gunther Kress and Roger Kneebone. 2011a. "Do You Have Another Johan?" Negotiating Meaning in the Operating Theatre. *Applied Linguistics Review* 2: 313–34.

Bezemer, Jeff, Ged Murtagh, Alexandra Cope, Gunther Kress and Roger Kneebone. 2011b. "Scissors, Please": The Practical Accomplishment of Surgical Work in the Operating Theater. *Symbolic Interaction* 34(3): 398–414.

Bezemer, Jeff, Terhi Korkiakangas, Sharon-Marie Weldon, Gunther Kress and Roger Kneebone. 2015. Unsettled Teamwork: Communication and Learning in the Operating Theatres of an Urban Hospital. *Journal of Advanced Nursing* (Early online).

Bromiley, Martin. 2008. Have You Ever Made a Mistake? *The Royal College of Anaesthetists Bulletin* 48: 2442–5.

Cullati, Stéphane, Sophie Le Du, Anne-Claire Raë, Martine Micallef, Ebrahim Khabiri, Aimad Ourahmoune, Armelle Boireaux, Marc Licker and Pierre Chopard. 2013. Is the Surgical Safety Checklist Successfully Conducted? An Observational Study of Social Interactions in the Operating Rooms of a Tertiary Hospital. *BMJ Quality & Safety* 22(8): 639–46.

Darzi, Ara. 2008. *High Quality Care for All: NHS Next Stage Review Final Report*. London: Department of Health.

Department of Health. 2006. *Safety First: A Report for Patients, Clinicians and Healthcare Managers.* London: The Stationery Office.

Endsley, Mica R. 1995. Toward a Theory of Situation Awareness in Dynamic Systems. *Human Factors: The Journal of the Human Factors and Ergonomics Society* 37(1): 32–64.

Gardezi, Fauzia, Lorelei Lingard, Sherry Espin, Sarah Whyte, Beverley Orser and G. Ross Baker. 2009. Silence, Power and Communication in the Operating Room. *Journal of Advanced Nursing* 65(7): 1390–9.

Goffman, Erving. 1983. The Interaction Order. *American Sociological Review* 48: 1–17.

Gupta, Babita, Pramendra Agrawal, Nita D'souza and Kapil Dev Soni. 2011. Start Time Delays in Operating Room: Different Perspectives. *Saudi Journal of Anaesthesia* 5(3): 286–8.

Haddington, Pentti, Tiina Keisanen, Lorenza Mondada and Maurice Nevile (eds). 2014. *Multiactivity in Social Interaction: Beyond Multitasking.* Amsterdam: John Benjamins Publishing Company.

Haig, Kathleen M., Staci Sutton and John Whittington. 2006. SBAR: A Shared Mental Model for Improving Communication between Clinicians. *Joint Commission Journal on Quality and Patient Safety* 32(3): 167–75.

Haynes, Alex B., Thomas G. Weiser, William R. Berry, Stuart R. Lipsitz, Abdel-Hadi S. Breizat, E. Patchen Dellinger, Teodoro Herbosa, Sudhir Joseph, Pascience L. Kibatala, Marie Carmela M. Lapitan, Alan F. Merry, Krishna Moorthy, Richard K. Reznick, Bryce Taylor and Atul A. Gawande. 2009. A Surgical Safety Checklist to Reduce Morbidity and Mortality in a Global Population. *New England Journal of Medicine* 360(5): 491–9.

Hazlehurst, Brian, Carmit K. McMullen and Paul N. Gorman. 2007. Distributed Cognition in the Heart Room: How Situation Awareness Arises from Coordinated Communications During Cardiac Surgery. *Journal of Biomedical Informatics* 40(5): 539–51.

Hindmarsh, Jon, and Alison Pilnick. 2002. The Tacit Order of Teamwork: Collaboration and Embodied Conduct in Anaesthesia. *The Sociological Quarterly* 43(2): 139–64.

Hindmarsh, Jon, and Alison Pilnick. 2007. Knowing Bodies at Work: Embodiment and Ephemeral Teamwork in Anaesthesia. *Organization Studies* 28(9): 1395–416.

Husebø, Sissel Eikeland, Hans Rystedt and Febe Friberg. 2011. Educating for Teamwork: Nursing Students' Coordination in Simulated Cardiac Arrest Situations. *Journal of Advanced Nursing* 67(10): 2239–55.

Iedema, Rick. 2009. New Approaches to Researching Patient Safety. *Social Science & Medicine* 69 (12): 1701–4.

Iedema, Rick, Eamon Thomas Merrick, Dorrilyn Rajbhandari, Alan Gardo, Anne Stirling and Robert Herkes. 2009. Viewing the Taken-for-Granted from under a Different Aspect: A Video-Based Method in Pursuit of Patient Safety. *International Journal of Multiple Research Approaches* 3(3): 290–301.

Isaac, Anne. 2007. Effective Communication in the Aviation Environment: Work in Progress. *Hindsight* 5: 31–4.

Korkiakangas, Terhi, Sharon-Marie Weldon, Jeff Bezemer and Roger Kneebone. 2014. Nurse–Surgeon Object Transfer: Video Analysis of Communication and Situation Awareness in the Operating Theatre. *International Journal of Nursing Studies* 51(9): 1195–206.

Korkiakangas, Terhi, Sharon-Marie Weldon, Jeff Bezemer and Roger Kneebone. 2015. Video-supported Simulation for Interactions in the Operating Theatre (ViSIOT). *Clinical Simulation in Nursing* 11(4): 203–7.

Koschmann, Timothy, Curtis LeBaron, Charles Goodwin and Paul Feltovich. 2011. "Can You See the Cystic Artery Yet?": A Simple Matter of Trust. *Journal of Pragmatics* 43(2): 521–41.

Leonard, Michael, Suzanne Graham and Doug Bonacum. 2004. The Human Factor: The Critical Importance of Effective Teamwork and Communication in Providing Safe Care. *Quality and Safety in Health Care* 13(Suppl 1): i85–90.

Lingard, Lorelei, Sherry Espin, Sarah Whyte, Glenn Regehr, G.R. Baker, Richard Reznick, J. Bohnen, B. Orser, D. Doran and E. Grober. 2004. Communication Failures in the Operating Room: an Observational Classification of Recurrent Types and Effects. *Quality and Safety in Health Care* 13(5): 330–4.

Lingard, Lorelei, Glenn Regehr, Sherry Espin and Sarah Whyte. 2006. A Theory-Based Instrument to Evaluate Team Communication in the Operating Room: Balancing Measurement Authenticity and Reliability. *Quality and Safety in Health Care* 15(6): 422–6.

Makary, Martin A., Arnab Mukherjee, J. Bryan Sexton, Dora Syin, Emmanuelle Goodrich, Emily Hartmann, Lisa Rowen, Drew C. Behrens, Michael Marohn and Peter J. Pronovost. 2007. Operating Room Briefings and Wrong-Site Surgery. *Journal of the American College of Surgeons* 204(2): 236–43.

Maxfield, David, Joseph Grenny, Ron McMillan, Kerry Patterson and Al Switzler. 2005. *Silence Kills: The Seven Crucial Conversations for Healthcare*. Provo, UT: VitalSmarts.

McFerran, Sharon, Julie Nunes, Duayna Pucci and Anita Zuniga. 2005. Perinatal Patient Safety Project: A Multicenter Approach to Improve Performance Reliability at Kaiser Permanente. *The Journal of Perinatal & Neonatal Nursing* 19(1): 37–45.

Mondada, Lorenza. 2011. The Organization of Concurrent Courses of Action in Surgical Demonstrations. In *Embodied Interaction: Language and Body in the Material World*, edited by Jürgen Streeck, Charles Goodwin and Curtis LeBaron, 207–26. New York: Cambridge University Press.

Mondada, Lorenza. 2014a. Instructions in the Operating Room: How the Surgeon Directs Their Assistant's Hands. *Discourse Studies* 16(2): 131–61.

Mondada, Lorenza. 2014b. Requesting Immediate Action in the Surgical Operating Room: Time, Embodied Resources and Praxeological Embeddedness. In *Requesting in Social Interaction*, edited by Paul Drew and Elizabeth Couper-Kuhlen, 269–302. Amsterdam: John Benjamins Publishing Company.

Moore, Alison, David Butt, Jodie Ellis-Clarke and John Cartmill. 2010. Linguistic Analysis of Verbal and Non-Verbal Communication in the Operating Room. *ANZ Journal of Surgery* 80(12): 925–9.

Newton, Lorelei, Janet L. Storch, K.S. Makaroff and Bernadette Pauly. 2012. "Stop the Noise!": From Voice to Silence. *Nursing Leadership (Toronto, Ont.)* 25(1): 90–104.

Sanchez Svensson, Marcus, Christian Heath and Paul Luff. 2007. Instrumental Action: The Timely Exchange of Implements during Surgical Operations. In *ECSCW 2007: Proceedings of the 10th European Conference on Computer Supported Cooperative Work*, edited by Liam J. Bannon, Ina Wagner, Carl Gutwin, Richard H.R. Harper and Kjeld Schmidt, 41–60. London: Springer.

Seiden, Samuel C., and Paul Barach. 2006. Wrong-Side/Wrong-Site, Wrong-Procedure, and Wrong-Patient Adverse Events: Are They Preventable? *Archives of Surgery* 141(9): 931–9.

Schegloff, Emanuel A. 2007. *Sequence Organization in Interaction. A Primer in Conversation Analysis I.* Cambridge: Cambridge University Press.

Vats, Amit, Charles Vincent, Kamal Nagpal, R.W. Davies, Ara Darzi and Krishna Moorthy. 2010. Practical Challenges of Introducing WHO Surgical Checklist: UK Pilot Experience. *British Medical Journal* 340(7738): 133–5.

Vincent, Charles. 2009. Social Scientists and Patient Safety: Critics or Contributors? *Social Science & Medicine* 69(12): 1777–9.

World Health Organization. 2008. *World Alliance for Patient Safety: Safe Surgery Saves Lives.* Geneva: WHO.

Terhi Korkiakangas is a social interaction researcher with background in psychology. She received her PhD from the University of Roehampton. Her principal research interests include multimodal interaction and conversation analysis in everyday and institutional settings. Terhi was a Research Associate in two Economic and Social Research Council funded projects, "Transient Teams in the Operating Theatre" (2012–13) and "Multimodal Methodologies for Researching Digital Data and Environments (MODE)" (2013–14). Currently, she is a British Academy Postdoctoral Fellow (2014–17) undertaking video-based research on interactions in the operating theatre. Terhi is the co-founder of ViSIOT™ training model for improving communication in the operating theatre using simulation and video.

Sharon-Marie Weldon is a Senior Research Officer/Nurse and a PhD candidate at the Department of Surgery and Cancer, Imperial College London. Her research focuses on Sequential Simulation (SqS), communication and public/patient/clinician engagement. Sharon started her nursing career as a theatre practitioner, and then joined the Health Protection Agency undertaking research into tuberculosis diagnostic tools. She was a Research Nurse in an Economic and Social Research Council funded project, "Transient Teams in the Operating Theatre" (2012–13), while completing an MSc in Public Health at the London School of Hygiene and Tropical Medicine. Sharon is the co-founder of ViSIOT™ training model for improving communication in the operating theatre using simulation and video.

Jeff Bezemer, PhD, is Reader in Learning and Communication and an ethnographic researcher at the University College London (UCL) Institute of Education, with a particular interest in learning, identity and communication. His publications deal with educational, medical and academic practice in a changing social, technological and representational landscape. Jeff has been Principal and Co-investigator on a number of research projects funded by the Economic and Social Research Council, including "Multimodal Methodologies for Researching Digital Data and Environments (MODE)" (2011–14), "Transient Teams in the Operating Theatre" (2012–13), "Digital Technologies in the Operating Theatre" (2011–14) and "Gains and Losses: Changes in Knowledge, Representation and Pedagogy" (2007–09).

Roger Kneebone, PhD, is a clinician and educationalist who leads a multidisciplinary research group at the Department of Surgery and Cancer, Imperial College London. His innovative work on contextualized simulation builds on his personal experience as a surgeon and a general practitioner, and his interest in domains of expertise beyond medicine. Roger has built an unorthodox and creative team of clinicians, computer scientists, design engineers, social scientists, artists and performers. In 2013 he took up a Wellcome Trust Engagement Fellowship.

11 Lovers, Wrestlers, Surgeons: A Contextually Motivated View of Interpersonal Engagement and Body Alignment in Surgical Interaction

Alison Rotha Moore

11.1 Introduction

Models for describing how body alignment contributes to the meaning-making of human social contexts have tended to yield elaborate but instance-bound "thick descriptions". While these approaches allow for very rich accounts of particular cases, they do not lend themselves to systematic empirical comparison – for instance, of how participants in a highly charged endeavour like surgery align their bodies to each other in ways that may convey different meanings under different conditions (e.g., different types of surgery, different phases of surgery, different levels of fatigue, engagement or personal involvement in the procedure at hand, when taking different agentive roles, when working with different teams or just working on different days).

The need for such empirical analyses in areas like surgery is increasing as we find more and more evidence that a team's sense of engagement is crucial to its capacity to avert and reduce errors (Wilson et al. 2005; Healey et al. 2006; Bezemer et al. 2011; Weldon et al. 2013).

Recently, systemically oriented accounts have been emerging which hold promise for dealing with these kinds of empirical analyses. In particular, Martinec (2001) has offered a framework for analysing the means of construction and expression of interpersonal relations through action, drawing on Hall's (1959, 1966) classic analysis of spatial distance between bodies, and incorporating his own analysis of reciprocal body angle. Yet what is missing from the leading models of body alignment is a systematic account of how the same distance and orientation selections may have quite different meanings even in subtly different contexts; that is, there is no systematic account of the dynamic role of context in the meanings attributed to movement and position.

In this chapter, I examine what we can gain by emphasizing the stratal rapport between context, semantics and expression choices in multimodal analyses, starting with the issue of how body alignment construes engagement in surgery, and drawing on recent developments in systemic functional linguistics (SFL) by Hasan (1999, 2009) and Butt (2004) regarding the constructs of *Field*, *Tenor* and *Mode*. Although this approach raises further issues (Butt and Wegener 2007; Bowcher 2013), it increases our explanatory power significantly. In the context of surgery, it explains why team members who work in close proximity are not contravening Hall's rules of thumb about appropriate intimacy; rather, they are operating within register-specific relations between context, semantics and expression. Such register-specific accounts of meaning systems at work can make the professional logic of a context more available for scrutiny by institutional members, and can contribute to organizational and professional development (Moore 2004, 2005; Moore & Tuckwell 2006).

11.2   The Research Context and Problem

The discussion of ways to model body alignment presented here grew out of a specific research need to understand how surgical teams engage and signal their engagement with one another during operative procedures. This concern was part of a broader study on communication and safety in surgical care (Butt, Moore and Cartmill 2003). The aim of the overall study was to make existing systems of communication, and how they may lead to adverse events, more explicit. With an estimated 18,000 deaths per year from adverse medical and surgical events in Australia (Wilson et al. 1995), or one death per year per 1000 population, and similar rates in other developed countries, this work is ultimately motivated by health outcomes.

Trying to reduce errors through better communication in contexts like surgery may sound anything but new, but a very brief account of the research on communication and medical error should help to explain why there is still a need for approaches like ours. Increasingly, in the medical error field, adverse events in operative care are considered systemic rather than as simply individual error or as a product of system breakdown (Reason 2000). Studies repeatedly identify "communication failure" as a factor in medical error, and many give the proportions of error caused by communication, as distinct from other causes (e.g., Gawande et al. [2003] attribute 43 per cent of errors in their study to communication breakdown). But somewhat curiously the "systemic turn" in medical error research has tended to treat communication as one of the "individual factors" in error, with allocation to "system factors" being reserved for causes of error that are (by implication) not communication factors. I argue that individual and system factors are merely different points of view of what is actually the same phenomenon, and that it is impossible to distribute the causes of adverse incidents into those related to communication and interpretation, and those where communication has no bearing (Moore et al. 2005, 2010). Related limitations in the existing research on communication and error which we hope this study will begin to address include the following:

(a) most studies of communication in medical contexts focus on ideational (representational) meaning only, and not on interpersonal or textual meaning (Halliday 1973);

(b) interpersonal and emotional factors are recognized as important in the surgical context but are either not treated as (relevant) communication, or not treated systematically;

(c) "nonverbal communication", in particular, is treated in an unsystematic way – there is little systems thinking here;

(d) the study of communication is limited to productive not receptive perspectives – the interpretive practices of a smoothly operating team are taken as irreducible, a kind of automatic product of experience;

(e) most studies focus on what "goes wrong", leaving little information available on how the routine achievements of surgery are produced and the interaction such achievements entail.

Against this background, our project was set up to describe surgery as a system of meaning-bearing systems, integrated from context to content to expression, and incorporating language and other symbolic systems. The project used a mixed methods approach, combining video-ethnography, participant observation, fieldnotes, interviews and collaborative engagement with key stakeholders (surgical, nursing, anaesthetic and administrative staff) at Nepean Hospital, Sydney, Australia. The linguist researchers (Butt and Moore) attended and observed 14 days of surgical lists, and video recordings were made of 10 of those days totalling approximately 50 hours of footage. The videoed lists involved a single senior surgical specialist, two registrars, two surgical residents, three scrub nurses, approximately ten scout nurses and other nurses, three senior anaesthetists and several medical students. All patients were receiving colorectal surgery, of varying degrees of complexity. Data were transcribed using ELAN software for multimodal analyses and SysAm software for linguistic analyses. Linguistic tools including system networks (Halliday 2003; Hasan 1996) were used to map meanings, expression and variation in engagement, showing the "ensemble effects" (Butt 1988) of choices in these systems and how they predispose towards or inhibit adverse outcomes. We wanted to test whether our approach – treating surgery as a set of integrated meaning-bearing systems (Butt 2006; Chapter 8, this volume) – could generate ideas on how to improve the safety of surgery for patients and professionals.

11.3   The Meaningfulness of Body Alignment

In our initial observations of surgery, we were struck by the coordinated, almost choreographed, movements of surgical team members. The more we looked, the more it became evident that all members of the surgical team were using systematic distinctions in body alignment as part of a suite of communicative resources that are used to get things done in surgery. In other words (we hypothesized) body alignment could be shown to be an important and **systemic** meaning-bearing system charged with specific roles in this context; if there were differences in people's understandings of this system of meanings, they would be a potential source of the kinds of miscues that can build up and produce "adverse events" in surgery. But to examine this further, it would be necessary to be able to say what kinds of meanings were being expressed and what distinctions in body alignment were being used to express them. Using our 50-hour corpus of videotaped observations of surgery, this chapter reports on such an approach, and in particular aims to:

(a) make explicit the kinds of meanings routinely being made in surgery through body alignment, with particular reference to the way bodies are used to signal the engagement of minds;

(b) make explicit the variation in such meanings that seems to be critical for smooth teamwork and ultimately for reducing/avoiding medical error.

11.3.1   Models of Body Alignment as Degree of Engagement

In order to engage in the empirical work proposed above, a method for describing and comparing different physical alignments of team members' bodies was needed, preferably one which lent itself to drawing out potential relationships between the meanings of different choices of body alignment and the meanings made by different choices in language which might accompany them or perhaps substitute for them. This section describes the general systemic framework used in the study, and briefly places it in the context of work on proxemics and gesture; issues to do with my own development of this model are discussed as the chapter progresses.

The field of scholarly research that discusses body alignment has its most important disciplinary origins in anthropology and ethnography. Much of the empirical work in this area has tended to develop very thick descriptions of individual instances of interaction. While the close description of individual instances is highly valuable, this approach tends to have a number of limitations for our goals of mapping the variations and consistencies in how bodies are aligned from one surgical phase to another, from one team to another, one day to another and so on, and linking the variations in their meanings with the kinds of meanings being expressed and understood by team members through the resource of language. One highly influential line of development is the work of the anthropologist Edward T. Hall (1959, 1966), and its further development by the linguist and semiotician Radan Martinec (2000, 2001, 2004), as part of his semiotics of action. As Martinec puts it, a systemic functional semiotics of action "classifies movements into different kinds on the basis of their observable characteristics. The aim is to have categories of movement, abstracted from specific instances, which enable one to identify patterns in texts that otherwise would be difficult to pinpoint" (2000: 314).

The kinds of movement I am concerned with teasing out in this chapter involve the category Martinec calls *presenting action*. Presenting action concerns the meaning that bodies make about the here and now, or perhaps the *here and next*, as the cognitive scientist and co-developer of the mirror neuron hypothesis Michael Arbib suggests (pers. comm.). Presenting action – more perhaps than other types of action – forms patterns that are hard to pinpoint in terms of the kinds of meaning it constructs, and is similar to what Halliday (1973) describes as *interpersonal meaning* in language. The hallmark of these kinds of meanings – whether conveyed through language or through movement – is that they construct and modify relationships between interactants. In particular, the key aspect of presenting action that we are interested in here is the system of *engagement*, which concerns "the social relations between interactants which are realized by the distance and angle of their bodies" (Martinec 2001: 118).

This *presenting* type of meaningful action must be distinguished from what Martinec calls *representing action*, which concerns an area of meaning that has been given more attention by theorists of language and of movement than interpersonal meaning (this is what philosophers of language call the "referential bias"). Representing action corresponds roughly with ideational meaning in SFL, and with the idea of referential meaning more generally: it functions to communicate about contexts that are potentially displaced from the here and now. It is similar to what Kendon (2004) calls gestures and what Ekman and Friesen (1969) call emblems.

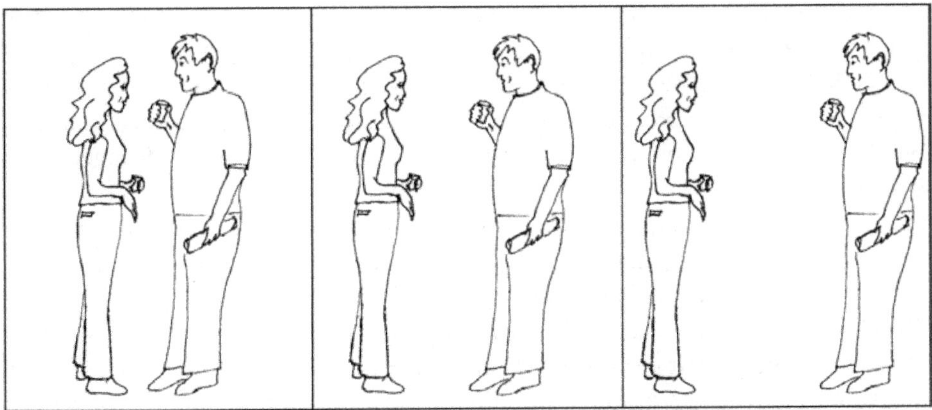

Figure 11.1: (a) Intimate, (b) personal and (c) social distance (after Hall 1966)

To distinguish *representing and presenting* action, Kendon's (2004: 7) distinction is useful: the kinds of visible body actions that count for others as an attempt to *give* information correspond to representing action, whereas those which *give off* information without intention (Goffman 1963: 13–14) correspond to presenting action. It is this latter type that we are concerned with in the present chapter (although such a sharp distinction may evaporate under models of representational meaning that adequately account for connotation, intertextuality and so on before we even begin to problematize the notion of *intention*).

One key way in which people *give off* interpersonal meaning is through their bodily proximity to each other. Hall (1966) brings to our attention sets of culturally constructed zones of space around individuals which cultures use to construe interaction as ranging from intimate (up to 18 inches apart – see Figure 11.1a), to personal distance (18 inches to 4 feet – Figure 11.1b) to social (4 to 12 feet – Figure 11.1c) and out to public space (12 to 25+ feet – not illustrated). Hall's ultimate purpose for his model is to make sure that spatial, architectural and urban planning needs are considered to be culturally relative, dependent on how space is bounded and construed. For instance, the spatial and architectural needs of cultures as close as Germany and America, or America and Britain, are shown to be quite different: for Germans, at least in the 1960s, an open-plan office represents intrusion on the personal space required to work and concentrate, and sets up "an unusually relaxed and unbusinesslike air", whereas when doors are closed Americans feel left out and sense "a conspiratorial air" (Hall 1966: 128).

11.3.2 Hall's Model as a Semiotic System

Before moving on to discuss recent developments, I want to describe in a little more detail Hall's model as a semiotic system. To illustrate the social power of these zones, Hall comments that a wife may stay inside her husband's close personal zone (in America, up to two and a half feet apart) with impunity, but for another woman to do so is "an entirely different story" (Hall 1966: 113). An important implication here is that, although he does not describe them as such, Hall's zones of proximity are presented as the expression plane in a Hjelmslevian semiotic system (Hjelmslev 1961), where the content plane corresponds to categories of social distance. That is, body proximity forms a set of meaningful contrasts which both reflect and construct social context: close-up is where you go if you want to increase the intimacy of the moment; but closeness is also where you *see* intimacy as an observer.

Like semiotic systems in general, the relationship between a particular expression choice and what it means is likely to vary from culture to culture, and also from context to context within each given culture. Hall's work captures both cultural and, to a lesser extent, situational variation in the hook-up between each expression option (distance setting) and its meaning. An example of cultural differences in meaning is the contrast Hall gives between German and American interpretations of space as outlined above. As a pointer to the ways in which situational variables may influence how a particular distance setting is interpreted, Hall suggests that 67 per cent of tasks in submarines take place in the zone of close personal distance (Hall [1966: 119], referring to U.S. naval research done by Dimmick and Farnsworth circa 1951), whereas in other situations the proportion of tasks taking place in this close personal zone is much smaller.

At the same time as he allows for cultural and situational differences, Hall provides good evidence for the relationship between distance and meaning not being entirely arbitrary, since increasing proximity gives increasing biological access to individuals of visual, thermal, olfactory and auditory sense experiences of each other and this inherently motivates the cline between intimacy and public social space, even if different cultures mark the intervals between interpersonal and public space in different ways.

Now, if standing farther apart construes lower intimacy between individuals, what then is construed by other changes in the alignment of bodies, such as turning one's body away from front-to-front body orientation (see Figure 11.2)?

Martinec (2001) builds such variation into a model based on the work of Hall discussed above. To Hall's carefully graded system of proximity and its contextual meaning, Martinec adds an additional carefully graded variable – the angle of bodies – to give the variable *engagement*. Engagement is represented as a semiotic system in which two simultaneous dimensions of choice apply. A social actor may simultaneously vary (1) how close they stand to another social actor (as above), and (2) the relative orientation or angle of their body with respect to another social actor. Are they facing the other, are they side-on to the person, or do they have their back to that person? The angle of orientation crucially changes the *valeur* of the distance: as orientation moves out from *front-to-front* to *side orientation* and then on to *back orientation*, this is held (by Martinec) to lower the degree of engagement that would otherwise have been attributed to the interactants' proximity.

Although both distance and orientation are in essence continuous variables (like height or weight), they are presented as categorical variables (like country of birth or eye colour), or at least as salient transition points on a cline. The three options in the angle of the body's orientation are cross-classified with six different distance levels. This produces 18 options of meaning which are presented in Martinec's model as degrees of engagement with the closest engagement being *close intimate* and the least engaged state being (as in Hall's model) *far public engagement*. Basically then, in Martinec's model, the kind of interpersonal meanings at stake remain the same as those in Hall – in Hjelmslevian terms the *content form* is the same in the two models; whereas the *expression form* in Martinec now involves variables in combination.

At this point, the question arises: is it always appropriate to model angle and distance as alternative (or cumulative) ways of increasing or decreasing interpersonal

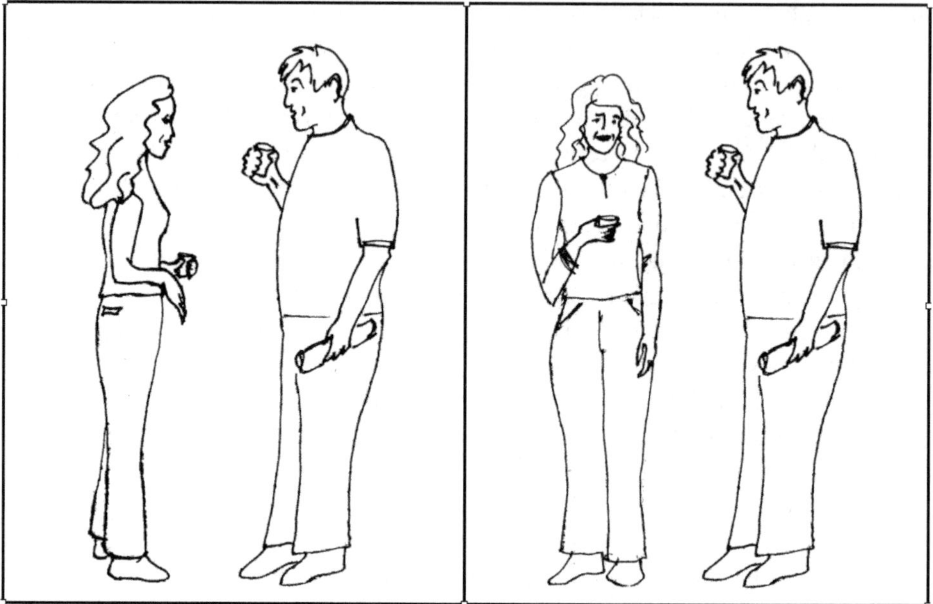

Figure 11.2: Moving from personal to social distance by changing angle of orientation (after Martinec 2001)

engagement? In the section below I show that, in the context of surgery, the angles and the distances between team members' bodies do *not* act alone as alternative or cumulative ways of increasing or decreasing engagement – an aspect of interpersonal meaning. Instead, both distance and angle need to be interpreted with reference to settings in *Field* (ideational meaning) and *Mode* (textual meaning), and also with reference to other aspects of interpersonal meaning such as agentive role, before we can settle on how we should interpret the contribution of body proximity and orientation to interpersonal meaning (*Tenor*). This is the case in surgery and, I suspect, more generally as well.

11.4 Surgery and the Need for a Registerially Sensitive Model of Body Alignment

In surgery, then, according to Martinec's model, two team members like those represented by the two solid-line participants shown in Figure 11.3a would count as having *maximally close* personal distance, since their heads (at least) are about six inches from each other and are spatially arranged in a *head-to-head* orientation. The participant sketched in dotted lines on the right of Figure 11.3a is further away and is not directly facing either of the other two participants – this person's engagement with each of the two solid-line figures would be gauged as lower under Martinec's model. But what of the participants in the next sketch (Figure 11.3b)? We can see that the first two from the left are in a position of *very close* proximity – again their heads, and this time other parts of their bodies, are within the 18-inch zone that denotes for Hall (1966) and Martinec (2001) a *context of intimacy*. According to Martinec's schema, this kind of configuration arguably represents a drop in engagement from *close intimate* to *personal distance*, since the participants, although close, are no longer oriented *head-to-head*. What these sketches represent, in practice, is that the surgeon and assistant may be working across the table from each other (Figure 11.3a) or may change to working on the same side of the table (Figure 11.3b).

Prima facie, it seems likely that moving from working across an operating table to working alongside each other on the same side would not always constitute a change in *degree* of engagement but could – at least sometimes – constitute a change in *kind* of engagement. But what might these kinds of engagement be? How are they signalled through the expressive resources of body position? When should we interpret options as meaning "less engaged" and when should we take them to mean "just as engaged, but in a different way"? To explore these issues I discuss several instances from our video corpus of 50 hours of colorectal surgery, including cases where engagement seems successfully managed, and one which reflects how meanings about engagement can be crucially misunderstood.

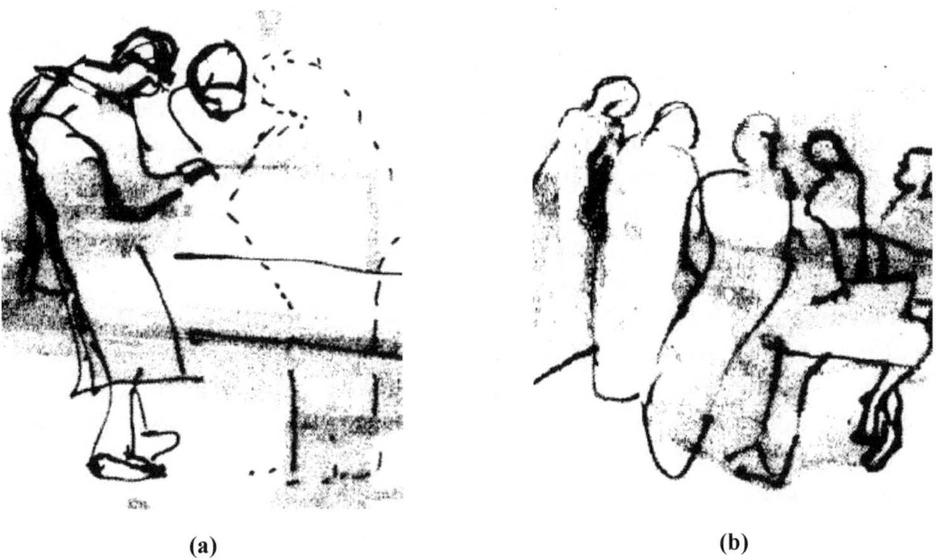

(a)(b)

Figure 11.3: (a) Across-table engagement in surgery; (b) along-table engagement in surgery

11.4.1 Working with Data from Surgery: The Taking-Over Episode

Having presented the idea of body alignment as a resource for negotiating engagement, along with the idea that this resource, like linguistic resources for meaning, must involve an alignment of contextual, semantic and expression-plane parameters, I now want to demonstrate this approach, using a transcript and some still shots from an episode of surgery which our team of researchers and research participants has dubbed "the taking-over episode".

In this episode, a "routine" procedure meets with some difficulties. The supervising staff specialist and his senior registrar (i.e., a fully qualified medical practitioner in the final year of training as a specialist surgeon) end up swapping agentive roles (i.e., the roles of who is "assisting" and who is "doing" the surgery) in order to complete the surgery in a timely way. A role swap like this is by no means unusual (Bezemer et al. 2014): it is a good example of the way that plans for routine surgical procedures must often be altered along the way, and it is an excellent example of the demands that surgical work routinely makes on staff, not just in technical facility, but also in what we might think of as agility in interpersonal meaning-making. Both the endpoint of this role swap and the process by which it is negotiated entail a number of adjustments to interpersonal engagement between the team members. In turn, in order to make a smooth role transition, all the parties need to reciprocally interpret each others' meanings about engagement in an appropriate way – that is, in a way that draws on the same systemic mapping between expression and content.

As we will see below, the surgical team members studied here do seem to work with such a shared system of meaning through body alignment. This shared system works in interdependence with the participants' shared system of linguistic meaning, but three caveats are important here. Firstly, the claim that body alignment is *systemic* communication does not preclude occasional, or even systematic and serious, differences and misunderstandings between individuals or groups, just as linguistic communication can entail important systematic differences (e.g., Bernstein's [1971] work on coding orientation). Secondly, a great deal of work is still needed before we can specify the dependencies that exist between speaking and body alignment, and there is room only for passing comments on this question in the present chapter (see below). Thirdly, a full linguistic analysis of this episode is also beyond the scope of this chapter, but it is important to give a transcript of the linguistic meanings that constitute the instance of interaction under scrutiny (see Lukin et al. [2011] for one account, which relates choices in lexicogrammar, semantics and context for the present episode).

Our episode starts some time into the surgical procedure. The registrar is finding it difficult to completely free up the bowel from its surrounding tissue, a preliminary to removing the diseased section. The dialogue begins with the specialist asking the registrar "Is it coming?" (see Excerpt). In this transcript, words shown in double parentheses are transcription comments, e.g., "((Tone 4))". Words shown in single parentheses are backchannels or completions from another speaker, e.g., "(yep)". The numbers inside the "text" column with no bracketing are ranking clause numbers; double vertical lines "||" indicate clause boundaries and double chevrons "<< >>" indicate interrupting clauses (Halliday and Matthiessen 2004). Dotted lines indicate contextual phase shifts in this episode of surgery, which have somewhat fuzzy boundaries. These contextual shifts are examined via the analyses of proxemic and linguistic patterns discussed below.

11.4.2 Phase 1: Moving to Continue the Current Context

As shown in the following transcript, the first four turns at talk (Clauses 1–12) can be seen as comprising one phase of the context of situation examined. From the point of view of linguistic meaning, this phase is marked by (a) the surgeon's use of interrogative mood (interpersonal *grammar*) to demand information (interpersonal *semantics*) from the registrar about progress and method, e.g., Clause 8 *Are your fingers down below it?*, and (b) the registrar's responses that give information using declarative mood, e.g., Clause 10 *My fingers are below it*. The registrar also uses imperative mood, as in Clause 4 *Grab that* and declarative mood (non-congruently) for demanding goods and services from her student assistant, as in Clause 3 *I'm just gonna move you in deeper*. In this phase, the specialist produces congruent demands for goods and services acting as advice, e.g., Clause 12 *Pull up on that band*.

Excerpt: Taking Over Episode in Colorectal Surgery

Speaker	Text
PHASE 1	
Specialist	((to Registrar)) 1 Is it coming?
Registrar	2 It is- ((Tone 4)) hmm. 3 Jackie, I'm just gonna move you in deeper. 4 Grab that. 5 Er ah ((exerting considerable force)) there, just there. 6 Oh how annoying. 7 I can feel it.
Specialist	8 Are your fingers down below it?
Registrar	9 Almost like a suction effect at the moment in the pelvis. 10 My fingers are below it.
Specialist	11 Ok well pull on em hard. 12 Pull up on that band. ((several seconds of no dialogue))
PHASE 2	--
Registrar	13 Naah, this is ... ((trails off))
Registrar	14 Nup!
Specialist	15 ...faffing, isn't it?
Registrar	16 It is faffing.
Specialist	17 Oh that's not the word, um. 18 It's all very stiff in there, just from his previous disease. 19 Let's just go straight down the middle of the front || 20 and see what we run into. ((to Scrub nurse)) 21 Can you get a little small sponge thanks Sally, or a medium sponge. 22 So we've just had a – || 23 roll it into a ball, into a roll – || 24 so we've been frustrated || 25 and we've been <<26 what?>> repelled (yep), || 27 so we're just gonna try another (way) .... || 28 So just roll that down – || 29 that might be too much actually – || 30 and get down there, || 31 pull on that bit || 32 and I'll see || 33 if Jackie and I can show you that. ((to Jackie, a medical student)) 34 Jackie can you help me? 35 We'll both hold a second. 36 You need to get more than one finger down there, || 37 so that you've got a little bit of a front.
Registrar	38 And an angle. ((12 seconds no dialogue))
Specialist	39 Let me move the retractor – || 40 you stay there.
Registrar	41 Suction.
Specialist	((to Registrar)) 42 That's nice. 43 Sweep it out to the side, || 44 that's great – nice one. 45 Yep, that's going good. 46 Let me move this again.
Registrar	47 Can you pull up a little bit?
Specialist	((to Student)) 48 Hold it up a little bit. ((to Registrar)) 49 Are we showing it to you? ((she nods, then several seconds no dialogue))
PHASE 3	--
Registrar	((to Specialist)) 50 Sorry. 51 I'm in the way, aren't I?
Specialist	52 No, I just can't stand it any more.

Speaker	Text
Registrar	53 I'm actually getting somewhere now.
Specialist	((supportively)) 54 No but you're doing- you're doing fine!
Registrar	55 You wanna take over, don't you?
Specialist	56 No, no.
Registrar	57 Yes you do!
Specialist	58 No, I absolutely don't want to take over!
Registrar	59 You do! 60 I feel!
Specialist	61 Well, no I don't, || 62 I don't.
Registrar	63 I didn't say || 64 I was going to let you! 65 I just said || 66 I feel.
Specialist	67 Don't suck up there Jackie! 68 The action's down here.
Student	69 Oh.
Specialist	70 That's all right. 71 Don't worry. ((3 seconds no dialogue))
Student	72 Are you getting frustrated? ((Tone 1))
Scrub	((laughs quietly and catches Specialist's eye, sharing some levity re Student's remark))
Specialist	73 No, I'm not - || 74 I'm very happy with the way it's proceeding. 75 If there was bleeding and stuff, || 76 I would not be happy, || 77 but I'm happy. 78 The other thing is that we don't need to get all much further down anteriorly, here, because we're gonna turn him over and we'll get the best view of it.
Registrar	79 Have a feel. 80 Have a feel, || 81 see what you feel, that I feel. 82 There's a lateral band here, || 83 that I've been having difficulty getting, || 84 do you feel that?
Specialist	85 Yeah.
Registrar	86 I'm just really awkward at getting that.
Specialist	((to Registrar)) 87 Can we swap sides || 88 and I'll have a go at it?
Registrar	89 Sure.
Specialist	90 And we'll just see what I-
	((to whole operating theatre team)) 91 Can we swap sides please? ((to Registrar)) 92 And I can, I can feel cancer, about in the same area. 93 So we'll swap sides.
Specialist	((to Scrub)) 94 Can we have fresh gloves Sally for when we um, yeah-
Scrub	95 Yeah. Yeah.
Specialist	96 As, as we finish the pelvic dissection || 97 I'd like fresh gloves.
Scrub	98 Fresh gloves.
PHASE 4	--
Specialist	((to another nurse, helping him disconnect headlamp lead)) 99 Thanks, Ned. ((each surgeon walks around to

Speaker	Text
	the other side of the operating table)) ((to Registrar)) 100 Now what happened there? 101 Did you abdicate || 102 or did I take over?
Scrub	((to a scout nurse)) 103 Seven and a half. ((to Specialist)) 104 Seven and a half?
Registrar	105 I can't get it.
Specialist	106 OK let's see if I can.
Registrar	107 And I've tried a few different ways || 108 and I still can't get it.
Specialist	109 Yep, ok.
Scrub	110 ((repeating request about glove size, to Specialist)) Seven and a half?
Specialist	((to Scrub)) 111 Ah Vicks thanks ((a retractor)). 112 Yeah, I'll have seven and a half, || 113 but not for a little while.
Scrub	114 No, no – I've got time.

The interpersonal grammatical and semantic patterns exhibited as this episode opens are a manifestation of the *Tenor* roles at play, including agentive role, hierarchy and social distance. In terms of *agentive role* the registrar is principal surgeon but this role is quite *mutable* (Butt 2004) as shown in the "taking over" that ensues; in terms of *social hierarchy*, the registrar is not the most senior surgical person in the room and this parameter is *not mutable* within the instance, although it may change over the years. The specialist's *agentive role* is assistant (mutable), but this role is layered with the role of supervisor and trainer (not mutable), thus incorporating the displayed need to give advice, but also motivating a complex and shifting set of *goal orientations* for the procedure in terms of *Field*. The student is hierarchically junior and, agentively, engaged in a role that is less *declared*; she is largely a silent helper who does as she is bid. The fourth team member observed here is very senior in terms of social hierarchy but, as a nurse, belongs to a different *seniority domain*; her agentive role is *complementary* to that of the primary surgeon but *not mutable*, and the person she is "scrubbing for" depends on negotiations made between the surgical staff, not on negotiations she is involved in herself; at the same time she coordinates the action and negotiates the relations of other nurses in the theatre. Across these participants, *social distance* (within *Tenor*) varies from *regular, multiplex contact* over many years between scrub and specialist; a *shorter history of contact* but a *shared professional coding orientation* between surgical specialist and registrar; down to *much less regular contact* between scrub nurse and medical student.

Very crudely, we can add that in terms of *Field*, the primary activity in this episode is the *material action* of mobilizing the bowel. From the point of view of *Mode*, language is *ancillary* to this primary material action: its role at this point is to help get the bowel mobilized.

Additionally, though, there is a kind of interpersonal colouring of gradually accumulating frustration that can be seen in the Tone 4 that undercuts the registrar's claims of progress in clause 2, in the appraisal token *annoying* in clause 6, and in the echoes of *Are we there yet?* when the specialist asks *Is it coming?* in clause 1.

The motif of frustration brings with it a sense that the *contextual configuration* is relatively unstable. If frustration has been developing for some time as we infer, we might expect a move from one or more participants to change something at this point: to try a different method or reconsider goals (adjusting *Field*), to change who is doing what, or to evaluate the process in a different way (adjusting *Tenor*). But such a move does not occur for a number of clauses yet. How do the participants co-construct the timing of this change? One aspect of co-constructing change is signalling that, at least on certain parameters, no change is being undertaken. Looking at the body movement that accompanies this part of the dialogue (Figure 11.4), we can see that the interlocutors' *distance, body orientation and gaze* changes. But rather than disrupting the primary contextual configuration, these changes arguably signal *no change*. This sequence also shows how these three features must be seen analytically as separate factors in construing engagement.

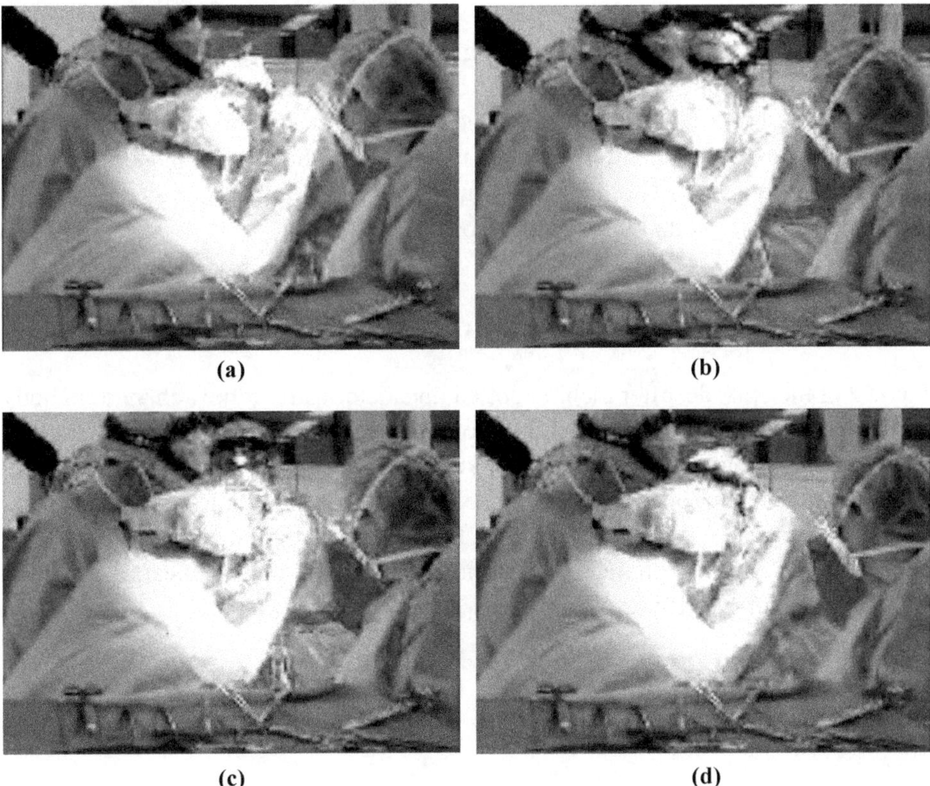

(a)   (b)
(c)   (d)

Figure 11.4: Moving to continue the current context

In *frame (a)* of Figure 11.4, the senior registrar is at the back, right. The registrar partly signals and enacts her role as the *primary surgical agent* by having her head down low, directly over the wound (the cut in the patient's abdomen through which surgery takes place).

What occurs next is one of those moments where one "holds the floor" without speaking. In *frames (b) and (c)* of Figure 11.4, we see the senior registrar's head pop up. While she does this her body is aligned in exactly the same direction and distance with respect to other team members – e.g., her left arm stays in the same anchoring position. Maintaining these aspects of body position, I argue, constitutes, *inter alia*, a message to other team members that she is retaining her agentive role as primary surgical agent (*Tenor*); and that the primary activity remains the material action of mobilizing the bowel (*Field*). In *frame (c)* especially, we can see how her neck and head are, by contrast, no longer oriented in the general direction of the staff specialist: now her body orientation makes a point of avoiding direct gaze with any of the team members. Primarily, this signals that she does not want to change the engagement from joint action to direct conversational exchange. This then is a signal about *Mode*, that there is no change from language being ancillary, to language being constitutive of the context, which is a contextual shift that *is* made a short time later.

In Figure 11.4, *frame (d)* we see the registrar's head returned to its default setting of low over the wound with denied gaze, as she continues with the task of mobilizing the bowel. Looking over all four frames we see little change in the mutual body alignment of the other team members. This arguably shows they have interpreted these movements as the "hold" in the context suggested, rather than as the substantial change in context that it might have been.

11.4.3   Phase 2: Moving to Change the Context

Phase 2 of the episode, after the first dotted line, demonstrates how changes in body alignment contribute to a successful re-configuration of the context. Linguistically, the move from Phase 1 to Phase 2 is marked by the specialist's shift into the declarative mood (interpersonal *grammar*), used to give information to the registrar and others (interpersonal *semantics*). Subtle shifts in body alignment (see Figure 11.5) appear to act as a vanguard for these interpersonal linguistic meanings, which appear very shortly afterwards, as discussed below.

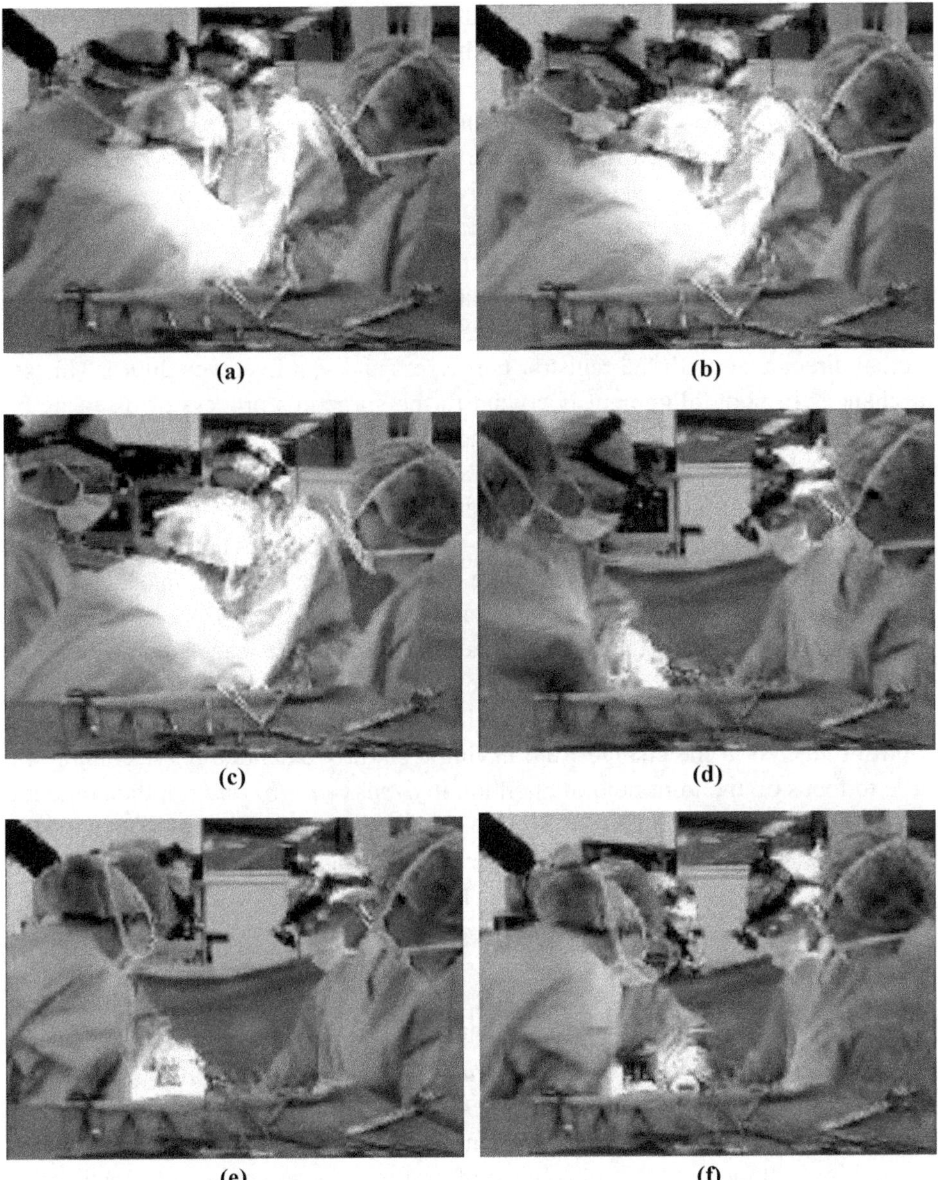

Figure 11.5: Changes in body alignment constituting a new phase in the surgical context

Frame (a) in Figure 11.5 shows the specialist as he utters clause 11, *Pull on em hard*, at the final turn of Phase 1. He is still in the role of assisting and guiding the registrar. The registrar's *body position* over the wound signifies her continuing role as primary surgical agent, despite the specialist's coaching. The specialist's head (back right) and the registrar's head (back left) almost touch. Both are focused on the *joint field of attention*, the wound, with the specialist giving the registrar *primary visual and manual access*. Consistent with its ancillary role with respect to material action, the linguistic exchange here takes place *without direct gaze* between the specialist and registrar. In *frame (b)*, before the specialist signals linguistically that he is no longer convinced they are on track, he begins to *distance his head and body* from the registrar and others, i.e., from the joint field of attention. Note there is no significant change in the body positions of the registrar (back left) or student (front left) or scrub nurse (front right) yet. By the time he begins Clause 13 *Naah, this is faffing, isn't it?*, the specialist is standing completely upright (*frame (c)*), his gaze taking in the wound and the registrar's face, offering – but not demanding – mutual direct gaze with the registrar (see Kress and van Leeuwen 2006). This set of changes in body alignment is crucial to the surgeon's process of disengaging himself from the agentive role of assisting the registrar to mobilize the bowel, and beginning a new configuration. Note how far the surgeon's head travels.

There is still no change in body position of registrar, student or scrub nurse in Figure 11.5, *frame (c)*. By *frame (d)*, however, bodily disengagement with the previous configuration is now complete for all team members, and this is construed linguistically too, with the registrar agreeing in clause 16 *It is faffing*. The registrar has moved back relative to the table (note the wall space now visible); the student has moved right back *behind* the specialist, leaving space for the leaders to reconfigure their engagement first. The scrub nurse's disengagement is (very subtly) reflected in the change from having a slightly extended neck, craning it a little to focus on the joint field of attention in *frames (a), (b) and (c)*, then relaxing it in *frame (d)*.

A new contextual configuration has been emerging, as shown by the reciprocal body positions. In *frame (e)* of Figure 11.5 the specialist can be seen to embody this change by beginning to *lower his head* and take up the space and visual access assigned to the *primary surgical agent*. As mentioned above the specialist produces a series of declaratives (clauses 17–18; 22, 24 etc.), construing himself rather than the registrar as information giver, and therefore primary agent, in *Tenor*, and at the same time adjusting the *role of language* in *Mode* from ancillary to *constitutive*, at least for the time being. *Frame (e)* corresponds to the specialist's switch to declaratives, in which he mitigates potential damage to the collegial tenor of the context by backing off from his choice of "faffing" as an apt term for evaluating the team's progress (clause 17). By *frame (f)* the specialist is using space and angle differently (lowest head position), along with different voice quality and intonation (for intonation analysis of this passage see Smith [2007]), signalling his new role as primary surgical agent while he works "first-hand" on the wound, taking the role of primary surgical agent. At this point he utters the next declarative, clause 18, *It's all very stiff in there*, moving the domain of appraisal (Martin and White 2005) from *judgement* of the registrar's/team's performance to *appreciation* of the quality of the patient's tissue.

Note that in *frames (d)–(f)* of Figure 11.5 the student's head follows closely the head of the specialist; she correctly interprets the change of primary surgical agent and the implication that her role now is to observe and assist the specialist not the registrar. Note also how the sequence of stills, with its coming together and moving apart of the heads and bodies of the team members, hints at the episodic rhythm of real-time surgery. In this case, the rhythmic unit is quite short – the specialist uses the above changes in *Tenor* and *Mode* to make some micro adjustments to *Field*, in clause 19: *Let's just go straight down the middle of the front*. He then goes back to acting as the registrar's assistant, as shown in the "advisory" demands for goods and services, *Roll it into a ball*, and the positive appraisal, *Nice one*, addressed to the registrar.

As Figure 11.5 illustrates, the turning point in this sequence occurs when the specialist *increases his distance* from the registrar. I would argue that this move *does* count as a disengagement of some sort, as Hall's (1966) and Martinec's (2001) modelling of distance would suggest. On the other hand, the simultaneous change of orientation to *head-to-head* might be expected to increase the degree of engagement, and therefore perhaps cancel out the decrease in proximity, but if we take the two dimensions of change together, what we really have is in fact a *different type of engagement*. In this new type of engagement, the two people concerned are engaged directly with each other in a primarily semiotic exchange rather than being engaged jointly in some action (here material action) on an object or a third party (here the patient). It is only in this semiotic type of engagement that the "maximal" engagement is very close, head-to-head alignment.

11.4.4 Degrees and Types of Engagement

If we consider the other members in the surgical team we can strengthen the argument for thinking in terms of different kinds, as well as different degrees, of engagement. Note how the student (in Figure 11.5) changes her orientation during the sequence: while the registrar is the primary surgical agent the student faces her in *frames (a)–(c)*, and thus the student's orientation to the specialist is somewhat oblique (turned away). In *frames (d)–(f)* the student now displays her shared understanding that the specialist is taking over the role of primary surgical agent. But, to construe *increasing engagement* with the specialist, instead of the student squaring off towards the specialist, i.e., towards a more head-to-head orientation which we would expect under Hall's (1966) or Martinec's (2001) models, the student's alignment with respect to the specialist becomes even more oblique than it had been. That is, she moves into more of a *shoulder-to-shoulder* position with respect to the specialist. It would be wrong to interpret such turning away as a lowering of engagement in this situation when, given the activity being undertaken, establishing a shoulder-to-shoulder position with respect to another team member signals that one is ready to take their point of view on the problem (literally) and to act jointly with them on the same shared phenomenon.

A helpful way of thinking about these two kinds of interpersonal engagement can be drawn from Colwyn Trevarthen's work on children's development. Trevarthen proposes the notions of *primary* and *secondary intersubjectivity*, identifying age reference points for when children tend to develop these important aspects of the sense of self (Trevarthen 1979). While the developmental timeline does not concern us here, the constructs and what they afford are important. Primary intersubjectivity manifests bodily in young infants in the kind of head-to-head alignment with direct gaze that represents Hall's and Martinec's maximal engagement (think of the "mirroring" of expressions between mother and baby). After about three months of age a baby will start to "become interested, not only to look about and try to get hold of objects for himself or herself...but also to follow the gaze of the other person who is occupied in seeking and acting on objects" (Trevarthen 2004: 13). This kind of behaviour becomes the basis of Trevarthen's "secondary intersubjectivity" which he also glosses as "cooperative awareness" and which he keeps strongly tied to bodily links between doing and showing. In a similar approach, Zlatev (2008) makes a further distinction between the *mutual gaze* of primary intersubjectivity (I see you), the *shared attention* (I see that you see X) and *joint attention* (I see that you see that I see X, and vice versa). This third case requires an understanding that the sign "has *the same meaning for the addressee as for the sender*" (Zlatev 2008: 229).

The point of these analogies with child development is that the type of embodied action that constructs and maintains a joint field of attention, and which implies shoulder-to-shoulder orientation, is, in some sense, the apex of mutual engagement. It is easy to see why it is important for surgical team members to be able to interpret, appreciate and deploy both *shoulder-to-shoulder* and *head-to-head* modes of body alignment in managing complex and shifting engagements in theatre (and outside). It is easy as a researcher to identify instances from the corpus, like the one above, that show team members tacitly but skilfully using their bodies – along with language – to enact and negotiate engagement. But it is also not difficult to spot occasions where body alignment as an expression plane option does not have the same meaning for all members of the team. This brings us to the final phase of the episode.

11.4.5 Phases 3 and 4: Swapping Sides

After further complex linguistic negotiations (Phase 3) which we discuss elsewhere, the specialist and registrar end up "swapping sides" and swapping primary surgical roles for the rest of the procedure (Phase 4). Figure 11.6 displays this change, showing the registrar still acting as surgeon in *frame (a)*. In *frames (b)–(d)*

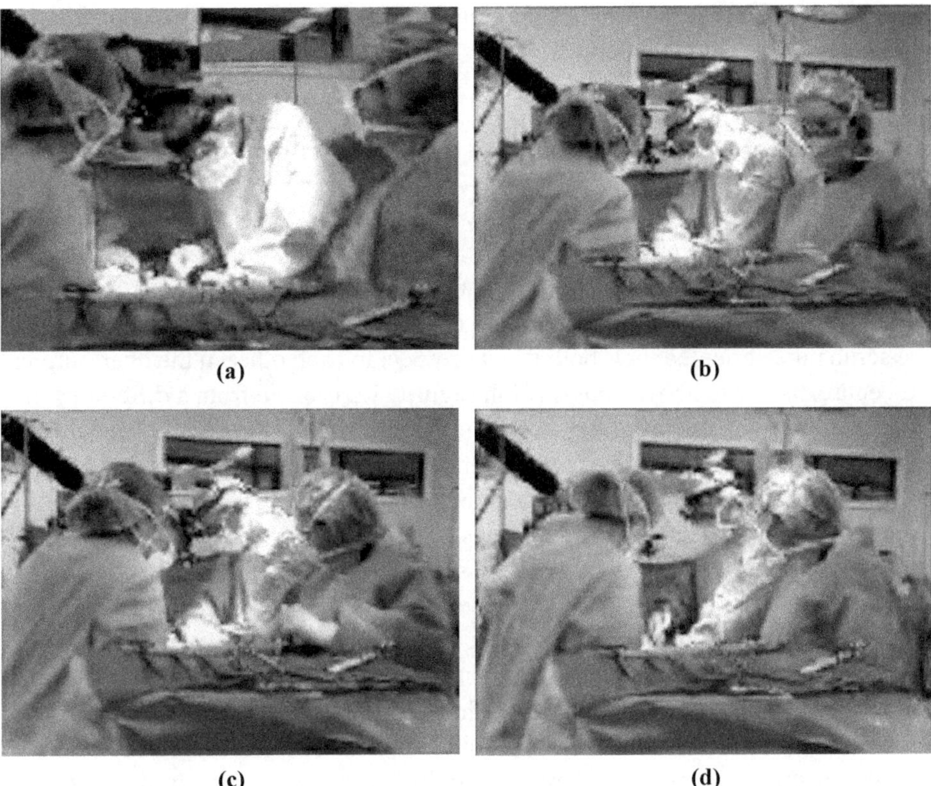

(a)   (b)

(c)   (d)

Figure 11.6: Scrub nurse orientation to surgeon with (a) registrar as primary surgeon and (b–d) specialist as primary surgeon

the specialist, now acting as surgeon, is on the right-hand side of the picture, with the registrar now tucked in on the left (note the headlamp protruding). The registrar is now engaged as surgical assistant (*agentive role in Tenor*).

Note that the scrub nurse (far right) orients herself somewhat differently with respect to the primary surgeon when this role is filled by the staff specialist, with whom she has worked over many years. The scrub nurse now tends to stand closer and more in the shoulder-to-shoulder alignment than she had when the registrar was acting as primary surgical agent – compare *frame (a)* in Figure 11.6 (and Figure 11.5) against *frames (b)–(d)*. As Figure 11.6 shows, after the staff specialist has "taken over", the scrub nurse still moves her head and neck to allow for different gazes, including taking in more of the surgeon's action at the wound, but she does not turn her whole body *towards* the surgeon as she had been doing while the registrar was acting as primary surgeon. Under the model proposed here, this dispreference for head-to-head orientation is seen not as disengagement but as the heightened engagement of "professional intimacy" (*Tenor*) given other specific parameters of the surgical context.

11.4.6   Different Modes of Surgery and Different Stratal Alignments

The final example, in Figure 11.7, shows the shift from *open surgery* in *frame (a)* to *laparoscopic surgery* in *frame (b)* in which telemonitors replace the wound itself as the most important field of attention. In Figure 11.7 *frame (a)* is a replica of the corresponding frame in Figure 11.6, reminding us of how the registrar and the scrub nurse oriented their bodies with respect to each other in the open surgical procedure discussed above; *frame (b)* in Figure 11.7 is taken from a different surgical procedure with the same key personnel working laparoscopically. Under these conditions the "rules of engagement" change quite considerably. Note that in *frame (b)* the surgeon and assistant (specialist and registrar) are on the same side of the table as each other, sharing similar views of, and access to, the wound. The scrub nurse is now on the other side from both surgical staff.

The most significant thing about this episode for the purpose of this chapter is that there are monitors on each side of the table, and the scrub nurse could arguably display engagement fully by facing the surgeon and taking in the monitor behind the surgeon at the same time, but she does not. Instead, the scrub nurse spends most of this procedure with her back or side towards the surgeon and the assistant, looking at the same monitor they are looking at. My argument is that she does this because maintaining a physically embodied joint field of attention is such an important, persistent and unconscious signifier of strong engagement – at least in the unmarked *contextual configuration* of surgery, which can be (crudely) depicted as entailing *material action* in *Field*, *regular contact* and *shared coding* in *Tenor*, and *language as ancillary* in *Mode*.

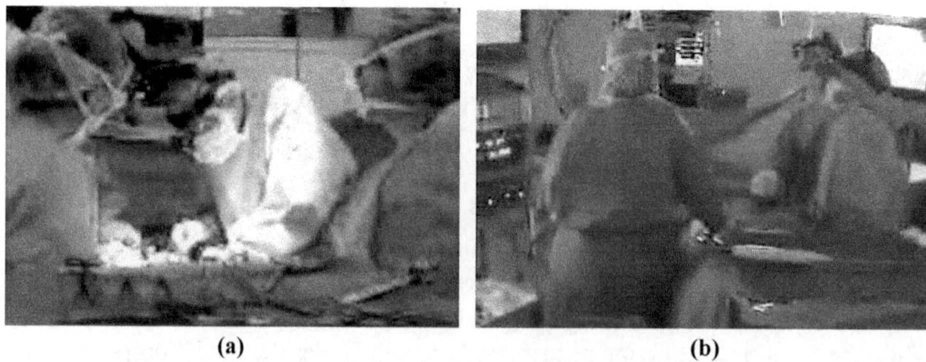

(a)   (b)

Figure 11.7: Scrub nurse orientation to surgeon in (a) open and (b) laparoscopic surgery

11.5 Mutual Understanding and Cross-Professional Understanding of Alignment Systems

Patterns of body alignment become critical to the success and the safety of the surgical operation both when they are understood and when they are misunderstood. For instance, as part of our interviews and debriefing sessions with surgical and nursing staff, we discussed a particular procedure, using the laparoscopic mode, when a surgeon "spat the dummy" (the surgeon's own term for this not uncommon occurrence in surgery). It became clear that one of the things that contributed to the surgeon's discomfort during that procedure was the fact that the surgeon felt as if the scrub nurse in question was not as engaged as they usually would have been, and perhaps as they should have been. It turned out that the scrub nurse was using a way of engaging with other team members that nurses, as a group, recognized as typical for laparoscopic surgery but not for open surgery. The surgeon in question was not aware that nurses used two different "default positions" for these two different types of surgery, and had interpreted the nurse's body orientation as a *drop in engagement* instead of the intended manifestation of a *different type of engagement*.

11.5.1 How Do These Instances Imply a System of Bodily Engagement?

As the above discussion of excerpts from the surgery corpus has demonstrated, changes in body position, angle and so on may constitute changes in context, and engagement shifts are often the semantic principle on which such changes in context are construed. Clearly though, there is no simple one-to-one correspondence between a certain distance and a certain value of engagement, or even of a certain distance plus a certain angle of orientation, and a specific value of engagement. This is because contextual parameters – settings in *Field, Tenor* and *Mode* – mediate the relation between body alignment as the *expression plane* and engagement as the *content plane* in a semiotic system that typically accompanies and enhances speech. I have not been able to generalize a system for how such mediation happens across different registers, but our current work is to generalize a system for the particular register of surgery as a kind of case study, along the lines of the discussion above, which has tried to establish mediating principles for a handful of instances.

11.5.2 A Proposed Analysis

The following tentative proposal can be made for generalizing these mediating relationships within the context of colorectal surgery, moving from instance to register. When a surgical team member changes their body alignment vis-a-vis another member or members, this may mean a change in the degree of engagement if:

- there is no *Field*-based reason for the bodily change, such as a change to *laparoscopic* surgery (see Figure 11.6); and
- there is no *Mode*-based reason, such as change from *language-as-ancillary* to *language-as-constitutive* of the social process (see Figure 11.5); and
- there are no other *Tenor* changes – e.g., when agentive roles change it is possible to keep the same *high degree of engagement* but the *type of engagement* or the *engagement target* may change (see, e.g., the student's *redirection of engagement* in Figure 11.5, where she remains fully engaged from the point of view of the surgical team as unit, but the focus of her attention switches from registrar to specialist, as the specialist takes over the primary agentive role of surgeon).

11.6   Concluding Remarks

In this chapter there has not been room to discuss the very important issue of how the different modes, speech and action, are related to each other in multimodal texts. I agree with van Leeuwen's proposal (van Leeuwen 2004) that speech and action – like text and image – must be seen as working together in single unified communicative acts; it is not the case that there is a speech act and a separate "body alignment act". Yet even if, as members and analysts, we perform action and speech together, it seems clear that each has its own system of relations between expression and content. It therefore makes sense to work on a description of semiotic action such as body alignment in a way that states its properties separately from statements about linguistic semiosis, but holds in mind all the while that these two performed modes are themselves integrated into one system (Kendon 1972; Argyle 1975) and share many principles of structure and production and probably evolutionary development (Arbib 2001). Compare Baldry and Thibault's (2006) *principle of resource integration.*

In developing a more registerially sensitive account of the bodily semiosis of engagement, an important step will be to develop the explanatory power of the concept of *Mode*. Halliday's classic gloss gives *Mode* as "what it is that the participants are expecting the language to do for them in the situation" (Halliday 1985: 12). As pointed out by Muntigl (2004: 40), this does imply that other semiotic systems might be involved but does not focus on the meaning-making role of *semiotic systems other than language*. If Muntigl is right to claim that *Mode* plays a pivotal role in organizing which semiotic systems become activated in social contexts (Muntigl 2004; Martin 1992), it is probably also true that it is the overall *contextual configuration* of an instance which determines how such modalities end up being co-deployed. So elaborating *Mode*, and its way of contributing to contextual configuration in multimodal texts, must be a high priority (cf. Norris [2004] on the notion of *modal density* and Kress [2010] on *modal affordance*).

Nor is it just the observable selection and co-deployment of modalities that is important – there is also a question of connotative relations between modalities that may need developing, and this point takes us back to the issue of whether surgical team members working in very close proximity can be said to be intimate. As Hall (1966) points out, the sense of intimacy that is associated with close personal proximity to another person is not merely a matter of conventional sign relations. The fact that close proximity is felt to entail intimacy is largely owing to the fact that a person who is in very close proximity can be perceived through the senses of touch and smell. As well, they can be seen with the distortion of features and detail that "up-close" focal length brings (including seeing pores, facial hair). So, although smell and touch, *as semiotic systems involving staff bodies as symbol sources*, may not be prominent or even activated at all in a particular context such as surgery, they underpin the semiotic systems that *do* appear to be prominent, including the system of body alignment which (in part) construes interpersonal engagement (cf. Hindmarsh and Pilnick's [2002] idea of "intercorporeal knowing" among anaesthetists).

In summary, then, although much more clarification is needed, the present chapter shows that the relationship between *body alignment as expression plane* and *engagement as content plane* is highly context-dependent. Promising models such as that proposed by Martinec (2001) must build this dependency in much more centrally, and empirical research would profit from proceeding on Firthian principles of one "restricted language" (Firth 1957) or one register at a time. With respect to research that applies linguistics to surgery, an important priority is to explicate the systemic nature of choices in body alignment and the stratal relation between these choices and the experience of engagement. Building such an explication into clinical training and professional development is an important step in enhancing teamwork in ways that are likely to improve patient and staff safety (cf. Weldon et al. 2013). Findings from the project discussed in the present chapter have been incorporated into the development of a new postgraduate surgical training facility and teaching hospital at Macquarie University.

Acknowledgements

The Australian Research Council kindly supported this research through an ARC Discovery Project DP344447, entitled "Systemic Safety: The Meanings of Behaviour in Contexts of Surgical Care" including an ARC postdoctoral research fellowship for myself, based at Macquarie University. Chief Investigators were

David Butt, John Cartmill and myself – my thanks go to David and John for generous intellectual and institutional support as well as comments on the present chapter. I am very grateful to Lorraine Squire and Jodie Ellis-Clarke for crucial institutional access, advice and discussion; to Rebekah Wegener for analytical assistance; and to the organizers of the European International Systemic Functional Linguistics Conference, Gorizia, 2006, where this material was first presented and invited for publication in a book on multimodal semiotics which although in press since 2007 unfortunately did not eventuate. Sincere thanks to the staff, students and patients at Nepean Hospital who allowed us to observe their surgical operations, and who must remain anonymous. Aspects of the work published here have been discussed in Moore et al. (2010) in the *Australian and New Zealand Journal of Surgery*. A linguistic analysis of the episode discussed here is presented in *Linguistics and the Human Sciences* (Lukin et al. 2011).

References

Arbib, Michael. 2001. Co-Evolution of Human Consciousness and Language. *Annals of the New York Academy of Sciences* 929: 195–220.

Argyle, Michael. 1975. *Bodily Communication.* London: Methuen.

Baldry, Anthony, and Paul J. Thibault. 2006. *Multimodal Transcription and Text Analysis: A Multimedia Toolkit and Coursebook.* London and New York: Equinox.

Bernstein, Basil. 1971. *Class, Codes and Control (Volume 1).* London: Routledge & Kegan Paul.

Bezemer, Jeff, Alexandra Cope, Gunther Kress and Roger Kneebone. 2014. Holding the Scalpel: Achieving Surgical Care in a Learning Environment. *Journal of Contemporary Ethnography* 43: 38–63.

Bezemer, Jeff, Ged Murtagh, Alexandra Cope, Gunther Kress and Roger Kneebone. 2011. "Scissors, Please": The Practical Accomplishment of Surgical Work in the Operating Theatre. *Symbolic Interaction* 34: 398–414.

Bowcher, Wendy. 2013. Material Action as Choice in Field. In *Choice: Critical Considerations in Systemic Functional Linguistics*, edited by Lise Fontaine, Tom Bartlett and Gerard O'Grady, 101–40. Cambridge: Cambridge University Press.

Butt, David. G. 1988. Randomness, Order and the Latent Patterning of Text. In *Functions of Style*, edited by David Birch and Michael O'Toole, 74–97. London and New York: Pinter.

Butt, David. G. 2004. *Parameters of Context: On Establishing the Similarities and Differences between Social Situations.* Sydney: Department of Linguistics, Macquarie University.

Butt, David G. 2006. The Robustness of Realizational Systems. Invited address to the Symposium on Meaning in Context: Implementing Intelligent Applications of Language Studies. To mark the official launch of The Halliday Centre for Intelligent Applications of Language Studies (HCLS), City University, Hong Kong, March 26–9, 2006. http://hallidaycentre.cityu.edu.hk/events/symp2006/profile/Dr-David.htm

Butt, David G., Alison Rotha Moore and John Cartmill. 2003. Systemic Safety: The Meanings of Behaviour in Contexts of Surgical Care. ARC research application. Sydney: Macquarie University.

Butt, David G., and Rebekah Wegener. 2007. The Work of Concepts: Context and Metafunction in the Systemic Functional Model. In *Continuing Discourse on Language: A Functional Perspective*, edited by R. Hasan, C. Matthiessen and J Webster, Vol. 2, 589–618. London: Equinox.

Ekman, Paul, and Wallace Friesen. 1969. The Repertoire of Nonverbal Behavior: Categories, Origins, Usage, and Coding. *Semiotica* 1: 49–98.

Firth, John Rupert. 1957. *Chapters in Linguistics 1934–1951*. London: Oxford University Press.

Gawande, Atul, Michael Zinner, David Studdert and Troyen Brennan. 2003. Analysis of Errors Reported by Surgeons at Three Teaching Hospitals. *Surgery* 133: 614–21.

Goffman, Erving. 1963. *Behavior in Public Places: Notes on the Social Organization of Gatherings*. New York: The Free Press.

Hall, Edward T. 1959. *The Silent Language*. New York: Doubleday.

Hall, Edward T. 1966. *The Hidden Dimension: Man's Use of Space in Public and Private*. London: Bodley Head.

Halliday, Michael A.K. 1973. *Explorations in the Functions of Language*. London: Edward Arnold.

Halliday, Michael A.K. 1985. Context of Situation. In *Language, Context, and Text: Aspects of Language in a Social-Semiotic Perspective*, edited by Michael A.K. Halliday and Ruqaiya Hasan, 3–14. Burwood, Victoria: Deakin University Press.

Halliday, Michael A.K. 2003. Introduction: On the "Architecture" of Human Language". In *On Language and Linguistics: Volume 3 in the Collected Works of M.A.K. Halliday*, edited by Jonathan Webster, 1–29. London and New York: Continuum.

Halliday, Michael A.K., and Christian M.I.M. Matthiessen. 2004. *An Introduction to Functional Grammar*. 3rd edition. London: Edward Arnold.

Hasan, Ruqaiya. 1996. Semantic Networks: A Tool for the Analysis of Meaning. In *Ways of Saying, Ways of Meaning: Selected Chapters of Ruqaiya Hasan*, edited by Carmel Cloran, David Butt and Geoff Williams, 104–31. London: Cassell.

Hasan, Ruqaiya. 1999. Speaking with Reference to Context. In *Text and Context in Functional Linguistics*, edited by Mohsen Ghadessy, 219–327. Amsterdam: John Benjamins.

Hasan, Ruqaiya. 2009. The Place of Context in a Systemic Functional Model. In *Continuum Companion to Systemic Functional Linguistics*, edited by Michael A.K. Halliday and Jonathan J. Webster, 166–78. London & New York: Continuum.

Healey, Andrew N., Shabnam Undre, and Charles A. Vincent. 2006. Defining the Technical Skills of Teamwork in Surgery. *Quality and Safety in Health Care* 15: 231–4.

Hindmarsh, Jon, and Alison Pilnick. 2002. The Tacit Order of Teamwork: Collaboration and Embodied Conduct in Anaesthesia. *Sociological Quarterly* 43: 139–64.

Hjelmslev, Louis 1961. *Prolegomena to a Theory of Language*. Trans. Francis J. Whitfield. Revised English edition. Madison, Milwaukee and London: The University of Wisconsin Press.

Kendon, Adam 1972. Some Relationships between Body Motion and Speech. In *Studies in Dyadic Communication*, edited by Aron Wolfe Siegman and Benjamin Pope, 177–216. New York: Pergamon Press.

Kendon, Adam. 2004. *Gesture: Visible Action as Utterance*. Cambridge: Cambridge University Press.

Kress, Gunther. 2010. *Multimodality: A Social Semiotic Approach to Contemporary Communication*. London: Routledge.

Kress, Gunther, and Theo van Leeuwen. 2006. *Reading Images: The Grammar of Visual Design*. London and New York: Routledge.

Lukin, Annabelle, Alison Moore, Maria Herke, Rebekah Wegener and Canzhong Wu. 2011. Halliday's Model of Register Revisited and Explored. *Linguistics and the Human Sciences* 4(2): 187–243.

Martin, James R. 1992. *English Text: System and Structure*. Amsterdam and Philadelphia: Benjamins.

Martin, James R., and Peter R.R. White. 2005. *The Language of Evaluation: Appraisal in English*. London and New York: Palgrave Macmillan.

Martinec, Radan. 2000. Construction of Identity in Michael Jackson's *Jam*. *Social Semiotics* 10: 313–29.

Martinec, Radan. 2001. Interpersonal Resources in Action. *Semiotica* 135: 117–45.

Martinec, Radan. 2004. Gestures that Co-Occur with Speech as a Systematic Resource: The Realization of Experiential Meanings in Indexes. *Social Semiotics* 14: 193–213.

Moore, Alison Rotha. 2004. The Discursive Construction of Treatment Decisions in the Management of HIV Disease. PhD thesis, Macquarie University, Australia. http://hdl.handle.net/1959.14/46321

Moore, Alison Rotha. 2005. Modelling Agency in HIV Decision-Making. *Australian Review of Applied Linguistics*, Special Edition S19: 103–22.

Moore, Alison Rotha, David G. Butt and John Cartmill. 2005. Systemic Safety in Surgery: Risk, Responsibility, System. Chapter presented to COMET-VELIM 05 – 3rd Interdisciplinary Conference on Communication, Medicine and Ethics. University of Sydney and Macquarie University, June 30–July 2, 2005.

Moore, Alison Rotha, David G. Butt, Jodie Ellis-Clarke and John Cartmill. 2010. Linguistic Analysis of Verbal and Non-Verbal Communication in the Operating Room. *ANZ Journal of Surgery* 80: 925–9.

Moore, Alison Rotha, and Kathryn Tuckwell. 2006. A Tenorless Genre? Forensic Generic Profiling of Workers' Compensation Dispute Resolution Discourse. *Linguistics and the Human Sciences* 2(2): 205–32.

Muntigl, Peter. 2004. Modelling Multiple Semiotic Systems. In *Perspectives on Multimodality*, edited by Eija Ventola, Cassily Charles and Martin Kaltenbacher, 31–50. Amsterdam: John Benjamins.

Norris, Sigrid. 2004. *Analyzing Multimodal Interaction: A Methodological Framework*. London and New York: Routledge.

Reason, James. 2000. Human Error: Models and Management. *British Medical Journal* 320: 768–70.

Smith, Bradley. 2007. Intonational Systems and Register: A Multidimensional Exploration. PhD thesis, Macquarie University, Australia. www.isfla.org/Systemics/Print/Theses/SmithBradPhD.pdf

Trevarthen, Colwyn W. 1979. Communication and Cooperation in Early Infancy: A Description of Primary Intersubjectivity. In *Before Speech: The Beginning of*

Interpersonal Communication, edited by Margaret Bullowa, 321–72. Cambridge: Cambridge University Press.

Trevarthen, Colwyn W. 2004. Learning about Ourselves, from Children: Why a Growing Brain Needs Interesting Companions. Research and Clinical Centre for Child Development, Annual Report 2002–03 (No. 26), 9–44. Graduate School of Education, Hokkaido University. Accessed online June 3, 2006. http://www.perception-in-action.ed.ac.uk/publications.htm

van Leeuwen, Theo. 2004. Ten Reasons Why Linguists Should Pay Attention to Visual Communication. In *Discourse and Technology: Multimodal Discourse Analysis*, edited by Philip Levine and Ron Scollon, 7–20. Washington: Georgetown University Press.

Weldon, Sharon Maree, Terhi Korkiakangas, Jeff Bezemer and Roger Kneebone. 2013. Communication in the Operation Theatre: Systematic Review. *British Journal of Surgery* 100: 1677–88.

Wilson, Katherine A., Shawn C. Burke, Heather A. Priest and Eduardo Salas. 2005. Promoting Health Care Safety through Training High Reliability Teams. *Quality and Safety in Health Care* 14: 303–9.

Wilson, Ross McL., William Runciman, Robert Gibberd, Bernadette Harrison, Liza Newby and John D. Hamilton. 1995. The Quality in Australian Health Care Study. *Medical Journal of Australia*, 163: 458–71.

Zlatev, Jordan. 2008. The Co-evolution of Intersubjectivity and Bodily Mimesis. In *The Shared Mind*, edited by Jordan Zlatev, Timothy P. Racine, Chris Sinha and Esa Itkonen, 215–44. Amsterdam: Benjamins.

Alison Rotha Moore, PhD, is a Senior Lecturer in English Language and Linguistics at the University of Wollongong and an Honorary Research Associate with the Language in Social Life Research Network at Macquarie University, Sydney, where she held an ARC Project on interaction within surgical teams, with John Cartmill and David Butt, among other joint endeavours. She currently publishes on medical discourse, animal studies and functional linguistics, in particular register theory.

12 Who's Who?: Role Performance during Minor Awake Procedures

Israel Berger and Sarah J. White

12.1 Introduction

Communication has a significant impact on operating theatre practices. A recent review of studies looking at communication in operating theatres found that job-related strategies and goals were prevalent and that even seemingly simple tasks were accomplished through sophisticated collaborative work (Weldon et al. 2012). In the same setting, utilizing social power to restrict communication and access to resources (*gatekeeping*) can negatively impact patient care (Weldon et al. 2013). Conversation Analysis (CA) allows for an in-depth analysis of many aspects of operating theatre communication, including physical movements, gaze, spoken language, vocalizations and combinations thereof. For example, although requests rarely identify a recipient through everyday practices such as gaze or naming, the recipient is implied based on the sterility and proximity of the requested item or action (Bezemer, Murtagh et al. 2011: 403). This chapter focuses on how people involved in minor awake procedures construct their roles and orient to the procedures.

Important differences that are relevant to interaction exist between awake procedures (i.e., when the patient is conscious and a local anaesthetic is used) and procedures under general anaesthesia (i.e., when the patient is "asleep"). The main and obvious difference between awake procedures and those performed under general anaesthesia is that in awake procedures, the patient is conscious and able to listen and/or speak, thus potentially limiting the topics that are discussed between health professionals and introducing the possibility that the patient could be involved in conversations. Awake procedures include those as major as some brain surgeries and most Caesarian sections all the way to quite minor procedures such as mole or cyst removal and haematoma drainage. Although most major awake procedures are arranged such that the patient cannot see the surgical field (whether due to a barrier or because the surgery involves the head), the patient may be able to see minor procedures depending on the location of the lesion. In minor awake procedures, the sterile field and team are much smaller (perhaps only a doctor or a nurse practitioner), and the patient may be accompanied by a friend or family member, a prospect that would be almost unheard of in most other surgical situations aside from Caesarian section. These findings are also evident in less formal surgical settings, such as for minor awake procedures.

Although conversation analytic research has examined communication in a variety of medical contexts, including surgery, it has not yet looked at the dynamics of awake procedures. In this chapter, we present an exploration into this setting by examining a corpus of publicly available minor awake procedures for ways in which diverse parties perform their roles. Data have been sourced from educational and patient-distributed videos of actual procedures involving a variety of health professionals, patients and presenting problems. We also compare these data to patient-distributed data of lay people performing sebaceous cyst removal and ear haematoma drainage to further explore whether the roles are situation-specific or qualification-specific (or perhaps a bit of both). We then consider how policies and communication may be affected by knowledge of parties' potential role-related behaviours and how to minimize harm whilst maximizing benefit to the patient's care and experience.

12.2 Multiple Roles and Role Performance

All the world's a stage,
And all the men and women merely players:
They have their exits and their entrances;
And one man in his time plays many parts...
– Jaques, *As You Like It* Act II Scene VII by William Shakespeare, c. 1600

The ideas that we *perform* the roles we have in a given interaction and that we have different roles in different contexts have their origins prior to the development of the social sciences. The above quote from Shakespeare's *As You Like It* illustrates this four centuries ago. Mead (1934) introduced the concept of *role* to the social scientific community. Although Mead did not explicitly define role at this time, he implied that roles are intrinsic to statuses and can be taken on by those who do not own those statuses, for example a child pretending to be a teacher. Merton (1957) goes on to distinguish between *status sets* and *role sets*, and it is Merton's work that forms the basis of modern role theories. Status sets (sometimes loosely called "multiple roles") involve disparate categories that do not necessarily significantly overlap. One person may have the status of a daughter, mother, PhD student, medical doctor, patient, driver, recreational pilot etc. in different areas of her life.

Within this status set, her role as a daughter does not make her a mother, driver etc. However, within her status as a medical doctor, she may have a role set consisting of her simultaneously being a surgeon, consultant, lecturer, tutor, medical library user, security card holder etc., each contingent on her status as a medical doctor. In addition to the roles she may occupy within the role set, the role set also includes the roles of those around her who are involved in the practice and teaching of medicine (e.g., nurses' roles as receptionists, theatre booking administrators, medical and nursing students in tutorial groups and as clinic or operating theatre visitors).

Goffman (1961: 135) argues that roles involve social relationships, which vary to the degree that they are "social" vs "business". Goffman does not distinguish between the normative framework of a role and the requirements associated with a particular job description. He recognizes, though, that one person may have competing requirements and sets out roles in a situated basis, for example in a given moment, whether a surgeon is being a operator (someone performing an operation) or a clinician (someone seeing patients clinically). In all of a person's roles, they demonstrate some sort of relationship to others (Coser 1966: 179). The requirements of one's role may be explicit (e.g., a job description), or they may be implicit. For example, the requirement for scrub nurses and scouts to understand surgeons' *idiolects* (idiosyncratic ways of speaking or of naming objects) is necessary for the smooth operation of the operating theatre (Bezemer, Cope et al. 2011), yet rarely (if ever) is this requirement formally documented. So pervasive, though, is this requirement that nurses may keep notebooks detailing surgeons' idiolects in addition to their instrument and set up preferences for different procedures (ibid.).

Perhaps the most famous discussion of roles in the social sciences is that of the *sick role* (Parsons 1951, 1968; Parsons and Fox 1952). Parsons (1951) postulated that people who are ill have a particular set of rights and obligations: that they are exempt from normal social roles, that they are not held responsible for their condition, that they should want to get well (i.e., define being ill as a bad thing) and that they should seek competent help and cooperate with that help. He defines "somatic illness" as the "incapacity for relevant task performance" and "mental illness" as the "incapacity for the role performance" (Parsons 1968: 262), thus implying that a sick person must adopt the sick role lest they develop the incapacity for proper role performance. However, the sick role is not often observed in real-life sick people and their households (Brown and Rawlinson 1975; Friedson 1961 cited in Siegler and Osmond 1973) despite widespread agreement with its rights and obligations in this setting (Arluke, Kennedy and Kessler 1979; Brown and Rawlinson 1975), and it is inconsistent with expectations for people with long-term illnesses or disabilities (Winter 2003). It can thus be said that whilst roles may exist in thought and to some extent in practice, they are not static, immutable things that drive unthinking and passive people to act in predetermined ways. Rather, roles help us think about what, based on cultural norms, is expected of people in different circumstances and situations.

Merton (1957: 114) argues that expectations around roles and role performance are readily observable aspects of social systems that allow for out-of-role behaviours. In contrast, Goffman (1961) views roles as statuses straddled somewhere between situated and semi-permanent with specific expectations. Embarrassment can be used to bring attention to failings in role performance, thus making visible the requirements of a role (Gross and Stone 1964), or as Goffman (1956) puts it, that an individual has projected incompatible definitions of themselves. What is deemed compatible with a role is with regard to reference-group behaviour, such that a given behaviour is either part of or not part of the "normative framework of a role" (Coser 1966: 174; Goffman 1961: 115). People may take on incompatible roles by using *role distance* to partially take on a role whilst denigrating that role or distancing oneself from it (Coser 1966). Such role distancing may be to test out potential roles or to gain acceptance in another role. People who do not practice role distance may be considered "too serious". For example, a surgeon who jokes during an operation may be considered by societal expectations to be acting outside the normative framework of the "surgeon" role in that they may appear less focused on the patient and their work. However, whilst this behaviour is not part of the role itself, neither is it deviant. Not joking may signal a problem socially or with the procedure itself, as joking communicates to others on the surgical team that they are a team player and "good humoured" (Coser 1966: 174). The surgeon is expected to lead the surgical team, to exercise control and to help others maintain their own confidence in their roles, and a combination of role distance and ritual (in the form of particular environment, clothing and behaviour) helps to achieve these goals (Coser 1966: 177). The surgeon in this case "gives up some prerogatives usually associated with his[/her] status the better to impress the fact that permissiveness rests with him[/her]" (Coser 1966: 183, masculine generic language corrected).

Similarly, the role of main surgeon may be changeable depending on the presence of others. Trainees, residents, surgical technicians, physician's assistants, nurses and surgical assistants may be assistants to a consultant surgeon (as in Svensson, Heath and Luff 2007), or an advanced trainee or fellow may be the main surgeon with a less experienced trainee acting as surgical assistant. A consultant may even act as assistant in order to aid a trainee in developing their skills (Moore et al. 2010). Yet, in all of these cases, the consultant has the right to take the role of main surgeon or to exercise decision-making even without scrubbing. Although the consultant may relinquish *control* in this way, they retain *command*.

12.3 Interactional Relevance of Roles

Although role has been discussed predominately as an overarching concept that lends reason and order to interactions and broad social organizations, Halkowski (1990) demonstrates how interactants draw on their and others' roles to both *make sense of* and *accomplish* social interactions in situ. This differs from dominant conceptualizations of roles such as role theory (e.g., Hardy and Conway 1978) in that it stresses the interactive and constructed nature of roles rather than as predetermined frameworks around which social actions are structured. Heritage (e.g., 1984, see also Heritage and Clayman 2010) argues that different contexts are "talked into being" through individual interactions and that simultaneously interactants mould their behaviour based on contexts. Institutional talk, including medical and surgical dialogue, is derived from the rules and resources that we use in everyday conversation.

Not every role is relevant in every interaction. The above doctor's colleagues and patients may not even know that she has a pilot's licence. Unsurprisingly, though, one area in which some roles are likely to be relevant are medical interactions, particularly roles such as patient, doctor, nurse, relative, friend etc. Role performance and its implications have especially been examined in paediatrics, where third parties (parents, caregivers) may be intimately involved in the consultation from opening to closing. The patient (in the case of paediatrics, the child) may do work to manage the third party's (the parent's) involvement (Clemente 2009). The implications of third party involvement in these cases can be great; for example parents/caregivers' desires (as perceived by the doctor) can have significant impact on prescribing practices, leading to unnecessary antibiotic prescribing (Stivers et al. 2003). Conversely, recognition of the various roles that a patient and third parties have in other aspects of their lives, along with their knowledge and values, is a key element of patient-centred care, in which clinicians attempt to bracket their own views in exchange for their interpretation of the patient's, and consumer-directed care, in which clinicians relinquish the power they traditionally hold to find out inductively what the patient wants (Aged & Community Services Australia, Council on the Ageing, and Leading Age Services 2013).

Power has a prime place in the discussion of roles in healthcare settings, and Merton (1957: 113) argues that differences in power serve to stabilize role sets. Under usual circumstances, the main surgeon or doctor is expected to set the tone for junior colleagues and other health professionals. They are thought to have more of a right to use humour and other potentially delicate devices than others, and the burden of conflict resolution within the immediate interactional environment (or between them and another member) ultimately rests with them (Coser 1966: 179). However, their position of power enables them to potentially create social fictions that put the blame on others or away from themselves when something goes wrong (e.g., Finn 2008: 122). Their social authority may not necessarily reflect their administrative authority, leadership skills or "team player" status. Finn found that within operating theatre teams, hierarchies were reproduced in how people talked about teamwork and being members of teams. Surgeons and anaesthetists utilized a technical-instrumental repertoire to discuss teams, legitimating their power and privileges, whereas nurses and operating department practitioners (ODPs) utilized a relational repertoire, emphasizing egalitarianism through social capital without directly challenging existing structures. Finn (2008: 105) goes on to argue that multi-professional teamwork has unintended divisive effects that maintains professional inequality. Conversely, Collin, Paloniemi and Mecklin (2010: 46) argue that strict delineations between workers' duties and identities are in direct conflict with promoting teamwork within the operating department. They argue that operating department workers grapple with the competing demands of creating a team environment and their respective disciplines, a situation that may be alleviated by having a "team leader" who promotes inclusiveness to help overcome the effects of cross-disciplinary status differences (see also Nembhard and Edmondson 2006).

The distinction between an operating department and an individual operating theatre is an important one when considering power and hierarchies. The reality of the operating department is that those managing the *department* are not people in traditional positions of authority in the operating theatre; they are administrators or nurses whose power is invested by the hospital rather than by their titles. Thus those with the authority to change theatre bookings or assign staff may not have authority in other areas such as surgical decision-making despite also being a part of an operating *theatre* team. Commonly, operating theatre teams are multi-professional, rather than inter-professional, in that hierarchies and sharp role delineations exist (Bleakley et al. 2006; see Collin, Paloniemi and Mecklin 2010: 50 for an example of mapping task divisions in surgical teams). However, as Collin and colleagues (2010: 56) argue, "despite strong agreement about the professional roles and duties of each participant, smooth teamwork also requires a helpful attitude and, if needed, practical help outside one's own professional scope", i.e., actions outside the normative framework of a role. A surgeon may help clean up, a porter may press a button on the diathermy machine, a student may bring items from the storeroom etc. By participating in these ways, members take on tasks outside the formal role requirements associated with their titles to stress their roles as members of a team, thus momentarily turning a predominately multi-professional environment into an inter-professional environment.

The role, in the predetermined sense, of many surgical patients is consistent with that of Parsons' sick role in that they are exempt from normal social roles (by virtue of being admitted to hospital), they may or may not be held responsible for their condition (someone having cosmetic surgery or surgery for a self-inflicted ailment *could – but not necessarily –* be held responsible for their incapacity), are expected to work towards getting back to normal activity levels, have sought competent help and are expected to follow aftercare instructions. Yet, they may not feel that society accepts them as belonging in the sick role if they are day surgery patients, despite their own needs (Mottram 2009). Even more so for someone having a minor awake procedure such as a cyst or mole removal may be expected to go back to work later that day and then go home and cook dinner for their family. They are probably not held responsible for their condition – unless the procedure was for a self-inflicted wound. They have sought competent help (which may not necessarily be a medical professional, e.g., peer ear haematoma drainage at a boxing match) and are expected to follow basic aftercare instructions such as changing the dressing and protecting the site from trauma. Thus, minor awake procedure patients fit some but not all of the rights and obligations (and perhaps not the key right of being exempt from other social roles) of the sick role. Yet, they are clearly in a vulnerable position as the subject of a procedure and also are actors in clinical encounters involving themselves. How, then, do we examine the building of such a unique role from an interactional perspective?

12.4   Method

12.4.1   Data

We have compiled a corpus of 20 publicly available videos of educational and patient-distributed minor awake procedures on a video self-publishing website in accordance with copyright laws and user agreements. See Berger (2012) for more information on the legal and ethical aspects of using data from self-publishing websites in research. Although the videos are publicly available, we have masked identifying details. Procedures include cyst removal, haematoma drainage, surgical drain removal and other procedures involving superficial structures.

The quality of procedures can vary greatly, however we do not evaluate the operators' skills, whether they are professionals or lay people; rather we focus on the communicative aspects of the situation. For example, although operators trained as surgeons are likely to avoid puncturing a sebaceous cyst in order to ensure the entire cyst is removed, many other health professionals and lay people will squeeze out the contents of the cyst prior to removing the sac (if the sac is removed at all). The likely outcome of an incompletely removed cyst is recurrence, yet assessing the quality of the procedure is beyond the scope of this chapter. Instead, we examine how parties are observed to orient to the procedure, each other and their roles.

12.4.2   Design

We used CA to examine how diverse parties perform their roles during the procedures. As described in Chapter 2 of this volume, CA examines the moment-by-moment unfolding of naturally occurring interaction captured in video or audio recordings. CA and other detailed interactional approaches have only recently begun to examine surgical settings, perhaps due to researcher access and recording logistics, with only a few research groups intimately involved in research involving naturally occurring operating theatre interactions and surgical consultations.

Surgical topics studied from a CA perspective thus far span a range of interesting and important issues. The overall structure of surgical consultations (e.g., White et al. 2013; see also Chapter 2, this volume), and aspects of how treatment recommendations are framed in orthopaedics consultations (Hudak, Clark and Raymond 2013; Chapter 7, this volume), object transfer in operating theatres (Svensson, Heath and Luff 2007) and group dynamics of operating theatres (e.g., Mondada 2001, 2006, 2011; Weldon et al. 2012) have been examined in detail. Mondada (2011) discusses the interactions among senior surgeons and junior surgeons acting as assistants revolving around use of electrocautery tools during laparoscopic surgery. She observes how the level of explication and instruction given by the same surgeon differs by both assistant and how potentially vulnerable to error the area being dissected is. That instructions are given almost exclusively by the senior surgeon is an unspoken indication of their role as main surgeon – someone who is ultimately responsible for the procedure and more experienced than others. The senior surgeon remains in command throughout but can relinquish aspects of control to other members of the operating team. Assistants may be responsible for retracting tissues and guiding the laparoscope, but they may (as in Mondada's data) also be allowed responsibility for dissection under the command of the senior surgeon. That some assistants may take initiative (and be given the go ahead by the surgeon) "since [they] know" (Mondada 2011: 214) and instruction-action resumes spontaneously upon arrival at more delicate areas, is indicative of participant orientation to both role and competence. Code-switching in terms of language (French vs English), technical/instructive content and questioning style is also seen when interacting with observers and assistants during surgical demonstrations, thus sharply delineating who the intended recipient is based on roles, co-presence and what they are expected to understand (Mondada 2001).

12.5 Analysis

In the data we examined, five key points with regard to differences and similarities between parties came to light:

(1) All parties time their talk to avoid delicate moments.
(2) The operator has relatively unlimited speaking rights.
(3) Patients and third parties avoid the turn space of health professionals.
(4) The operator speaks with authority, regardless of qualification.
(5) Third parties may play an especially social role in minor awake procedures.

In the following sections, we will provide detailed analyses of key extracts to illustrate these concepts. We will refer to the person performing the procedure as the operator (O), the one receiving the procedure as the patient (P), with third parties named according to their relationship to the patient or their job title: student (St), nurse (N), friend (F), mother (M), and sister (Sr). For ease of reading the transcripts, a simplified Jeffersonian transcription style (see Chapter 2) is used throughout and physical movements are only described when relevant to the particular analytic point.

12.5.1 All Parties Time Their Talk to Avoid Delicate Moments

Because minor awake procedures are often relatively quick, delicate moments tend to be entire phases of the operation rather than temporary handling or approach to fragile tissues as in other procedures. Delicate moments may include the initial incision in the skin or the bulk of a procedure near an important structure. For example, one cyst removal involving a large sebaceous cyst near the patient's spine and that initially had insufficient pain management was mostly silent from the initial incision until the sac was empty (Extract 1). The entire procedure is approximately five minutes, with three minutes of the doctor squeezing out the contents of the cyst and all parties being silent.

Extract 1 [Sebaceous Cyst on Back]

```
01 P:    not numb yet
02 O:    nope here we go big sting
03 O:    ((injects local anaesthetic and withdraws needle,
04       some cyst content comes out of injection sites))
05 F1:   man that looks nasty
06 F2:   huhhuhuhhuh
07 O:    okay
08 O:    ((pokes into cyst with scalpel))
09 P:    It's hurtin
10 O:    ((continues making incision))
11 P:    ow
12 O:    ((withdraws scalpel and examines
13       incision with slight squeezing))
14 F2:   °°Squeeze squeeze squeeze squeeze°°
15 O:    ((continues examining incision))
16 O:    Sting sorry ((injecting local anaesthetic))
17 P:    ((flinches))
18 O:    ((lengthens incision))
19 O:    ((squeezes))
20 O:    ((lengthens incision))
21 O:    ((deepens incision))
22 O:    ((squeezes contents out of incision))
23 O:    ((wipes and examines contents))
24 O:    ((squeezes contents out of incision, periodically
25       wiping with finger))
26 O:    alright I think that's ((squeezes contents out of
27       incision))that's an empty sac there ((removes
28       remaining contents from skin with fingers))
```

In lines 1–4, the operator is preparing to and then injecting the local anaesthetic into the area around the cyst on the patient's back. Immediately after this is completed, one of the patient's friends responds to the leakage of cyst contents out of an injection site, "man that looks nasty" (line 5) and the other laughs (line 6). The operator then prepares to begin the incision ("okay", line 7) and makes an initial incision (lines 8–13). Only after the scalpel has been removed does one of the friends speak again (line 14, "squeeze squeeze squeeze squeeze"). The operator continues examining the incision and then injects additional local anaesthetic at line 16, warning the patient that it will sting. The patient flinches (line 17), and the operator begins a series of incisions, squeezing, wiping and examining the expressed contents (lines 18–25). He signals that the procedure is almost over (line 26, "alright I think that's") but then squeezes what turns out to be the final contents from the sac. In line 27, he states that the sac is empty (and thus that the procedure is over) and wipes the skin with his finger. As we can see in lines 3–4 and 18–28, all parties are silent during delicate moments of the procedure. In lines 2 and 16, the operator warns the patient of potential pain, and in lines 26–8, the operator explicitly states that the bulk of the procedure is over as he removes the last of the sac contents. His role as operator allows him to speak at these points to signpost to others, in particular the patient, the immediate trajectory of the procedure.

12.5.2 The Operator Has Relatively Unlimited Speaking Rights

Although health professionals performing minor procedures in the office (and many lay operators) are largely silent during minor awake procedures compared to other parties present, when they do speak, they are superordinate speakers, becoming particularly focal to all parties. During points in the procedure when others are silent, such as when the operator injects local anaesthetic into the patient's back (Extract 1, above), the operator may talk to the patient. Talk at these points may be to warn the patient of potential discomfort, as in Extract 1. It may also be to distract them from psychological or physical discomfort or from pain when pain management cannot be better addressed and may include a request that the patient reciprocate the talk, as in Extract 2. The patient in this extract is a man who has had a large cyst for several years, and his girlfriend is removing it at home for him.[1]

---

1   Simple procedures such as this performed by lay people are frequently encountered in the United States, where healthcare is funded through individuals rather than through the tax system. A single cyst removal performed in the doctor's office can cost up to $2000 (or more if in a delicate location) without insurance, including the surgeon's fees and pathology. If imaging is required, the cost can be more, and insurance coverage for surgical procedures and diagnostics varies. When lay people perform minor awake surgeries, there is commonly no local anaesthetic used due to their prescription only status (a topical substitute may be available but of limited usefulness). When local anaesthesia is used, pain is a patient-mentionable phenomenon rather than something that must be continuously monitored by the surgeon.

Extract 2 [Cyst Removal at Home]

```
01 O:    you okay
02       (0.8)
03 P:    °yeah°
04       (13.9)
05 O:    is that hurtin
06       (1.4)
07 O:    honey
08 P:    °I'm fine°
09 O:    well keep talkin to me so I kno:w (0.5)
10       that you're not passin out on me
```

The operator has just opened the cyst and received a minimal, delayed response to her talk (lines 1–3). She asks the patient in line 5 whether he is experiencing pain and receives no response (line 6). After pursuing a response in line 7 ("honey"), the patient provides another quiet response, this time more explicit – "I'm fine" does not answer the question of whether it hurts, but rather it answers that the patient is able to handle any pain he may be experiencing (line 8). The operator then explicitly requests that the patient keeps talking so she knows he is not overwhelmed with pain (lines 9–10). As this extract demonstrates, the operator has unlimited speaking rights during the procedure. Delicate moments may have phases that are less delicate, or when the operator does not require quite as much concentration. That it is normative for the operator to speak during ostensibly delicate moments, while others still do not, marks their role as distinct from other parties in that they are able to transgress this silence and thereby identify the less delicate phases in which full concentration is not required and communication with the patient takes precedence.

12.5.3 Patients and Third Parties Avoid the Turn Space of Health Professionals

Despite their authority to speak at any point during the procedure, the operator during a minor awake procedure speaks less than others present. Because the operator tends to speak much less than others, it is difficult to say with certainty that they are privileged with regard to turn-taking. However, in the data we examined, sequences involving the operator occurred with either gaps or precision-timing of talk during routine points in procedures, and minimal overlap occurred during communication difficulties (see Nevile 2006 on a similar phenomenon among air traffic controllers and flight crews, with the exception of silence, which without non-vocal cues can lead to simultaneous starts, 2007). There were no cases of significant overlap with the operators' speech except for an ear haematoma drainage performed by lay people at a boxing match using a needle and syringe to drain the blood without an incision (Extract 3). In this case, the operator was asking the patient whether he was ready for the procedure to begin, to which he subsequently responded that he was not.

Extract 3 [Ear Haematoma at Boxing Match]

```
01 F1:    I see how does it feel
02 O:     feel that it feels hard
03        ((F1 squeezes ear gently))
04 O:     feel t[hat
05 P:          [it feels disgusting
06 O:     WOOO
07 O:     rea[dy
08 P:        [it just feels like=
09 O:     alright
10 P:     =I have like=
11 O:     come on [y'ready
12 P:            =[some kind of cotton thing in my ear
13 O:     alright you ready
14 P:     wuh wait
15 O:     dude it's like a balloon
16 F2:    just do it
17 P:     HEY HEY ((pulls O's hand away))
18 O:     I'm not going to squeeze it I'm just
19        sticking a needle in
20 O:     one ((puts needle in haematoma blister))
21 O:     that thing's already started to deflate
22 P:     I didn't even feel it that's how big it is
```

Extract 3 begins with an onlooker asking about how the haematoma feels (line 1). The operator describes it as hard and instructs the onlooker to feel the ear (line 2). The onlooker feels the ear, and the operator seeks confirmation that he feels the hard texture (line 4). The onlooker's face is off-camera, so he may have responded non-vocally. The patient responds to the onlooker's question as a subjective question – how does the injury itself feel – in line 5 ("it feels disgusting"). The operator makes a vocalization "WOOO" at line 6 and asks whether the patient is ready for him to insert the needle ("ready", line 7) – that if he is ready the insertion of the needle is imminent. The patient begins a new turn on the topic of how his ear feels to him, "it just feels like..." (line 8). The operator re-issues his turn as "alright" (line 9), which makes relevant progression of the procedure and the at least temporary end to the conversation; the patient continues speaking, "...I have like..." (line 10). The operator produces a third, stronger attempt at line 11, "come on y'ready", both with a direct summons "come on" and recycling "ready" from line 7, this time as "y'ready". The patient overlaps with "y'ready", continuing his turn "...some kind of cotton thing in my ear" (line 12). In line 13, the operator again recycles his previous attempts, this time as "alright y'ready". Again, "alright" draws attention to the need to continue the procedure and at least temporarily stop conversing. "Y'ready" again highlights to imminent insertion of the needle. At this point, the patient halts the procedure "wuh wait" (line 14). The operator cites the size of the patient's ear as indicating the necessity to progress the procedure, "dude it's like a balloon" (line 15). Another onlooker urges the operator to "just do it" (line 16), and the patient pulls the operator's hand away yelling "HEY HEY" (line 17). The operator reassures the patient that he is not going to squeeze the ear and that he is just sticking a needle in to draw up the blood into a syringe (lines 18–19). The patient visibly relaxes and is silent, and at line 20, the operator begins a count of one and inserts the needle into the haematoma blister. He then observes that the ear has "already started to deflate" (line 21), and the patient announces that he could not even feel the needle because the ear is so large (line 22). Overlap between the operator and others, notably the patient, occurred here during a problem with the progressivity of the procedure – the patient was not ready for the procedure to begin and instead engaged in troubles telling about the injury. Further pressure from the operator and an onlooker resulted in the patient panicking. However, after reassurance and a brief description of the procedure in the service of reassurance, the patient relaxed and the operator began the procedure. They both then chatted about the earlier topic from a new perspective – that of the actual drainage – and without overlap. Usually there is no overlap with the operator, who appears to occupy a privileged status with regard to turn-taking. The stark difference between sequences in this extract illustrates well how overlap with the operator can be a sign that there is a problem (in this case, with the procedure itself).

Even in a busy emergency department (also an ear haematoma drainage), other parties (the patient, a nurse, a student and a friend of the patient) avoided overlap with the operator, practising precision-timing or allowing gaps to form. Minimal overlap did occur during a communication problem during this procedure (Extract 4), with an interesting duplication of two sequential environments involving very different practices the first and second times. We would like to call readers' attention especially to comparing lines 3/4 and 18/19 as well as 26/27 and 32/33. Extract 4 begins near the end of the procedure for an ear haematoma that was performed in an emergency department. The operator is suturing bolsters to the ear so that it does not fill up with blood again before it heals.

Extract 4 [Ear Haematoma at Emergency Department]

```
01 N:    does he need to go home on any antibiotics
02       (1.4)
03 O:>>  u[m
04 P:>>   [I'm actually already taking some now
05 N:    what are you taking
06 P:    uhh (0.8) amoxicillin (.) anti-inflammatories
07       and antibiotics
08 N:    amoxicillin (0.2) when did you start taking those
09       (0.8)
10 P:    yesterday
11 N:    okay (0.2) your doctor gave them to you
12 P:    yeah he wanted me to
13 N:    oh cuz (he knows)
14 P:    he wanted me to fill it better (than
15       being infected exactly)
16 N:    right
17 N:    do you want him to keep taking the
18       amoxicillin or:::
19       (2.2)
20 O:>>  uhm (1.6)
21 P:>>  I got a little (0.9) pad that has like (0.8)
22       y'know a bunch of different pills
```

```
23        and it tapers do̲w:n
24 N:     is it a zee pack are you sure it's amoxicillin
25        and no[t azithromycin
26 P:          [well that's the anti-inflammatory I'
27        talkin about the amoxicillin is a bottle of pills
28 N:     steroid maybe[:?
29 O:                  [it's probably a Medrol Dosepak
30        I would stop that
31 P:     stop th'uh: (.) anti-inflammatory
32 N:     the pack
33        (0.7)
34 N:>> y[°eah°
35 O:>>   [the Medrol Dosepak
36 O:     take the antibiotics
37 P:     o[kay
38 N:      [okay
39 (1.5)
40 P:     °no problem°
```

A nurse has come into the bay and asks the operator whether the patient needs a prescription for antibiotics (line 1). After a gap at line 2, the operator (who has been focused on performing the procedure, see Chapter 13 regarding surgeons' interaction with tissue) says "um" (line 3), which is partially overlapped with the patient, who adds information that might affect his aftercare – that he is already on an antibiotic (line 4). After an insertion sequence between the nurse and patient about what medications he is on (lines 5–16), she asks the operator again, reformulating her initial question from "antibiotics" and a new prescription to "amoxicillin" and "keep taking" (lines 17–18). After a gap at line 19, the operator again begins to respond with "uhm" (line 20). This time, the patient waits to provide additional information, allowing the operator a 1.6-second pause (line 20) before further describing the medication he is on (lines 21–3).

After some discussion between the nurse and patient about the medication, the operator (line 29) overlaps terminally with the nurse's prior turn (line 28). During her turn, the nurse maintains her prosody and volume. The operator instructs the patient to stop the medication pack he described, "I would stop that" (line 30). The patient initiates an other-repair on the operator's "that", specifying "the anti-inflammatory" (line 31). The nurse offers another other-repair, "the pack" at line 32, followed by a gap, and confirms her own repair at line 34, "yeah". However, as soon as she begins, the operator provides an insertion repair on her "the pack" as "the Medrol Dosepak" (line 35) and specifies in a positive instruction "take the antibiotics" (line 36). The nurse does not maintain her prosody and volume, rather she immediately lowers her volume and ends this word quietly. The patient and nurse claim understanding ("okay", lines 37–8), and the patient adds additional claim to his intention to adhere to the proposed regimen (line 39, "no problem").

In the first set of duplicate sequential environments, the nurse has asked the operator a question regarding the patient's post-operative treatment. The patient provides additional information about his current medications. In the first instance, this occurs after a gap and the operator has begun to say "um". In the second instance, this occurs after a gap, the operator has said "uhm", *and a pause has occurred*. In the second set of duplicate sequential environments, the nurse has provided an other-repair on something the patient has said, and the operator says something to the contrary in terminal overlap with her (NB: in the second instance, the overlap occurs not on her original repair but on her self-confirmation of the repair). In the first instance, the nurse maintains her volume and prosody, yet in the second instance, she immediately lowers her volume. Not only is the end quiet, but it is actually the majority of the word and the turn. She has effectively dropped out in favour of the operator's turn. It is important to note that it is the patient and the nurse who quickly learn to anticipate the operator's speech and allow him to speak rather than the other way around, which could have occurred just as easily.

12.5.4 The Operator Speaks with Authority, Regardless of Qualification

Operators tend to speak calmly and with authority, whether they are health professionals or lay people. They may use minor jargon to describe the procedure or pathology, they may offer reassurance, and/or they may instruct the patient or other parties (as in Extract 2, above). Both of the former are present in Extract 5, a later portion from the same procedure as Extract 2 involving a man having a sebaceous cyst removed by his girlfriend at home. In this case, the operator is using minor jargon and describing the procedure in the service of reassurance.

Extract 5 [Cyst Removal at Home]

```
01 O:>> you have (2.7) like (1.5) I don't know how
02    >> to explain it (3.2) you had a lot of juice
03       comin on out (1.6) and there's not that
04       much blood (2.9) but it looks like I'm gonna
05       have to cut a li::ddle bit more (1.4) to
06    >> allow fo:r: (0.7) the mass to come out is
07       that okay
08 O:    ((lengthening incision)) I'm gonna allow a
09       liddle bit more of a hole it's not bleeding
10       that much which is good but as you know you
11       have really tough skin and I'm trying not
12       to poke on you too much
```

The operator has just attempted to squeeze the contents of the cyst, which has become semi-solid, through the initial incision without success. In line 1, she begins to explain the current state of the procedure by describing the pathology. She acknowledges her difficulty articulating what she sees, describing serous collection as "juice" (line 2). She goes on to tell him that there is not much bleeding (lines 3–4) but that she needs to enlarge the incision "a little" (line 5). By mitigating the need to enlarge the incision (i.e., just "a little bit"), she is reassuring the patient. She goes on to explain why the incision needs to be lengthened (line 6, "to allow for the mass to come out"). She then asks for consent to enlarge the incision (which could cause pain) at lines 6–7, "is that okay". There is no obvious response and no sign of protest from the patient during this explanation. Given his overall minimal responses and silence, a lack of protest can be read as consent in this case, and is done so by the operator. The operator proceeds to lengthen the incision in line 8 and reassures the patient that "it's not bleeding that much which is good", as the procedure continues. Despite her acknowledgement of difficulty describing the pathology (revealing her lay status) at line 1, and use of colloquial language ("juice", line 2), the operator uses minor jargon in describing the cyst as a "mass" in line 6. She goes on to further describe what she is doing as a reassurance technique in lines 8–10 as well as explicitly say she is trying not to "poke on [him] too much" (lines 11–12). Both her description, particularly the use of minor jargon, and her calm speaking style position her as authoritative, thus displaying her role as a trustworthy and reassuring operator on whom that the patient can rely.

12.5.5 Third Parties May Play an Especially Social Role in Minor Awake Procedures

Third parties may be very active participants in the minor awake procedure. They may demonstrate (1) their relationship to the patient through teasing, (2) their roles as lay people by commenting on the "grossness" or extreme nature of the procedure, and (3) the minor nature of the procedure through both of these approaches.

<u>Third parties' demonstration of their relationship to the patient</u>

Although we may know a third party's relationship to the patient because they have stated who they are, e.g., the patient's mother, they may demonstrate their relationship in other ways. One way they may demonstrate their personal connection to the patient is through teasing. Teasing shows a casual approach to the patient (as well as the situation, see below) that would be inappropriate for a stranger (and usually professionals) to take. Although the patient may challenge the teasing to some degree, they do not initiate a dialogue about it nor go so far as to ask the third party to leave (which would show disregard for the third party's assumed concern for the patient). The focus of the interaction remains on the procedure, and the patient may even expand on the topic of teasing, as in Extract 6.

Extract 6 [Wood Chunk]

```
01 Sr:   can you ↑feel it
02       (1.4)
03 Sr:   if you can feel it let 'em know
04       (1.0)
05 P:    I can't feel anything
06       (2.6)
07 M:>>  oh my gosh that's a huge piece of woo:d Andy
```

```
08    >>  oh my goodness it's like a giant a::w you're
09    >>  GUSHIn out look my holy ↑cow:
10 P:     sh(h)ut up
11 Sr:>   okay got little splinters in there it's like
12    >>  an inch long
13        (2.3)
14 Sr:>   it's a good thing we came here
15        (4.0)
16 P:     Mom's like I think I see the tendons
17 M:>>   ↑that's what we thought was the tendons
18    >>  it's a piece of woo:d↑
19        (2.2)
20 Sr:    wow
```

Extract 6 follows the injection of local anaesthetic and the beginning of efforts to clean out a penetrating wound of a young man's thigh that resulted from a BMX bike accident on a wooded trail. They have come to a nearby urgent care centre (a sub-emergency outpatient clinic common in the United States) to have him examined and treated. The patient's mother and sister are present in addition to a nurse and the doctor who is performing the procedure. In line 1, the patient's sister asks him if he can feel the procedure, to which he does not respond. She changes this from a question to an instruction ("if you can feel it, let 'em know", line 3), downgrading the response relevance of her turn, to which he does respond "I can't feel anything" (line 5). In line 6, the operator removes the largest of the pieces of wood (about an inch long) with very minimal bleeding. The patient's mother comments on the size of the wood in line 7 and goes on to tease the patient in lines 8–9 "oh my goodness it's like a giant aw you're gushin' out … holy cow". The patient challenges the teasing (which may be more due to the gory nature of the teasing than the teasing itself, which he addresses explicitly later in the procedure, see Extract 9) in line 10 ("shut up"). His sister then describes the piece of wood that was removed using dry language "okay got little splinters in there it's like an inch long". Moving further away from the teasing, she then says in line 14 "it's a good thing we came here", softening the tease to say that treating the injury certainly needed medical assistance. The patient then teases his mother back in line 16 "Mom's like I think I see the tendons". She then laughs about the nature of the injury "that's what we thought was the tendons it's a piece of wood" (lines 17–18), ending this phase of teasing. She also uses "we" instead of the patient's earlier reference to just her, thereby implicating the family as a whole in the mistaken identity of what was visible (a process Lerner and Kitzinger 2007 term *aggregation*). The patient's sister then draws attention to a new stage in the procedure with "wow" (line 20), in which the operator is measuring how far the piece of wood originally went into the patient's thigh. As this extract shows in lines 7–18, third parties may demonstrate their close relationship to the patient through teasing but also by using collective self-reference.

Occasionally, health professionals, including the operator, may also comment jokingly on the procedure as well, for example the large volume of some cysts. This approach may be more difficult for professionals to carry out given the potential for it to be interpreted as making light of the patient's condition.[2] The operator only used this approach in one instance of the data we examined (Extract 7) despite it being a recurring theme among third parties. It occurred in a Midwestern U.S. practice, and the interaction can be characterized as very casual and egalitarian. Extract 7 involves a man having a sebaceous cyst on his neck removed with two friends present. The operator has made his incision and is preparing to squeeze the contents of the cyst out through the incision.

Extract 7 [Sebaceous Cyst on Neck]

```
01 O:    kay ready for all this junk to come out
02 F1:   oh man
03 F2:   °(   )°
04 F1:   ((S squeezing cyst)) ohh(0.2) ohhhh
05       (1.5) ohhhohhhoo[ohhohohohohoho]
06 F2:                  [nice yeah wow ] lotta stuff
07 F1:   hh .hhthis is better than youtube
08 F2:   ↑hehehe
09 O:    you might get a million hits on this one
10 F1:   oh easy
11       (1.5)
12 O:    sorry I'm pushing on you
13       (0.5)
14 P:    you're alright ((S begins removing the sac))
15 F1:   ohhh
16 F2:   hehe wow
17       (2.7)
18 F1:   eeeohhh
19 O:    oh now we're getting somewhere
20 F1:   oh ho ho
21 F2:   heheh[eh
22 O:>>       [it's like I'm freaking pulling his guts out
23 F2:   heh .hh
24 F1:   FOR REAL
25 P:    I'm excited
26 F2:   (absolutely)
27 O:    you're gonna watch the whole thing
28       (1.4)
29 O:    that's most the sac right there
30 F1:   yeah
31 F2:   that's a lot
32       (1.8)
33 O:    it's a little easier when it's more
34       obvious and comes out in one piece
35       I've gotta take this out in (1.2)
36 F1:   pieces
37 O:    °bits and chunks a little bit°
38 F2:   is that the biggest one you've ever seen
39 O:    close yeah (.) on the neck for sure
```

---

2 Although Levinson and colleagues (1997) found that greater use of laughter and humour was one feature that differentiated general practitioners, general surgeons and orthopaedic surgeons who had no malpractice claims from those who did, some medical schools and hospitals continue to advise students and trainees not to laugh or joke at all on the grounds that it could offend patients.

In line 1, the operator announces that he is about to squeeze, "kay ready for all this junk to come out". This is followed by vocalizations and an assessment of the contents by the friends (lines 2–6). One of the patient's friends then assesses the procedure positively, "this is better than youtube" (line 7), and the other laughs (line 8). The operator upgrades the assessment at line 9, "you might get a million hits on this one", to which the original assessor responds favourably, "oh easy" (line 10). He continues to squeeze the cyst and then addresses the patient "sorry I'm pushing on you" (line 12), to which the patient responds "you're alright" (line 14). The operator begins removing the sac in line 14, accompanied by vocalizations and laughter from the friends (lines 15–21). The operator then comments on the sac removal, "it's like I'm freaking pulling his guts out" (line 22), to which one of the friends laughs (line 23) and the other agrees "for real" (line 24). The patient offers a further assessment as a statement of his looking forward to seeing the video, "I'm excited" (line 25), and one of the friends assesses his announcement, "absolutely" (line 26). The operator then asks the patient, "you're gonna watch the whole thing" (line 27), followed by an announcement that he has gotten the entire sac (line 29). The same friend then assesses the sac and contents, "that's a lot" (line 31). The operator explains that the procedure is easier when the sac comes out in one piece but that this one was not so simple (lines 33–7). She then asks him in line 38 whether this was the biggest cyst he had ever seen, to which he responds "close yeah on the neck for sure" (line 39). The "event" nature of this procedure, with two friends brought along to document the cyst, their joy in watching it be removed, and the size of the cyst all contribute to the operator being able to prac-tice role distance from the traditional expectations surrounding his profession. The characteristically casual region where he is practising may also contribute to the flexibility to join with the patient and his friends in this way despite its unusual occurrence more broadly.

Third parties' demonstration of their roles as lay people

Third parties may claim lack of prior knowledge (as in Extract 6, line 17, above, "that's what we thought was the tendons it's a piece of wood"), giving away their lay status explicitly. They may also demonstrate their lay status through "real" orientation to the grossness of the procedure. Teasing may claim that the procedure is extreme or gross, yet it is recognizable as non-serious. "Realistic" claims or demonstrations of being "grossed out", shocked or otherwise perturbed, fit the role of lay person by marking the procedure as outside their usual frame of reference. Extract 8 is a continuation of Extract 6, and the operator is estimating the length of the path of the piece of wood by inserting a small needle holder into the wound. Up until this point, the patient's mother and sister have both been giving a running commentary on the procedure.

Extract 8 [Wood Chunk]

```
01 M:>>  .hh>no I can't I don't wanna look at that part
02       (1.3)
03 P:    I could never be a doctor
04       (2.5)
05 M:>>  ↑oo my gosh he's goin way up there
06       (2.1)
07 M:>>  .hh↑aaaw[w
08 N:           [you gonna faint
09       (0.8)
10 P:    no
11 M:    no
12 N:    don't scare me
13       (2.0)
14 O:    it's (1.4) two point five say three centimeters
15       up this way
16 Sr:   oh my gosh Andy you musta really landed on a
17       piece of wood (1.7) it went right through his jeans
```

In line 1, the patient's mother has ceased her lighthearted comments and teasing and states that the current phase of the procedure is too much for her to watch. The patient agrees with "I could never be a doctor" (line 3). His mother exclaims that the needle holder is very far into the wound, "oo my gosh he's goin way up there" (line 5) and produces a "grossed out" vocalization at line 7. The nurse reponds to her vocalization by asking whether she is going to faint (line 8), to which both she and the patient (who could also reasonably be a recipient) respond "no" (lines 10–11). The nurse closes the sequence, "don't scare me" (line 12). The operator continues with the procedure, withdrawing the needle holder and dictating the findings of his exploration, "it's two point five say three centimeters up this way" (lines 9–10). The sister comments on the length and how hard he must have hit the branch, "oh my gosh Andy you musta really landed on a piece of wood it went right through his jeans" (lines 16–17). As shown in lines 1–7, third parties (and in this case also the patient) may demonstrate their roles as lay people through their orientation to the procedure as gross or extreme. In this extract, the operator stays in his role as operator by continuing the procedure, whilst the nurse demonstrates her role by orienting to the possibility of having to care for another patient – the mother, should she faint.

Third parties' orientation to the minor nature of a procedure

Both by teasing the patient and by commenting on the gross or extreme nature of the procedure, third parties can demonstrate orientation to the actual minor nature of the procedure. These approaches are sanctioned by professionals and other parties in the setting of minor awake procedures yet would be inappropriate if the patient were actually at risk. Teasing and comments about the repulsiveness or extremeness of the procedure thus, whilst potentially distressing, ultimately communicate that the procedure is comparatively trivial. Third parties may also explicitly acknowledge how minor the procedure is. In Extract 9 (from the same procedure as Extracts 6 and 8), the patient's mother describes how at first she was afraid his injury could be life-threatening and then upon examination realized that it was a relatively superficial wound.

Extract 9 [Wood Chunk]

```
01 M:    so I was out in the garden he comes home
02       and he's furious with me (0.9) cuz I wasn't
03       (0.6) answering the telephone well I'm like
04       how did you get home if you ↑can't walk
05 N:    mhm
06       (0.8)
07 M:    he's like I dunno but I'm here now he just
08       laid on the ground and I'm like .hhh! that could
09       be a main artery you're bleedin right through
10       yer pants [(huh) I] said let's go I had to=
11 O:             [mhm    ]
12 M:    =go upstairs (0.6) and have him take it o- oh good
13       it's not a main artery cuzyer not bleeding
14       anymore(h)huhuhuhh(h) I wasn't su(h)r:e.hh
15 Sr:   °°( )°° oh my god that's why I can't
16       look [anymore
17 M:         [is that all pieces of wood
18 O:    mm nn
19 Sr:   it's fat
20 O:    °this is° ((points with scissors))
21       (0.7)
22 Sr:   skin
23       (1.2)
24 O:    this i[s
25 M:          [the skin that got pushed in
26 P:    okay okay I can still hear I can hear this
27 (2.1)
28 Sr:   I think you can (0.3) have this: without the audio
29       too (        ) the same way
30 P:    (   )
31 O:    heh I like the commentary in this video though
32 M:    it's uh he's diggin in there Andy
33 M:    woo look at all this stuff look at all
34       this pieces of guck he got out of there
35 P:    mm
36 Sr:   °°(                                  )°°
37 M:    oh my goodness it reminds me of CSI you know
38       how they dig in the body and go in there with
39       that three D lookin
40 P:    hhh okay
41 M:    hehhehheh
```

Extract 9 begins with the patient's mother recounting how she originally thought that the injury was much more severe than it was, that she originally thought it was a "main artery" but that it couldn't be since the bleeding had stopped by the time he got himself home (lines 1–14). In lines 15–16, the patient's sister again notes the repulsiveness of the procedure, this time stating that *she* "can't look" (in Extract 8 his mother says she cannot look). This time the mother is engaged with the procedure and asks about what she is seeing (line 17), "is that all pieces of wood", to which the operator responds in the negative, "mm nn" (line 18). The surgical field is of course not *all* pieces of wood, although this is what the operator was removing at the time. The sister names the just removed tissue as fat (line 19). The operator specifies "this is", pointing with his scissors (line 20). At line 22, the sister then names the general structure the operator is working on, to which the operator again says "this is" without pointing (line 24). The mother then asks a follow-up question "the skin that got pushed in" (during the impact) at line 25. The patient cites the discussion as too gory in line 26, "okay okay I can still hear this". The sister notes in lines 28–29 that the operator might want to have the video without the audio and that this should be possible. The patient produces a short, inaudible response in line 30, and the operator also responds to the sister "heh I like the commentary in this video though" (line 31). The patient's mother then begins teasing the patient again in line 32, "it's uh he's digging in there Andy" and continues with "woo look at all this stuff look at all this pieces of guck he got out of there" in lines 33–4. The patient responds with an irritated "mm" at line 35. His sister continues inaudibly at line 36, and in lines 37–9, his mother compares the procedure to the autopsies they do on the television show *CSI*. At this point, the patient produces a loud outbreath and "okay" (line 40), to which the mother laughs (line 41).

The events that play out in Extract 9 include a number of practices that demonstrate orientation to the procedure as minor, i.e., that the patient is not in danger. These practices, discussed below, include (a) explicit recognition of the injury as minor rather than life-threatening (lines 1–14), (b) potentially distressing discussion of the procedure itself (lines 17–25), and (c) teasing (lines 32–9). The operator also explicitly sanctions the commentary that the mother and sister have been providing throughout the procedure (line 31).

(a) Although we may downplay the seriousness of a procedure for the benefit of a patient remaining calm, the patient's mother acknowledges that she *was* concerned that there was a life-threatening injury but upon inspection realized that the wound was relatively superficial. This is a nod to her role as concerned parent, yet being a concerned parent in this instance could lead to anxiety in the patient or operator. Her acknowledgement of the wound as not life-threatening differs from the practice of minimizing by telling a patient who is about to undergo a routine but life-saving procedure (such as an appendectomy or oophorectomy) that the procedure is nothing to worry about or that the operator does several a week. The fact that he is ostensibly safe makes the discussion acceptable.

(b) As with discussion about death with a patient about to undergo invasive surgery, discussion about how gory the surgery is would be socially unacceptable. The discussion in lines 17–25 about the tissues does indeed distress the patient. His distress is not severe enough to warrant the operator or nurse intervening, however, further demonstrating that the procedure is minor.

(c) The patient's mother plays off his distress with further description of the procedure and subsequent comparison to *CSI* autopsies. Again, teasing of this sort would warrant intervention if the procedure or injuries posed significant risk to the patient. Instead, the patient expresses further irritation with his mother and she ends the teasing by laughing (lines 37–41).

12.6 Conclusion

Although third parties appear to time their talk such that it does not disrupt the procedure, the content of their talk may be aimed at embarrassing the patient or may highlight details that the patient is not prepared to discuss during the operation. In addition to adding to our knowledge of how roles are performed in medical and quasi-medical settings, these findings have implications of direct relevance to health professionals.

The fact that third parties may demonstrate their roles as family members, friends and/or lay people in ways that may negatively affect the patient could impact whether inclusion of friends and family members in minor awake procedures is appropriate. These issues around third party behaviour raise the question of what it means to gain consent for them to be present. However, the fact that third parties do tease or make seemingly inappropriate comments communicates that the problem leading to the intervention is not a "serious" health problem and that the procedure itself does not have major consequences. Further research is needed to examine how gaining consent for them to be present is accomplished interactionally and whether restricting their comments impacts on patient anxiety or experience of the procedure.

It is interesting and important to note that the person performing the procedure has relatively unlimited speaking rights. This has implications for turn-taking and sequence organization, and a larger-scale analysis of this phenomenon across surgical contexts could potentially identify more clearly how this adaptation from existing conversational resources occurs. The fact that they have the authority to speak regardless of whether they are a nurse, doctor or lay person may be important for the patient experience of the procedure and reducing patient anxiety. A priori research is needed to examine whether varying speaking practices impacts patient anxiety or experience of the procedure, or whether in situ the "low anxiety procedure" is entirely co-constructed.

Transcription Notation

See Chapter 2, this volume.

References

Aged & Community Services Australia, Council on the Ageing, and Leading Age Services. 2013. Consumer Directed Care (CDC) Capacity Building Service Defining Characteristics of CDC. Rhodes, NSW: Aged & Community Services Australia.

Arluke, Arnold, Louanne Kennedy and Ronald C. Kessler. 1979. Reexamining the Sick-Role Concept: An Empirical Assessment. *Journal of Health and Social Behavior* 20(1): 30–6.

Berger, Israel. 2012. YouTube as a Source of Data. *PsyPAG Quarterly* 83: 9–12.

Bezemer, Jeff, Alexandra Cope, Gunther Kress and Roger Kneebone. 2011. "Do You Have Another Johan?": Negotiating Meaning in the Operating Theatre. *Applied Linguistics Review* 2: 313–34.

Bezemer, Jeff, Ged Murtagh, Alexandra Cope, Gunther Kress and Roger Kneebone. 2011. "Scissors, Please": The Practical Accomplishment of Surgical Work in the Operating Theater. *Symbolic Interaction* 34(3): 398–414.

Bleakley, Alan, James Boyden, Adrian Hobbs, Linda Walsh and Jon Allard. 2006. Improving Teamwork Climate in Operating Theatres: The Shift from Multiprofessionalism to Interprofessionalism. *Journal of Interprofessional Care* 20(5): 461–70.

Brown, Julia S., and May Rawlinson. 1975. Relinquishing the Sick Role Following Open-Heart Surgery. *Journal of Health and Social Behavior* 16(1): 12–27.

Clemente, Ignasi. 2009. Progressivity and Participation: Children's Management of Parental Assistance in Paediatric Chronic Pain Encounters. In *Communication in Healthcare Settings: Policy, Participation and New Technologies*, edited by Alison Pilnick, Jon Hindmarsh and Virginia T. Gill, 83–98. Chichester, UK: Wiley.

Collin, Kaija, Susanna Paloniemi and Jukka-Pekka Mecklin. 2010. Promoting Inter-Professional Teamwork and Learning: The Case of a Surgical Operating Theatre. *Journal of Education and Work* 23(1): 43–63.

Coser, Rose Laub. 1966. Role Distance, Sociological Ambivalence, and Transitional Status Systems. *American Journal of Sociology* 72(2): 173. doi: 10.1086/224276

Finn, Rachael. 2008. The Language of Teamwork: Reproducing Professional Divisions in the Operating Theatre. *Human Relations* 61(1): 103–30. doi: 10.1177/0018726707085947

Freidson, Eliot. 1961. *Patients' Views of Medical Practice*. New York: Russell Sage.

Goffman, Erving. 1956. Embarrassment and Social Organization. *American Journal of Sociology* 62 (3): 264. doi: 10.1086/222003

Goffman, Erving. 1961. *Encounters: Two Studies in the Sociology of Interaction*. Indianapolis: Bobbs-Merrill.

Gross, Edward, and Gregory P. Stone. 1964. Embarrassment and the Analysis of Role Requirements. *American Journal of Sociology* 70(1): 1–15.

Halkowski, Timothy. 1990. "Role" as an Interactional Device. *Social Problems* 37(4): 564–77.

Hardy, Margaret E., and Mary E. Conway. 1978. *Role Theory: Perspectives for Health Professionals*. Norwalk: Appleton-Century-Crofts.

Heritage, John. 1984. *Garfinkel and Ethnomethodology*. Cambridge: Polity Press.

Heritage, John, and Steven Clayman. 2010. *Talk in Action: Interactions, Identities, and Institutions*, edited by P. Trudgill, *Language in Society*. West Sussex: Wiley-Blackwell.

Hudak, Pamela L., Shannon J. Clark and Geoffrey Raymond. 2013. The Omni-Relevance of Surgery: How Medical Specialization Shapes Orthopedic Surgeons & Apos: Treatment Recommendations. *Health Communication* 28(6): 533–45. doi: 10.1080/10410236.2012.702642

Lerner, Gene H., and Celia Kitzinger. 2007. Extraction and Aggregation in the Repair of Individual and Collective Self-Reference. *Discourse Studies* 9(4): 526–57. doi: 10.1177/1461445607079165

Levinson, Wendy, Debra L. Roter, John P. Mullooly, Valerie T. Dull and Richard M. Frankel. 1997. Physician-Patient Communication: The Relationship with Malpractice Claims among Primary Care Physicians and Surgeons. *JAMA* 7: 553–9.

Mead, George Herbert. 1934. *Mind, Self & Society from the Standpoint of a Social Behaviorist*. Chicago, Ill : The University of Chicago Press.

Merton, Robert K. 1957. The Role-Set: Problems in Sociological Theory. *British Journal of Sociology*: 106–20.

Moore, Alison Rotha, David G. Butt, Jodie Ellis-Clarke and John Cartmill. 2010. Linguistic Analysis of Verbal and Non-Verbal Communication in the Operating. *ANZ Journal of Surgery* 80: 925–9.

Mondada, Lorenza. 2001. Intervenir à distance dans une opération chirurgicale: l'organisation interactive d'espaces de participation. *Bulletin suisse de linguistique appliquée* 74: 33–56.

Mondada, Lorenza. 2006. La compétence comme dimension située et contingente, localement évaluée par les participants. *Bulletin VALS-ASLA (Association suisse de linguistique appliquée)* 84: 83–119.

Mondada, Lorenza. 2011. The Organization of Concurrent Courses of Action in Surgical Demonstrations. In *Embodied Interaction: Language and Body in the Material World*, edited by Jürgen Streeck, Charles Goodwin and Curtis LeBaron. Cambridge: Cambridge University Press.

Mottram, Anne. 2009. Being in for a Day Doesn't Count: Patient Experiences of Day Surgery. British Sociological Association Annual Conference, Cardiff.

Nembhard, Ingrid M., and Amy C. Edmondson. 2006. Making it Safe: The Effects of Leader Inclusiveness and Professional Status on Psychological Safety and Improvement Efforts in Health Care Teams. *Journal of Organizational Behavior* 27(7): 941–66. doi: 10.1002/job.413.

Nevile, Maurice. 2006. Communication in Context: A Conversation Analysis Tool for Examining Recorded Voice Data in Investigations of Aviation Occurrences. Canberra: Australian Transport Safety Bureau.

Nevile, Maurice. 2007. Talking without Overlap in the Airline Cockpit: Precision Timing at Work. *Text & Amp; Talk – An Interdisciplinary Journal of Language, Discourse Communication Studies* 27(2): 225–49. doi: 10.1515/text.2007.009.

Parsons, Talcott. 1951. *The Social System*. New York: The Free Press.

Parsons, Talcott. 1968. *The Structure of Social Action: A Study in Social Theory and Special Reference to a Group of Recent European Writers*. New York: Free Press.

Parsons, Talcott, and Renée Fox. 1952. Illness, Therapy and the Modern Urban American Family. *Journal of Social Issues* 8(4): 31–44. doi: 10.1111/j.1540-4560.1952.tb01861.x.

Siegler, Miriam, and Humphry Osmond. 1973. The "Sick Role" Revisited. *The Concept of Health* 1(3): 41–58.

Stivers, Tanya, Rita Mangione-Smith, Marc N. Elliott, Laurie McDonald and John Heritage. 2003. Why Do Physicians Think Parents Expect Antibiotics? What Parents Report vs What Physicians Believe. *The Journal of Family Practice* 52(2): 140.

Svensson, Marcus Sanchez, Christian Heath and Paul Luff. 2007. Instrumental Action: the Timely Exchange of Implements during Surgical Operations. ECSCW '07: The Tenth European Conference on Computer Supported Cooperative Work, Limerick, Ireland.

Weldon, Sharon-Marie, Tehri Korkiakangas, Jeff Bezemer and Roger Kneebone. 2013. Communication in the Operating Theatre. *British Journal of Surgery* 100: 1677–88. doi: 10.1002/bjs.9332.

Weldon, Sharon-Marie, Tehri Korkiakangas, Jeff Bezemer, Roger Kneebone, K. Nicholson and Gunther Kress. 2012. Transient Teams in the Operating Theatre. *The Operating Theatre Journal* 261(1): 2.

White, Sarah J., Maria H. Stubbe, Kevin P. Dew, Lindsay M. Macdonald, Anthony C. Dowell and Rod Gardner. 2013. Understanding Communication between Surgeon and Patient in Outpatient Consultations. *ANZ Journal of Surgery* 83(5): 307–11. doi: 10.1111/ans.12126.

Winter, Jerry Alan. 2003. The Development of the Disability Rights Movement as a Social Problem Solver. *Disability Studies Quarterly* 23(1): 33–61.

Israel Berger completed his PhD in psychology at the University of Roehampton, London. He is a final year medical student at Sydney Medical School, University of Sydney, with a view toward surgery. He has taught research methods to undergraduate and postgraduate students in the UK and Australia. In his own research, he uses a variety of qualitative and quantitative methodologies to explore public health and service provision issues and is interested in healthcare interactions as a conversation analyst.

Sarah J. White is a qualitative health researcher and linguist with a particular interest in using conversation analysis to understand communication in surgical practice. She is a Senior Lecturer at the Faculty of Medicine and Health Sciences at Macquarie University, Sydney. Sarah was awarded her PhD from the University of Otago, Wellington in 2011 and has professional and academic experience in clinical communication, quality and safety in healthcare, and medical education.

13 Toward a Language of Operative Surgery

John A. Cartmill and David G. Butt

There are five duties of surgery: to remove what is superfluous, to restore what has been dislocated, to separate what has grown together, to reunite what has been divided, and to redress the defects of nature.
– Ambroise Paré (1510–90)

In this chapter the doing of surgery, the craft, is analysed from a linguistic perspective. A Surgeon (JC) presents observations that are answered and expanded in counterpoint by a Systemic Functional Linguist (DB).

13.1 Introduction

JC: This chapter directs attention beyond communication (spoken or unspoken) as it is conventionally understood, and applies linguistic concepts to the underlying interaction between operator and tissue, that of the surgical work itself, suggesting surgical technique as an applied form of gesture. I submit that the act of surgery, surgical meaning-making, "is" communication and not merely "like" communication; an interaction rather than a conversation but communication in the truest sense, transacted at the level of the tissue and the contextual layers of biological, anatomical and pathological complexity that constitute it.

I suggest that techniques of linguistic analysis be used, at least metaphorically, to break down and analyse operative surgery so it can be better understood, more readily learned and more effectively practised.

DB: There is a linguistic, or semiotic, framework within which what you are claiming receives considerable support: the American polymath, C.S. Peirce (see Hookway 1985), suggested first of all that a sign can be known by the fact that it can be misinterpreted; but, most relevant beyond that, is a class of signs – indexical signs – which are based not merely on convention but on the interaction with natural objects. They are readings from nature, and from the "nature of things": clouds can mean rain, obvious enough; but also symptoms can mean tissue damage, or tumour. It is eminently clear that specialists read anatomy, and that part of such a process is the responsiveness of tissue to touch.

13.2 Surgical Notation

JC: This project began as a practical exercise to record and formalize surgical technique, to develop a notation for the moves and sequences that constitute surgical action. As a pragmatically trained surgeon I was only vaguely aware of traditions of philosophy and linguistics, of the newer fields of neuropsychology and mirror neurones or the theories of language development and primate tool use that might have helped. I was unaware that Aristotle had identified the challenge over 2000 years ago by distinguishing *praxis* (the doing) from thinking and talking. Notation has been limited in fields of physical expression like dance and other art forms that, like surgery, express meaning in ways other than words and have instead been passed on from generation to generation in the style of implicit imitation: an under-explored process of emulation. We now have technologies that, paired with tools of thought (linguistics and the study of meaning-making), might make analysis of such emulation possible. Digital recording will be to *praxis* what the written word, paper and publishing have been for thought, logic, ethics and mathematics. It is paradoxical that I have to *write* now about the *doing* of surgery.

DB: Notation certainly isolates structure in behaviour, but with some cost. Writing systems dominate our reflections on spoken language – with the effect of turning a flow into a stream of events conceived of as isolates. The question is, what is the tool value of notation? Do we consider musical notation as a tool? The question for me is then how would clinicians (or other professions) benefit from a more explicit account of the silent discriminations of their craft – the knowledge of insiders in the "guild"?

JC: Language has evolved from the gestural to the spoken and beyond to the written with successive levels of nuance, abstraction and power. This chapter suggests that gesture, especially applied gesture as expressed in operative surgery, has also evolved remarkably along its path of physical expression albeit with no method of recording and therefore none of the benefits of analysis that have been available to spoken and written language. The surgical reader, aware that the term linguistics, like language, is derived from *lingua*, might wonder what linguistics has to do with operative surgery. But just as language may be considered an evolutionary extension of gesture, so might tools for the analysis of language, linguistic tools, be applied to the surgical field of applied gesture.

DB: The Greek word for this applied "art cum craft" was "techne": a word argued over by Socrates (Roochnik, 1996) and taken up by Aristotle in relation to action and morality, but involving "mastery" of a form of experience. The art of medicine became a particular point of debate around what was or was not a form of "mastery" (Angier 2010: 7–12). Readings on the history of sciences certainly show how far medicine had to "evolve" to gain the status of something that needed to be "mastered" – a craft of knowledge or what Richard Gregory discussed many years ago as a "mental tool" (1981). The historian of sciences in Greece and China, G.E.R. Lloyd (1970, 2002), noted that the axiomatic method (as in Euclid's geometry) was even tried...Something laughable today; but I wonder whether the determinism of our era will not seem simplistic to specialists in even 50 years (viz. Shapiro's work Evolution: A View from the 21st Century *[2011] and the work of Lewontin [1993, 2000] and others). But back to your point about an expressive language of surgical gesture...*

JC: There is admittedly a rich vocabulary and literature used to describe surgery and its results and yet the language of anatomy, of cutting and joining, is only barely able to describe the ultimate result of an operation and only hints at the nuanced and coordinated action involved in achieving it. Even with the benefit of its formal Latin and Greek roots, its hundreds of years of anatomy and physiology, and more recent refinements of biomechanics and cellular biology, there is no method of notation that begins to approach the *praxis*, the doing of it. It is possible to record a camera's perspective and surgeons will often use a simple line cartoon in addition to descriptors of convention, "proceeding by careful sharp and blunt dissection". But these are little more than catalogue entries, summaries that ultimately describe little, and are reminders of the hopeless inadequacy of our current notation.

Central to this argument is the concept of "meaning-making". John Dewey, the 19th-century philosopher, psychologist and educator developed, with William James, the concept of meaning-making as anything that "changes the world". Like Peirce, mentioned at the outset, these Pragmatists looked at how ideas do or don't make a difference. And a surgeon's actions, as an operator, do change the world, not with a sound, but with a movement, an act, an action.

DB: To quote my own teachers in linguistics:
"There can be no semiotic act that leaves the world exactly as it was."

JC: Earlier studies (Svensson, Heath and Luff 2007, 2009; Moore et al. 2010; Mondada 2003; Bezemer et al. 2011) have drawn attention to linguistic interactions *within* a surgical team. Here we explore an interpretation of operative surgery as a "conversation", as meaning-making between surgeon and tissue (Figure 13.1).

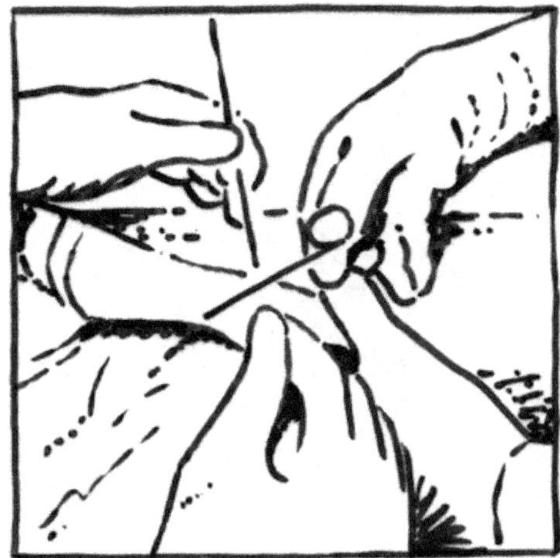

Figure 13.1: The doing of surgery; a "conversation" between surgeon and tissue
Treating the technical act of surgery as a language allows well established techniques of (linguistic) analysis to be brought to bear on the teaching, learning and doing (performance) of surgery.

Such an analysis can enrich the learning, the teaching and the practice of operative surgery. We hope to bring to surgical technique the benefits of a systematic analysis, by analogy with those of linguistics. Such an approach might allow the tools of systemic functional linguistics (from context to grammar and intonation), conversation analysis and pragmatics to bear on a field that even now relies on descriptors as unsophisticated as "good hands".

It is possible that just as I fail to fully appreciate the nuances of systemic functional linguistics or Jefferson notation, equally, the "non-surgical" reader may not fully appreciate the level of sensorimotor engagement that surgery entails; the all-consuming "in the moment" of touch and texture, torque, feedback and precise motor control. Prolonged interactions of the various dimensions of the encounter are mediated by inflammation, healing and repair, and the potential for complications add to complexity that is analogous to the contextual layers of a language. While alluding to primate gesture and primitive tool use as a protolanguage or prelude to language, modern operative surgery is conceptually as far from just grasping a nut as any other realm of developed human endeavour which needs to be interpreted. Operative surgery is a system of meaning-making comprising a vocabulary of moves, a grammar or syntax, and a hierarchy of contextual sequences; a system of actions rather than a system of words; but a system none the less – with affordances, choices, conventions and with implicit and explicit structures analogous in their architecture with the meaning-making levels of spoken and written language. The irreversible consequences of surgery may impart an even more precise or rigorous need for order and hierarchy of moves and manoeuvres than the

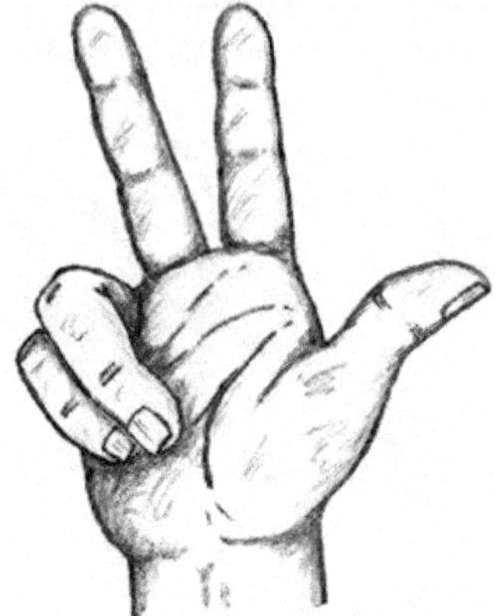

Figure 13.2: Scissor action: unspoken request for an instrument

spoken or written where there is some room for fuzzy interpretations. In surgery, it really does matter whether the artery is tied before the vein or not, and whether the first tie is proximal or distal. Thus there is an intrinsic order (motivated by the nature of the human body and the tools we apply) – hence a natural hierarchy of moves. But also, there are higher orders of arrangement, born of convention and hard-won experience about technique.

13.3   The Surgical Vocabulary

JC: The surgical reader will have experienced that realm where the spoken and gestural fuse and become indistinguishable. A surgeon may fall silent when they are challenged by a particular technical or pathological aspect of an operation, literally losing the word for the simplest of instruments and having to resort instead to an emblematic or indexical scissor action for example (Figure 13.2). Mistaken by the naive observer as arrogance, it is in fact the humblest of requests for help, an echo of the desired action of the end effector. David McNeill (1992: 2) suggests that "gestures and language are one system".

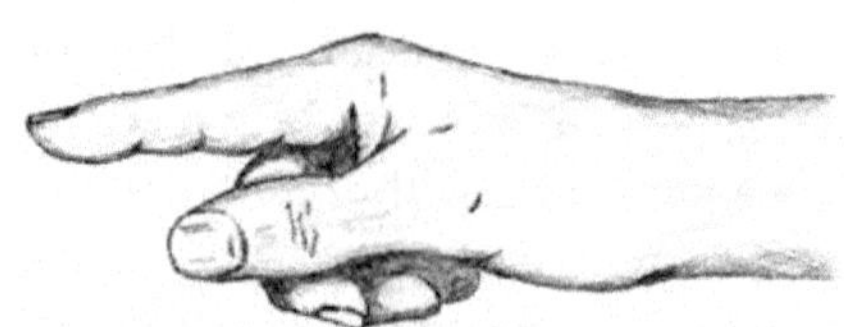

Figure 13.3: Indexical sign, here with no context; it could mean anything

It is self-evident that gesture (Figure 13.3) is a (powerful) dimension of communication, of "signing". And yet the hand makes only a limited number of signs, just as the voice can make only a limited number of sounds or utterances (or words). The essence of a language is that it takes that limited stock of units and combines them into a potentially infinite number of meanings through hierarchically organized sequences. For a linguist a critical component of the meaning being made is context. Context, or more correctly, layered, varied and prioritized contexts allow one meaning (one voice or one gesture) to be distinguished from another. Figures 13.4 through 13.7 illustrate the conceptual transformation of this gesture from the non-specific though directed meaning-making signal of the pointed index finger to that same finger making meaning in a surgical field (context) through the accurate placement and tensioning of a suture.

DB: All very intriguing to this observer of your guild! There are aspects of meaning-making in surgery that appear to be driven, or motivated, by a natural order that cannot be renegotiated. In language, there may be some also: the spectrum of hearing, how we use face-to-face signalling, and "how we mean" when we are not in view of each other. But how we allocate the potential from community to community looks much more plastic and conventional in vocal language. The linguistic potential becomes more powerful by cross-alignments – i.e., "this" intonation with "that" grammatical sequence, and then with a different one, with resulting changes to meaning. My teachers' teacher was J.R. Firth (1890–1960). His views would enfold your views of meaning quite felicitously: every expression is a form of contextualization, and all contextualizations flow like a prosody – an ensemble in which a polyphony of action and vocalizations become a repertoire of community personae (1957 [1950]). Hence, your semantic identity. Surgeons weave their own "tango" into this: they "touch" with purpose and permission, rather than with the conspiratorial, illicit, bodily readings of the structured dance.

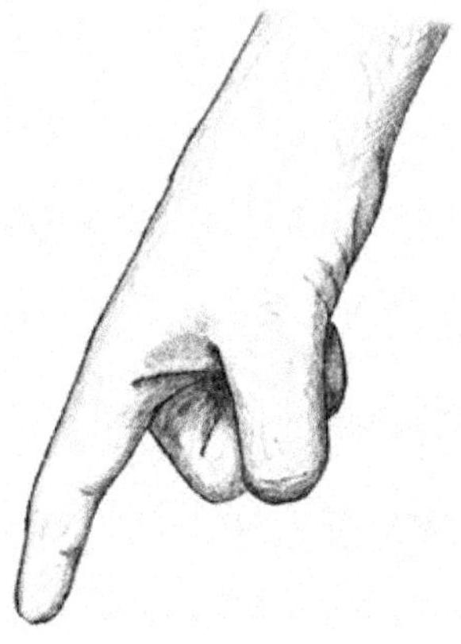

Figure 13.4: The same gesture with meaning altered as it engages with the surgical field

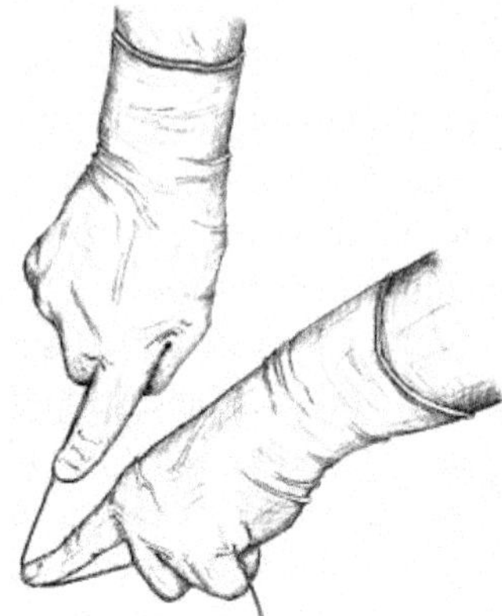

Figure 13.5: Positions...

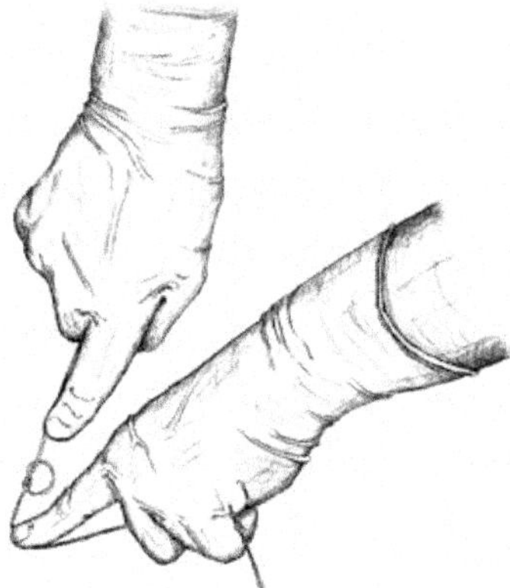

Figure 13.6: ...and tensions a surgical tie...

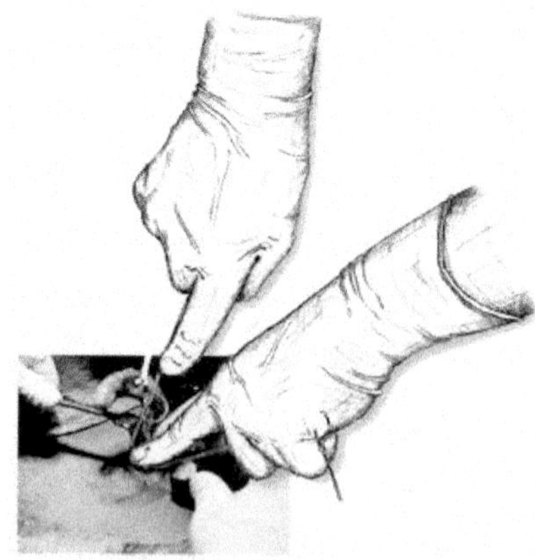

Figure 13.7: ...in a surgical context

JC: In Figure 13.7 surgical "context" is added; the index finger and hands are beginning to make, to signal, a surgical knot in the context of an appendicectomy. The same knot in the context of preparing for open heart surgery would have a different significance, a different meaning again.

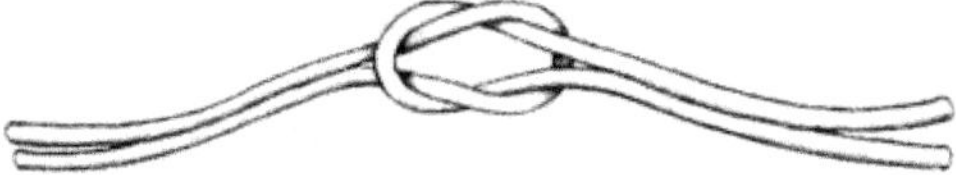

Figure 13.8: The reef knot, a well characterized surgical sign

Further developing the indexical suture tightening example by "stringing" several of these actions or surgical signs together develops the equivalent of a phrase or sentence or paragraph and with it a more evolved surgical meaning. The gestures leave a record. The square knot (Figure 13.8) is emblematic of fine surgical technique and enjoys a symbolic, even totemic value of quality and security. For a surgeon, tying a square knot feels good, looks good and is emphatic: it works. It is a sign, in this case a surgical sign or signal.

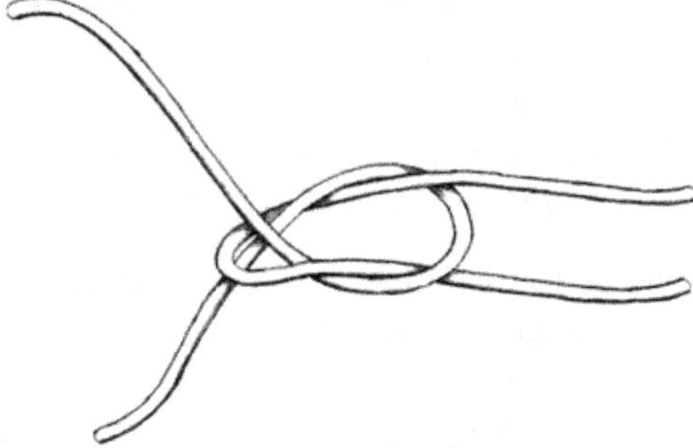

Figure 13.9: The grannie or slip knot

On the other hand, the knot shown in Figure 13.9 is not square and is disparaged as a "grannie" knot. With its predisposition to slip, it could be considered a poor choice of "words", or an example of bad operative surgical "grammar". However the slip knot has a place too, and there is a sophisticated level of surgical application where its ability to slide into position with a finely judged degree of angle and tension is prized. A surgical novice using this knot will be chastised for sloppy technique but the knot has a place analogous to a rhetorical device in a well-rounded surgical vocabulary; as long as it is deployed knowingly, in context, and "finished" square.

DB: Well, yes: with some specialists, "mastery" is evident at every level of technique; others may have an uneven repertoire. I recall some great theoretical

scientists – Pauli, for instance – being notorious for their disastrous experimental technique: hence the "Pauli effect" in the laboratory (Gilder 2008). There is no division in practical medicine between theory and praxis, as you mentioned. Technique has to be embodied in the team and then, ultimately, in the patient!

13.4 Surgical Grammar

JC: The "language" of operative surgery seems only to have an object and a verb; the subject (the surgeon) becomes invisible, lost in the flow, the moment, the immediate reality of the operating. This may be an argument for relegating the act of surgery to the level of a protolanguage but that analysis, critical perhaps to a neuropsychologist or linguist, is irrelevant to a surgeon who may not be concerned whether his "doing" is transitive or intransitive, who may not even be aware of the difference.

DB: Your sense of surgeon/subject works well for languages as well. In the majority of the world's languages, the Subject is implicit – from being embedded in human actions, in context, this seems a sound economy in making sense. English is at an extreme, in this regard. In addition, you DO gain by thinking about transitive/intransitive: transitive means there is a going over from one participant to another; intransitive means that process affects only the doer. Surely you would want the concept of transitive in your analytic framework – what could be more going over to another than the actions of the Operating Team?

JC: Arbib (2012; also see forthcoming) draws attention to the anatomical homology between the area where mirror neurons were discovered in other primates and Broca's area in humans; and while it is beyond this chapter to expound a particular theory of language development, the congruence between studies of tool use (read operative surgery) and primate language development are striking. Operative surgical language is utterly concrete rather than abstract, but exhibits a sophistication and effectiveness (invisible to most) reflecting its possible lead on the spoken in evolutionary development.

The "noun" in the surgical context could be applied to an anatomical continuum modulated by pathological context and by the vulnerability and proximity of adjacent structures. Formal anatomical description hints at surgical anatomy but misses its multidimensional cline (gradient) of subtle tissue variations: of elasticity and lines of tension, the changes of age and pathology and previous surgery. The "subject" is a fused connection of surgeon's self and instrument (the displaced end effector in neuropsychology) although the surgeon as subject may disappear entirely in the all-consuming, challenging haze of object and verb, hope and intent. So there is a noun (the acted on) and a verb (the process unfolding). But it is the higher orders of language description that are more helpful.

Surgeons open and close, divide and join, with each of these sequences in turn composed of sub-sequences and nuanced response to context – that is, to the emerging and changing qualities of the living surgical field. Cao's work (1999) recognizing and decomposing complex laparoscopic procedures into hierarchical sequences (sets and subsets of simpler moves) could be seen as anticipating work in the field of mirror neurons that suggests an implicit coding of hierarchical structure in both manual activities and verbal communication. For the surgical learner, emulation requires an understanding, somehow, of this implicit coding of hierarchical structure and its integration moment by moment into the flow of surgical process.

DB: You seem to be capturing the double perspective one can have on skilled behaviour – it flows like a rhythmic pattern that you do not need to break up into units; yet it is structured out of distinct achievements of structural elements. In linguistics, we might use the term "Prosodic" for the extended flow, and "Constituent" for the fact that there are discernible elements. The other factor you highlight is that it is finely tuned to changes in the context at a micro scale – the emerging details of the surgical field. All in all this goes to the core of your vision, I think – Process and Structure are entwined in the surgical performance; and both perspectives are necessary to understand surgical craft or mastery. The word "mystery" was used in the middle ages for a specialist craft to which you needed long years of apprenticeship. Auden (1966) uses it for poetry: to his dead friend/poet Louis MacNiece, he begins: "seeing you know our mystery from the inside". You seem to be reaching for what it is like to be a surgeon "from the inside".

JC: The next example of a grammatical sequence describes a relatively simple conventional sequential use of haemostats, simple hinged, lockable stainless-steel clips of universal design (usually intended for the right hand). In an era of robotic surgery and phenomenal technological investment in surgical instrumentation, the shape of these simple, effective instruments endures in the same way that in the West we still value and intuitively use a knife and fork. Evolved to reflect and augment (even sympathize) with the gentle curve of a hand at rest (Figure 13.10), the shape of these instruments itself determines aspects of surgical technique and grammar.

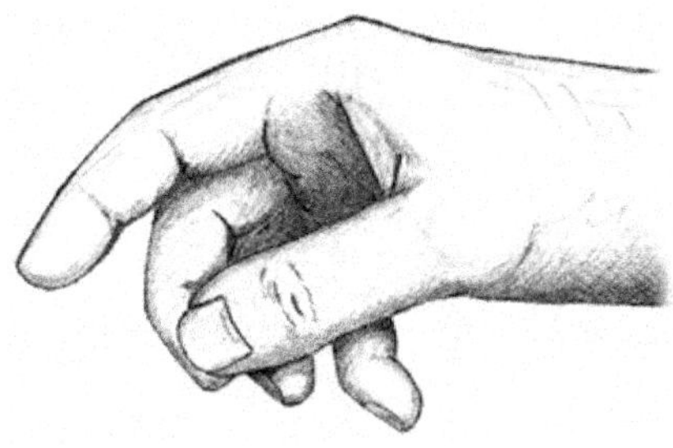

Figure 13.10: The hand at rest

The (grammatical) surgical sequence in Figures 13.11 through 13.14 depicts a method of formally and safely dividing a structure expected to bleed, and is known as "clip clip cut." The clipped structure is divided and the ends can then be tied using the knot sequence described above. The curved tips of the haemostatic forceps can be curved toward the specimen, away from the specimen, or toward or away from each other. There is a "correct" way of doing this that varies by training institution, hence by convention. Each convention has advantages and disadvantages that can be argued (and are argued) to the extent that the variations might even be considered "dialects". Figure 13.15 however shows a sequence that does not make sense: the instruments are applied in an order of clumsy interference that could be considered an error of grammar or at least an error of ergonomics which is the same thing as grammar at this silent level of sequenced movement. It is a good example of how one movement dictates the next or at least limits the options available for subsequent moves. The grammatical or ergonomic rule is called "working toward one's (right-handed) self" and applies as well to lighting the candles on a birthday cake.

Good surgical technique like good surgical knots (square or deliberately slipping, tied left- or right-handed using one or two hands, placed with precision and finger-tips rather than thumbs) are an important foundation to surgery just as a good

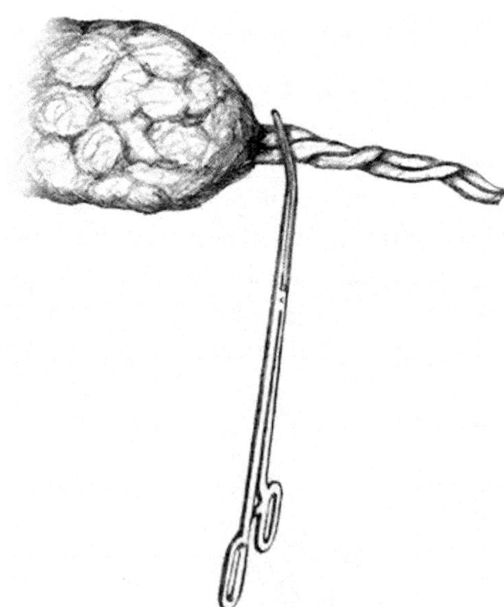

Figure 13.11: Haemostat applied with curve toward the specimen

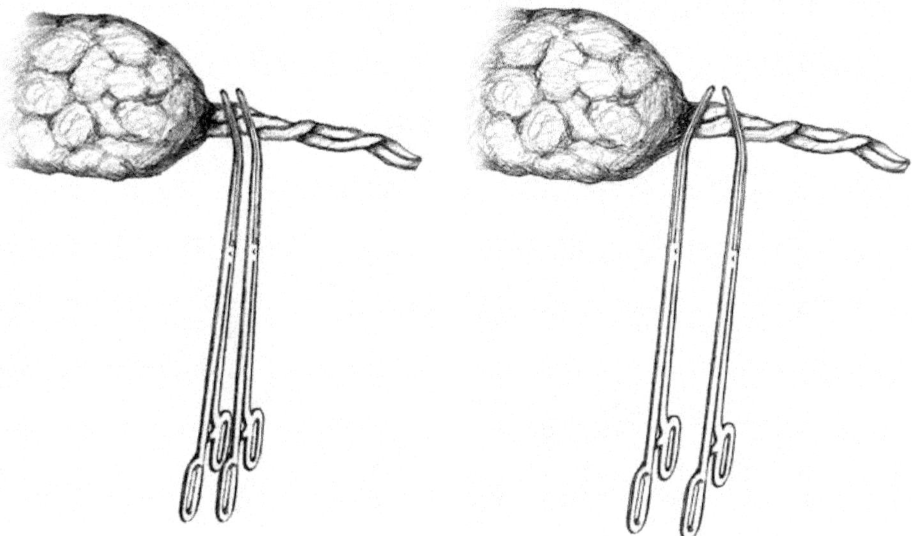

Figure 13.12: Second haemostat sympathetic to the curve of the first (and anticipating the curve of the scissors about to be used)

Figure 13.13: Second haemostat placed to facilitate subsequent ties
The difference between the alignment of forceps in Figure 13.12 and here is not subtle and carries significant surgical meaning. A pattern of such habits can constitute a surgical dialect strong enough to identify a training institution.

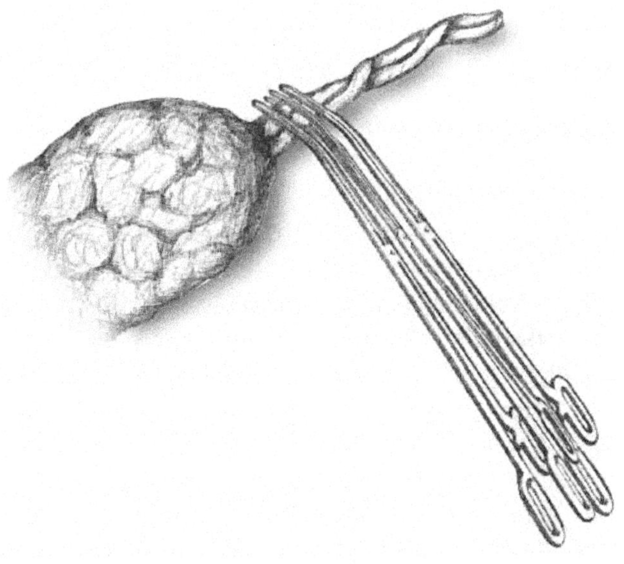

Figure 13.14: Clip clip cut

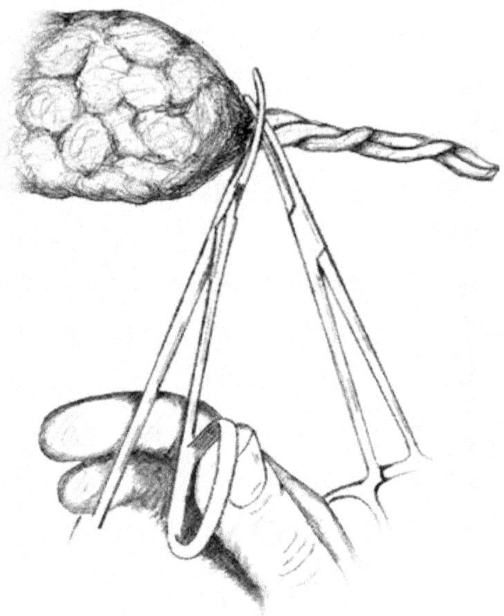

Figure 13.15: Awkward interference
The second clamp would have been more elegantly placed to the right of the initial clamp
avoiding the grammatical error of the knuckles getting in the way of a parallel clamp.

vocabulary and sense of grammar, tense and genre are good foundations that allow someone to express themselves effectively in voice or in print. Some surgeons can tie a knot that works in the depths of the chest or pelvis, and some cannot.

13.5   The Surgical Field Responds, Talks Back

JC: It is not a stretch of imagination to consider that the surgeon interrogates the tissue; inspecting by touching and feeling, deforming, retracting, cutting, separating and joining. Redo surgery demands a different register than surgery on virgin tissue; surgery for a complication, a different register again.

And the tissue talks back. Operative surgery is more than mere confrontation with the tissue. The surgical field "replies" in a language that is recognized tacitly; passed from surgical generation to generation, learned through experience and invisible to most observers; sensed through intuition, it has tactile qualities, colour, texture and smell. An operation is an extended negotiation with tissue; with stress, relaxation and tension, with bleeding and clotting in the short term, and with a protracted "tail" of the biological implications of what is known as inflammation, healing and repair (or not, in complicated cases) transacted over days or weeks.

The talking back varies in tone, tenor and mode, ultimately repairing, regenerating, scarring, remodelling, and regaining functional integrity. The surgeon observes and manages this process closely, intervening where necessary with pain-killers, anti-inflammatory drugs and antibiotics as well as splints, dressings and physical therapies.

The surgeon can make the sign, signal the intention, but what is being intended or signified doesn't necessarily happen; the bowel slithers around the retractor, the suture slips, the graft needs an embolectomy. This "to and fro" is communication, persuasion, even negotiation. There is no place for the verbal, no place for talk; at the level of the tissue, talk is relevant only in so much that the others in the theatre may call the surgeon out of this concentration – updates on strategy and results. So too the tissue is mute but the exchange of meaning is rich in many directions.

In surgery, many of the layers of context are continuously variable – not just biological layers (appreciated as increasingly complex, nuanced and individualized with advances in molecular biology) but social, financial and educational layers also determine the meaning-making of operative surgery (see the earlier diagrams of professional stratification in Chapter 8, this volume). Social and cultural layers determine the experience and training of the surgeon; finance constrains the range of instruments available and whether or not there is operating time available.

*DB: What you have brought out so vividly here are the semiotic currents that shape meaning – figuratively, we can think of meaning having its own morphologies – its recognizable contours; its regularities of sequence and accumulation. **Users** shape the language to the task in context, just as context demands resources of meaning. One point quite remarkable to me is how the fields within medicine are so intensely symbolic, so dependent on structures of interpretation and persuasion (viz., the rhetorical effort to convince a colleague to accept new patients into Departments under constant siege for places). What you have characterized for me is a **register**, a variant of language according to "use" – the form that language takes under the immediate socio-semantic pressures of getting some particular action done. We then cross this with the variation that emerges when different groups are involved: variation according to the "user".*

13.6 Cooperation

JC: While this chapter primarily addresses the interaction between surgeon and tissue, it is a travesty to exclude the role of the scrub nurse and surgical assistants (the anaesthetic interaction is in another plane again). An operation is not choreographed as would be a dance, nor annotated as would a musical duet, but evolves in the moment as an emerging realization of circumstance, opportunity and choice. The participants in the surgical field literally cooperate and with that intimacy comes a peculiar sense of recognition and flow as one move is supporting another in anticipation of a total, goal-directed performance.

DB: Nothing to dispute here: a move from duet to chamber orchestra, perhaps. The ensemble of participants with the polyphony of layers or levels, I suppose – continuing the earlier metaphors.

13.7 Surgical Style: Variations According to Participants

JC: Surgical language, and the communication it mediates, is more nuanced than the written or spoken. It has heft and weight, material mechanical properties, and torque and angle and force, anticipation, a before and after. If the surgeon is fortunate then it is mirrored by the scrub and amplified by the assistant, but there are no words to describe these critical phenomena. The language of machines, of radians, torque and vectors, underspecifies surgical technique although there have been partially successful attempts to apply them. The phenomenon of torque signature (Rosen et al. 1999) can clearly differentiate novice surgeon from expert. Another metaphorical approach is through that of literary styles. Surgeons can reliably recollect the surgical styles of their important mentors; styles they wish to emulate (or avoid). A spare, emphatic, deliberate style of operating perhaps, no wasted moves, as Ernest Hemingway made meaning. Others might operate like Wilbur Smith; adventure, blood, excitement, never too sure what will happen next. The best we can do with our current descriptive vocabulary is announce that a surgeon or trainee has "good hands" or exhibits "economy of movement"; but that is not enough. With this metaphor a trainee can work on, and be critiqued on, their syntagms – by assembling sequences, learning good technical rhetoric and smooth, coordinated and effective moves.

DB: Here I am at odds with you – the more "nuanced"; the "failure of words"; the machine metaphors also failing; the parallels with literary styles. The likelihood seems to me that actions within codes are differently "nuanced", if you like. Physical feedback is not required in the mastery of Chess or Go; but it is in dance, piano playing and judo. Language has time, depth and physical, even visceral, consequences: it carries the weight of meaning through time and the choices of generations (consider "techne"; or "eros"). While it enables choices in cortical systems, it engages deep experiences of childhood which have registered in subcortical systems (viz., Panksepp and Biven 2012; Malloch and Trevarthen 2008; and Trevarthen 1987). The musicality of language is participatory: it draws one into an intersubjective circle: first with your mother (pre-birth), then with the "collective consciousness" so central to Saussure's linguistics, and Durkheim's idea of a social fact. Social facts take on the concreteness of matter in the living of life (Saussure 1959 [1916]).

JC: Linguists have studied people "doing" before, and work at the surgeon tissue interface is akin to the work of artists and others who work with "material" rather than with abstract symbols or language. Sculptors, artists, musicians all make meaning that is available to techniques such as kinesics and proxemics; the study of movement and distance. For ballet this has classically been Laban notation and Benesh choreology, although video analysis is inevitably replacing these notations. Surgeons understand their material tacitly but describe it and explain it poorly, having no (abstract) tool more sophisticated than the "war story" or cartoon with which to represent tissue and the surgical field. Idealized diagrams in texts and the surgical literature and even video underspecify the reality, and surgeons rely instead on the single dimension of visuality – of showing one another and those who wish to learn. But there are so many dimensions of proprioceptive feedback, and dynamics that can only be implied.

*DB: I am back with you now; at least by the drift of your analogies. But consider the artists you mention: sculptors take a material that is natural and give it a new level of meaning. Poets take a material that already carries the complexity of the world – a language – and put it through a second articulation of meaning. This is not the physical experience in itself; but do words really fail? Sappho is credited with giving the most accurate brief account of the bodily reaction of being struck by adoration, in the moment. My colleague, Astika Kappagoda, himself a doctor, has argued (2004) that Thucydides' account of the plague in Athens can be diagnosed today because of the forensic method the historian gave to his verbal account – it was akin to SARS, not bubonic plague. Thucydides also used metaphor as a sixth sense of heuristic thinking. I would suggest to you, from your own rhapsodic verbal response to surgical experience, the surgical nuance **is** special in that it is extremely cross-modal, engaging so many levels of sensory and symbolic "information", all of which need to be reconciled into active response. Not a single move; nor more words.*

JC: There is a system to the unspoken, silent language passed from surgical generation to generation that has been heretofore hidden from analysis – not for any malevolent reason – but simply because non-participatory technologies have not been sophisticated enough to capture the nuance and complexity of operative surgery and reflect it back physically, or multi-modally, for analysis. Surgical praxis evolves, buoyed by its heritage and a tradition that is (literally) handed from generation to generation, unfettered by the limitations of what can be described by the spoken or written. Unfettered, but at the same time limited because there has been no tool to render it abstract enough for analysis. Digital recording is still far from the real thing but it is better than what we have had before and it is hoped that video technology will provide for surgical reflection, analysis and development the advantages that the written word has provided.

CODA

JC: It is possible that the relationships described here between language and operating are more than metaphorical. Perhaps surgery is a language, meaning-making at its most consequential and emphatic. As important as, in fact, the same thing as talk and communication; the readily understood model we share for making sense of our world, for learning it, for navigating it, for changing it. Tools developed to analyse the spoken and written language must then be applicable to that surgical praxis which precedes it and which challenges spoken and written language in its nuance, subtlety, grace, beauty and utility.

Acknowledgement

JC: To my father, Tim Cartmill AO, FRACS for challenging and helping develop these ideas.

References

Angier, Tom. 2010. *Technē in Aristotle's Ethics: Crafting the Moral Life*. New York: Continuum.

Arbib, Michael A. 2012. *How the Brain Got Language: The Mirror System Hypothesis*. Vol. 16. Oxford: Oxford University Press.

Arbib, Michael A. forthcoming. From Action to Typology? A Neuro-Evolutionary Perspective. *Language & Linguistics Compass*.

Auden, W.H. 1966. *About the House*. London: Faber and Faber.

Bezemer, Jeff, Ged Murtagh, Alexandra Cope, Gunther Kress and Roger Kneebone. 2011. "Scissors, Please": The Practical Accomplishment of Surgical Work in the Operating Theater. *Symbolic Interaction* 34(3): 398–414.

Cao, Caroline G.L., C.L. MacKenzie, J.A. Ibbotson, L.J. Turner, N.P. Blair and A.G. Nagy. 1999. Hierarchical Decomposition of Laparoscopic Procedures. In *Medicine Meets Virtual Reality: 7*, edited by J.D. Westwood, H.M. Hoffman, R.A. Robb and D. Stredney, 83–9. IOS Press, Washington, DC.

Firth, John R. 1957 [1950]. Personality and Language in Society. In *Papers in Linguistics 1934–1951*, 177–89. London: Oxford University Press.

Gilder, Louisa. 2008. *The Age of Entanglement: When Quantum Physics Was Reborn*. New York: Vintage.

Gregory, Richard L. 1981. *Mind in Science: A History of Explanations of Psychology and Physics*. London: Weidenfeld and Nicolson; New York: Cambridge University Press; paperback, Peregrine.

Hookway, Christopher. 1985. *Peirce*. London: Routledge & Kegan Paul.

Kappagoda, Astika K. 2004. Semiosis as the Sixth Sense: Theorising the Unperceived in Ancient Greek. Doctoral thesis, Macquarie University.

Lewontin, Richard. 1993. *Biology as Ideology: The Doctrine of DNA*. London: Penguin.

Lewontin, Richard. 2000. *It Ain't Necessarily So: The Dream of the Human Genome and Other Illusions*. London: Granta Books.

Lloyd, Geoffrey E.R. 1970. *Early Greek Science: Thales to Aristotle*. New York, London: W.W. Norton & Co.

Lloyd, Geoffrey E.R. 2002. *The Ambitions of Curiosity. Understanding the World in Ancient Greece and China*. Cambridge: Cambridge University Press.

McNeill, David. 1992. *Hand and Mind: What Gestures Reveal about Thought*. Chicago: University of Chicago Press.

Malloch, Stephen and Colwyn Trevarthen. 2008. *Communicative Musicality. Exploring the Basis of Human Companionship*. Oxford: Oxford University Press.

Mondada, Lorenza. 2003. Working with Video: How Surgeons Produce Video Records of Their Actions. *Visual Studies* 18(1): 58–73.

Moore, Alison, David Butt, Jodie Ellis-Clarke and John Cartmill. 2010. Linguistic Analysis of Verbal and Non-Verbal Communication in the Operating Room. *ANZ Journal of Surgery* 80(12): 925–9. doi: 10.1111/j.1445-2197.2010.05531.x

Panksepp, Jaak and Lucy Biven. 2012. *The Archaeology of Mind: Neuroevolutionary Origins of Human Emotions*. The Norton Series of Interpersonal Biology. New York, London: W.W. Norton & Company.

Rosen, Jacob, Mark MacFarlane, Christina Richards, Blake Hannaford and Mika Sinanan. 1999. Surgeon-Tool Force/Torque Signatures-Evaluation of Surgical Skills in Minimally Invasive Surgery. *Studies in Health Technology and Informatics* 62: 290–6.

Roochnik, David. 1996. *Of Art and Wisdom: Plato's Understanding of Techne*. Pennsylvania: The Pennsylvania State University Press.

Saussure, Ferdinand. 1959 [1916]. *Course in General Linguistics*. Trans. W. Baskin. London: Peter Owen Ltd.

Shapiro, James. 2011. *Evolution: A View from the 21st Century*. New Jersey: FT Press Science.

Svensson, Marcus Sanchez, Christian Heath, and Paul Luff. 2007. Instrumental Action: The Timely Exchange of Implements during Surgical Operations. In *ECSCW 2007*, 41–60. Dordrecht: Springer.

Svensson, Marcus Sanchez, Paul Luff and Christian Heath. 2009. Embedding Instruction in Practice: Contingency and Collaboration during Surgical Training. *Sociology of Health & Illness* 31(6): 889–906.

Trevarthen, Colwyn. 1987. Sharing Makes Sense: Intersubjectivity and the Making of an Infant's Meaning. In *Language Topics: Essays in Honour of M.A.K. Halliday*, edited by Rossand Steele and Terry Threadgold, 177–200. PLACE: John Benjamins.

Further Reading

Bullowa, Margaret (ed.). 1979. *Before Speech: The Beginning of Interpersonal Communication*. Cambridge: Cambridge University Press.

Butt, David G. 2008. The Robustness of Realizational Systems. In *Meaning in Context: Implementing Intelligent Applications of Language Studies*, edited by J.J. Webster, 59–83. London & New York: Continuum.

Halliday, Michael A.K. 2005. On Matter and Meaning: The Two Realms of Human Experience. *Linguistics and the Human Sciences* 1(1): 59–82.

Meares, Russell. 2005. *The Metaphor of Play: Origin and Breakdown of Personal Being.* Third edition. London and New York: Routledge.

David G. Butt, PhD, is an Associate Professor of Linguistics at Macquarie University, Sydney. He has published widely on systemic functional linguistic theory and applications including literary stylistics, educational linguistics and health discourses – in particular surgery, oncology and psychotherapy. He began discussions with John Cartmill at the recommendation of Professor Miles Little; and this connection led to their focus on the semantic complexity of institutional systems.

John A. Cartmill is a senior consultant surgeon at Nepean Public and Macquarie University Private Hospitals and a founding Professor in the Faculty of Medicine and Health Sciences at Macquarie University, Sydney. Professor Cartmill has played a leading role in developing the emerging area of postgraduate surgical education in Australia. A fortunate introduction to David Butt and Alison Moore has led to a fascination with the power of linguistics to unlock many of the (hitherto) intangibles of the specialty he enjoys so much.

Drawings by **Marcus Cremonese**, biomedical illustrator. The authors wish to acknowledge Marcus's ability to portray concepts that lie beyond the realm of articulation.

SECTION III
THE AFTERMATH

14 Inter-Professional Clinical Handover in Surgical Practice

Peter Roger, Maria R. Dahm, John A. Cartmill and Lynda Yates

14.1 Introduction and Literature Review

Clinical handover has recently attracted research attention, as a point at which responsibility for patient care is transferred. Handovers are obvious crucial points where there is the potential for information to be miscommunicated or lost altogether, with possible serious consequences for patient safety, effective care and outcomes. A primary driver of handover research has thus been the desire to improve information transfer, and this has led to studies (e.g., Haig, Sutton and Whittington 2006) assessing the role of proforma protocols in an attempt to ensure that "all bases are covered" when the patient care baton is passed. Such approaches face limitations, however, as they can underestimate the value of *interaction* between the parties concerned, particularly where the professional or team receiving the handover briefing wishes to check or clarify details that are presented, or question the rationale behind particular treatment decisions in order to understand the line of thinking that underpinned these decisions.

Much of the literature focuses on handover sessions that are formally recognized as such, in that they happen at a regular point in the daily routine of a clinical unit (usually involving a shift change) or coincide with the physical transfer of a patient from one place to another (e.g., an ambulance arrival at an emergency department). Handover events in hospital settings are more ubiquitous than this, however, and can happen at any point where two or more members of staff interact with a view to allowing one professional to move away (temporarily or permanently) from the care of a particular patient, while another picks up and continues the care. As Jorm, White and Kaneen (2009) point out, clinicians may not recognize that much of the inter-professional clinical communication that is part of their daily work is in fact a form of handover. Increased complications and even mortality rates have been linked to poor briefing and information-sharing practices during post-operative handovers (Mazzocco et al. 2009). Jorm and colleagues (2009) also highlight the tragic consequences that can result when channels of communication do not function as they should at critical "transfer of care" junctures.

It is important to recognize that the handover interaction is not concerned solely with information transfer, but also fulfils a number of other key functions (Symons et al. 2012). For instance, one party involved may ask the other for advice, or one party may flag particular tasks that need to be completed, either before the handover is complete, or afterwards. Such tasks could include contacting relatives, ordering or following up investigations, prescribing or ordering medications, or arranging for other medical or allied health professionals to assess the patient (consults). Randell, Wilson and Woodward (2011) also point to a "surveillance" element to handovers that has been identified in the literature, where incoming staff can consider critically what has been done so far, and outgoing staff can reflect on aspects of the management that has occurred on their watch. This means that a handover does not simply culminate in a list of unfinished actions (a "to do" list for the incoming team or clinician), but provides an opportunity for reflection on where to go from here.

Where handover interactions involve "parallel" teams or individuals from the same profession with equivalent roles and responsibilities, it is most usual that those tasks "to be completed" are passed on to the incoming individual or team, who can follow them up (or make adjustments to them) as part of continuing patient care. When handover encounters occur between members of different health professions (medical and nursing staff, for example) or between professionals of different seniority levels (e.g., specialist and resident medical officer), the handover acquires a new level of complexity. This is because of individual perceptions, and institutional policies, about who is responsible for what (and indeed who is *allowed* to do what) under the rules of the hospital and broader healthcare system. In such situations, clinical handovers can become interactionally more complex, as participants must (usually tacitly) negotiate potentially thorny professional and seniority boundaries as they work towards the effective continuity of patient care.

In stressing the central importance of handover encounters to the quality and continuity of care, Iedema and colleagues (2009: 291) characterize clinical handovers as representing "the intersection between shifts, units, organizations, professions, ranks, and different professional functions, including teaching, caring and curing". It follows that these differences in profession, role and seniority will at times lead to mismatched ideas about the way in which clinical handover communication should ideally occur. Mismatches such as these represent differences in the *expectations* that those involved in handover interactions have, and uncovering these differences is an important step in improving the quality of clinical handovers.

In the case of nursing shift handovers that occur regularly and thus acquire an established and predictable structure characteristic of the particular institution (or unit), regular participants in the handover are likely to share an understanding of what they are doing. However, hospitals in the 21st century are complex and diverse institutions. While there are many professionals who work consistently as part of a close-knit team or unit over a sustained period, the presence of casual nursing staff, as well as resident medical staff rotating through different areas, means that clinical communication often occurs between individuals who have not met before, or do not know each other well. Junior doctors have been found in some studies to be less than satisfied with their own handover skills (Cleland et al. 2009; Manser and Foster 2011). Added to this is the fact that a large percentage of the medical work-force in countries such as Australia has trained overseas. This means that issues of intercultural communication and the processes of acculturation into a different healthcare system also enter the equation (Dahm 2011).

In trying to understand how communication works in handover encounters, it seems logical to begin with the fundamental question of whether or not participants agree on *exactly what they are doing* when they participate in such encounters. While it is no doubt valuable to focus on issues such as the quality of information transfer, the ways in which clinicians listen actively to each other during handovers and the ways in which they show respect for their colleagues in handover interactions, these elements presume that participants share the same idea of the purpose of the encounter, and *what is going on* as they participate in it.

The aim of the current chapter is to examine the ways in which six medical practitioners with varying amounts and types of clinical experience approach a standardized handover interaction with a nurse. In particular, it aims to trace the participants' apparent understanding of what they are doing, as reflected in their contributions to the interaction. The context is the discussion of a paediatric surgical case in an emergency department.

14.2   Theoretical Framework

The central question that this chapter seeks to address is whether participants in handover encounters share the same understanding of the purpose of these interactions. Put another way, do their contributions suggest that they have the same idea of what they are doing at particular moments in the encounter? This fundamental question is effectively addressed through a discourse analytic approach known as "interactive framing", which is a technique associated with the broad field of interactional sociolinguistics. The key elements and theoretical underpinnings of this approach are outlined below.

The concept of framing, as it is applied here, can be traced to the work of Bateson (1955), who pointed out that individuals need to understand "what is going on" at any given moment in an interaction, in order to interpret the messages (verbal and nonverbal) of the other participants. Bateson observed interactions between monkeys, and noted that when the monkeys bit each other, the act of biting appeared to be interpreted very differently depending on whether the monkeys were "playing" or "fighting" at the time. In the 1970s, the sociologist Erving Goffman set out a comprehensive theory in his book entitled *Frame Analysis* (1974), using the question "what is it that's going on here?" as his point of departure. Hymes (1974) conceptualized framing in a similar manner, using it in his analysis of the ethnography of speaking in different cultures. The terms "frame" and "framing" as used in interactional sociolinguistics refer to the activity that is taking place at any given point in an interaction. The way in which participants perceive (consciously or subconsciously) this activity – or frame – will determine the way in which they interpret the utterances and actions of others, and the way in which they construct their own contributions to the interaction.

When participating in a wide range of social and professional interactions with others on a daily basis, how do individuals know which frames to invoke as these interactions proceed? As Tannen and Wallat (1993) emphasize, we draw on an accumulation of past experiences to form expectations about the ways in which our encounters with others will unfold.

Expectations that allow us to intuitively understand what frame is in operation at any given moment are built up over time with basic socialization processes in a particular culture, as well as experience in specific socio-cultural and professional contexts. Such expectations in effect constitute a stock of implicit knowledge, so that Tannen and Wallat (1993: 60) use the term *knowledge schemas* to refer to "participants' expectations about people, objects, events and settings in the world". Knowledge schemas include implicit and explicit general knowledge about the world, particular societies and cultures and individuals. They also include knowledge that particular individuals hold by virtue of their experience in a particular profession or occupation. Importantly, these knowledge schemas are not limited to factual knowledge and conceptual understanding, but also extend to knowledge of the typical features of a wide range of interaction types (interactional knowledge). Knowledge schemas are built in part from formal study and training, but also from basic life experience and socialization throughout an individual's lifespan.

When involved in any verbal interaction with others, we therefore draw on our accumulated experiences (and thus knowledge schemas) to intuit the frame in operation. But what is the mechanism that allows us to use our experiences in making these apparently intuitive judgements that are so essential to smooth communication? The mediating factor is what Gumperz (1982) calls *contextualization cues*. These cues are "...constellations of surface features of the message form that are the means by which speakers signal and listeners interpret what the activity is, how semantic content is to be understood and how each sentence relates to which precedes or follows..." (ibid.: 131). Contextualization cues can thus signal what "frame" is in operation at a particular time. They can include a wide range of verbal behaviours, including word choice, voice quality and volume, pitch, emphasis, intonation, and even the adoption of particular colloquialisms, accents or dialectal features. They also include nonverbal elements, such as gaze, facial expression, posture and gestures. Many of these contextualization cues are not universal in the meanings that they carry, leading to instances of miscommunication where inter-actants' life experiences and knowledge schemas, and therefore their expectations, diverge substantially.

Research that has drawn on forms of frame analysis to examine interactions in clinical settings has tended to focus on aspects of the exchanges between the health professional and patient/client. A variety of clinical settings have been the subject of research including aged care (Coupland, Robinson and Coupland 1994), audiology (Coupland and Jaworski 1997), gynaecology (Beck and Ragan 1992), medical doctor training (Thomassen 2009), paediatrics (Tannen and Wallat 1993), psychiatry (Ribeiro 1993) and speech-language pathology (Candlin and Roger 2013; Roger and Code forthcoming). In examining inter-professional communication, as we do in this chapter, we use this approach to explore the fundamental question of the degree to which participants share the same idea of "what they are doing" in these clinical handover encounters.

14.3 Methodology

The data were collected as part of a larger pilot study for which an opportunistic sample of participants was recruited through the Royal Australian College of General Practitioners, a large public hospital and a university medical school. Six medically-trained participants were recruited, representing a wide range of experience levels (from recent graduates to experienced specialists) and areas of medicine (see Table 14.1). The sample also included both participants who had completed their medical training in Australia, and participants who had complete their medical training and all of their practice experience in other parts of the world.

Table 14.1: Participant demographics

Pseudonym	Medical training and practice experience	Medical specialty	Clinical experience
Ali	South Asia	Respiratory Medicine	>10 years
Anne	Australia	Intensive Care	>10 years
Bron	Eastern Europe	Research	0 years
Fara	Central Asia	Internal Medicine	>10 years
Nina	Australia	Rotating internship/residency	2 years
Rebecca	Australia	General Medicine	>5 years

While studies that examine authentic clinical interactions can make claims to strong ecological validity, such studies are less suited to making comparisons between individual clinicians' performances. This is because of the inevitable differences in situational variables. For this study, we opted to use a standardized role-play scenario design more conducive to such comparisons (see, for instance, Bataller and Shively 2011), where each of the six participants was briefed in an identical manner before engaging first with a nurse, and then with the grandfather of the "patient". The roles of the nurse and grandfather were played by actors with extensive experience in medical training role-plays, and the actor who played the nurse is in fact also a registered nurse.

The two-part scenario itself was developed by an organization with extensive experience in designing "standardized" scenarios for the purposes of medical communication training programmes. It involved a paediatric surgical case, in which a young child, "Aaron", had been admitted with a fractured femur after being struck by a car. He had been staying with his grandparents at the time of the accident, and had had an adverse reaction to the intravenous contrast used for his CT scan. The first role-play, on which this chapter is based, involved a handover. The participants played the role of a resident doctor in the emergency department, who had just come on duty. Each participant received a very short briefing from another doctor, who was then "called away" and therefore instructed the participant to have a talk with "Sandra", the nurse, to find out more about the case, in order to update the grandfather in the second role-play.

In addition to being a handover scenario, it was decided that the two interactants should also have a request for the other to complete a specific task. This was done to introduce a "request for action" element into what might otherwise have simply been an information-sharing interaction. It also took account of the fact that the two interactants were from different professions, with different professional roles and responsibilities in the institution. The nurse was briefed to ask the doctor-participants, at some point during the encounter, to write up some antibiotics for Aaron. The doctor-participants were briefed that they should ask the nurse to organize an "anaesthetics consult" but it would transpire that the nurse had finished her shift and needed to leave the hospital shortly. The nurse-actor and doctor-participants were left to negotiate the completion of this task as they saw fit.

The role-plays were conducted in a medical simulation laboratory that was set up to look like a room in an emergency department. Participants were video-recorded by unobtrusive ceiling cameras and fixed lapel microphones. The role-play data were transcribed and analysed, with a focus on the ways in which the participants sought to frame the encounters at key junctures.

14.4 Findings

14.4.1 Getting Down to Business

Each interaction began with the doctor entering the room, where the nurse was seated at a small desk, writing. All participants engaged in conventional greetings and introductions with the nurse (as they had not met before) and then moved after a few turns to a discussion of the patient. This could be characterized as a shift from a "greeting" frame into a "clinical information" frame. Despite the fact that each participant received the same information going into the role-play, the participants' moves to contextualize and frame the interaction varied, as illustrated by the extracts below.

Extract 1

```
1 Rebecca   Hi are you Sandra?
2 S         Yes hello.
3 Rebecca   Hi I'm Rebecca. I'm the doctor this evening.
4 S         Oh ((gets up from chair, shakes hand)) hi doctor, how are you? =
5 Rebecca   =the last
6 S         =nice to meet you
7 Rebecca   The last doctor just handed over to me [yes] about a patient called
           Aaron [yeah] who was brought into hospital [yeah] I know his parents
           are outside [yeah] and uhm ( )
8 S         Well actually his grandfather is in ( )
9 Rebecca   Grandfather?
10 S        Yeah
11 Rebecca  Okay [yeah yeah] they want me go ( ) he's been waiting for some
           results from his accident this morning [yes] this morning, this
           afternoon so I just wanted to get a bit more information about
           what's happened [yeah] because I wasn't here [yeah] so that I can go
           in [yeah] nice and prepared
```

In Extract 1, Rebecca moves to frame the encounter explicitly, indicating what she hopes to learn ("I just wanted to get a bit more information") as well as the reason ("so that I can go in...nice and prepared"). Before doing this, however, Rebecca opens with a summary of what she knows already, prompting a correction from Sandra, who points out that it is the grandfather of the patient who is waiting in the next room, not the child's parents. Rebecca's move to "display" what she already knows thus serves a useful function.

Extract 2

```
1 Anne   Hi!
2 S      Hi! ((stands up from chair))
3 Anne   Sandra?
4 S      Yeah.
5 Anne   My name is Anne ((shakes hand))
6 S      Hi, Anne?
7 Anne   Yes!
8 S      Hi Anne, how are you?
```

    9 Anne   Good good. I'm the resident for the afternoon [okay]. I've taken over
             fro::m John [yes] who was the resident [yeah] beforehand. And I hear
             that you were uhm accompanying Aaron [yes] to the CT? [yup] Alright,
             could I just take a seat?
    10 S   yeah ((gestures towards the covered operating table just behind Anne))
    11 Anne Is there another seat?
    10 S   No ( ) ((looks around room quickly))
    11 Anne Yeah I just lean against this [yeah] okay ((as S sits down again, Anne
             leans against the covered operating table)) so uhm Sandra what happened
             with Aaron?

Anne's approach (in Extract 2) to contextualizing the interaction is unique among the six participants, in that she moves to frame the encounter both verbally and physically. At line 9, she explains her role ("I'm the resident for the afternoon"), focuses the discussion on Aaron ("I hear that you were accompanying Aaron to the CT"), and then asks if she may sit down, in effect inviting Sandra to resume her own seat for the discussion. This move could be seen as a contextualization cue that serves to create an unhurried atmosphere in which they can focus on the case at hand, rather than a conversation between people who are on their way to somewhere else. Her next utterance is congruent with the move to sit down, as she asks "So um Sandra what happened with Aaron?" The open question suggests that she is seeking a "story" from Sandra, and prefers to hear it as a sequence, rather than eliciting answers to specific questions at this point.

Quite a different approach is seen with Fara. An experienced international specialist trained in another medical system, she had not worked in an Australian hospital before. This put her in quite a different position, as the division of roles, responsibilities and typical inter-professional relationships may well have been different from those to which she was accustomed. The interaction between Fara and Sandra opens with the exchanges in Extract 3.

Extract 3

    1 S   Hi! How are you?
    2 Fara   Good morning, how about you?
    3 S   Hi [hi] I'm Sandra the nurse
    4 Fara   Okay (0.5) nice to meet you. ((shakes hand))
    5 S   Nice to meet you.
    6 Fara   Nice to meet you. Okay what's the problem?
    7 S   Ah, well I just, apparently they they: you're taking over from the
             other:, the other doctor is about to go home [oh okay, yeah] and you
             are taking over the care of Aaron?
    8 Fara   Yes yes.
    9 S   Yes. Uhm so did they tell you about, anything about Aaron?
    10 Fara Uh uh no, not very well but uh they mentioned because the shift change
             [yes] I have the responsibility after her [yes yes] and I want to see
             the patient [yup] and I want to know about him [okay] what they did and
             how is the condition of the patient now [okay]. First of all, to be she
             he is (a) stable or not?
    11 S   Yes uh well yeah he's good.
    12 Fara Is it a girl or a boy?

```
13 S    It's a boy [a boy]. He's a little six-year old boy [six-year old] yeah.
        So basically what happened [yeah]he was riding a bike [okay] in a quiet
        street at his grandfather's house and he was hit by car [okay] and he
        fell (his bike)[mm okay] and the car wasn't going very fast [mmh] but
        uh he did sustain a fracture to his left femur [oh okay ((very softly))]
        and just and some minor lacerations.
```

Following the greeting sequence, Fara moves to shift frames to talk about the clinical issue at hand. She does this, however, by asking "What's the problem?" (line 6) and without any prior contextualizing information. This implies that she has been called to address a particular problem, the nature of which she does not know. Sandra does not continue in the frame initiated by Fara, but responds by checking her understanding of Fara's role ("you are taking over from the other... doctor...and you are taking over the care of Aaron?"). In doing so, she establishes whether there is common understanding of the reasons for their encounter. Fara moves then to re-frame the encounter, this time highlighting the kind of information that she is seeking.

At this point, it is noteworthy that the respective roles of the interactants and the purpose of their interaction are managed (with one exception) through the provision of contextualizing information by the nurse and doctor participants in the initial turns of the encounter. The exception is the interaction between Sandra and Fara where Fara's move to initiate a "clinical information" frame (Extract 3, line 6) before either party has shared this contextualizing information prompts Sandra to invoke a "roles and responsibilities" frame (line 7) to clarify this. We also have some initial indications that Fara is operating in an unfamiliar cultural and linguistic environment, as the references to "Aaron" have left her unsure as to whether the patient is a boy or a girl.

14.4.2 Framing Clinical Responsibilities

An examination of the handover transcripts reveals that Aaron's current medical status was an important focus in all of the handover interactions. This was entirely expected, as the medical stability of the patient is obviously essential information to be shared during a clinical handover that takes place in an emergency department. Five of the six participants managed this within the "clinical information" frame, through a combination of "backchannel" responses (e.g., yeah, OK, yep, mm hm) in response to Sandra's recount of events and management, and some specific follow-up questions. The interaction between Sandra and Fara, however, was unique in that the interactants invoked what could be called the "roles and responsibilities" frame on more than one occasion to address the issue of the patient's medical stability. An examination of the following extract shows that Fara and the nurse are no longer "sharing medical information" and that the discussion has shifted to focus on Fara's responsibilities.

Extract 4

```
80 Fara     But uh let's uh first of all I have to check myself the patients
            [yes] to see what is the c- [okay] going on [alright]. Uhm At first
            I will uh see the vital signs the same like before [yes] as the
            breathings has okay [yeah] or auscultation [yeah] the auscultation
            because if there is uh some allergy (condition) [yeah] it can come
            back [yes sure] that's why it's so important.
81 S        Uhm before you see Aaron though, Aaron is stable [yeah]. His breath-
            ing's normal, he's all good [uh-hm] but his grandfather hasn't, his
            grandfather does not know [uh-hm] what happened up in the CT [uh-
            hm]. It's been two hours since the grandfather saw him [mm-hm] and
            the grandfather [uh-hm] doesn't know about the results of the CT and
            he doesn't know about the: reaction [mm-hm ((soft))] So could you
            see the grandfather before you see Aaron? If you don't mind?
82 Fara     Uh but if (it is) the patient is stable, it is safe for the patient
            first for the (safety) of the patient I have to uhm check the (Aaron)
            first =
83 S        =well
84 Fara     = it is my first=
85 S        =uh
86 Fara     =prio-
87 S        = yeah absolutely ( )
88 Fara     =(priority)
89 S        But I'm informing you that the patient is well
90 Fara     is okay if you (informed)
91 S        =patient is totally fine
92 Fara     = the doctor, doesn't
93 S        I can show you his observations charts [okay that's fine] He's
            totally fine [okay ((soft))] uhm but the grandfather is quite dis-
            tressed [uh-hm] because he hasn't seen Aaron and you know he is he's
            feeling guilty because Aaron has been staying with him [mm-hm] for
            a holiday [oh yeah]
94 Fara     But uh no one explained them? You didn't explain to the (grandfather)?
95 S        Well it's really not my role to explain to the grandfather about the
            reaction [okay ((soft))] and I literally we just got back [yeah]
            so I didn't, I feel it's the doctor's role to explain to the to
            the grandfather about Aaron's condition [okay]. I mean that's just
            our protocol [okay] here is that the doctor needs to explain test
            results and
96 Fara     Okay if the patients is as you say is uhm is uh stable [yes] and is
            uhm in a good condition [yeah, he is good] and comfortable [yes] at
            this time I can talk with the uh the p- parent [excellent] and family
```

In Extract 4, Fara invokes what we might call the "roles and responsibilities" frame. Sandra is obviously keen for her to speak to the waiting grandfather, while Fara insists that her first duty is to satisfy herself first-hand that the patient is stable. This leads to a number of exchanges in which Sandra tries to assure Fara that Aaron is indeed stable, and Fara tries to explain why it would be in order for her to assess Aaron first. Sandra highlights the fact that the grandfather will be waiting for some information, which leads Fara to question the fact that no one has yet spoken to the grandfather. Sandra follows with a discussion of local hospital protocols and her own feelings about her roles and responsibilities. After some discussion, Fara then agrees to speak with the family.

As the encounter unfolds further, however, it becomes clear that Fara still has reservations. After more discussion about whether or not the patient should be kept "nil by mouth" and the question of antibiotics, Sandra prepares to explain where the grandfather is waiting. Fara has not asked where his parents are (and indeed continues to refer to the person waiting as "the parent"), so Sandra explains this as well in Extract 5.

Extract 5

137 S   Okay. So can you, I show you where the grandfather is [yeah yeah] and you can see the grandfather [yeah]. You might need to know also the reason that he is with his grandfather, his parents are on holidays in Queensland
138 Fara   Okay but at the time when I'm talking with the parent is there anyone to take of the, what's the, the patient?
139 S   Oh of course he's around in=
140 Fara   =the ( )
141 S   In bay three there's other nurse around there, [okay] yeah
142 Fara   I should be sure there are some people observing the patient [absolutely] because of if it is rash and there is some
143 S   Doctor =you know I would not
144 Fara   =I'm I should be careful =because
145 S   =Trust me!
146 Fara   this is my responsibility
147 S   I understand=
148 Fara   =and you are really
149 S   =but it is also ( )
150 Fara   Your responsibility as well?
151 S   It's my responsibility as well [yeah] and I would not leave the patient if I was concerned that the patient wasn't well [okay ((soft))]. So the patient is in bay three and there are nurses around there that [okay] are keeping an eye on him [okay, that's right] okay?
152 Fara   Yeah, yes.

In all of the interactions, it is only the encounter involving Sandra and Fara where the "roles and responsibilities" frame is invoked. By way of comparison, we see that Australian-trained Anne's line of questioning assumes shared knowledge about the kind of hospital system in which the interaction is taking place. Evidence for this can be seen, for instance, when Anne refers to "the medical team" who would normally respond to emergencies such as this (Extract 6, line 19). Sandra's response suggests that she knows what Anne is referring to, and she confirms that the "medical team" was not called in this instance.

Extract 6

18 S   So he basically had the contrast [yup] and literally within a few minutes developed (0.6) the rash [okay] came up quite quickly [yup] and he had a bit of uhm shortness of breath [okay]. He was given hydrocortisone [yup] which, and he responded really quickly to that [yup] so =he's
19 Anne   =the medical team came? From= from ED? Or?
20 S   = ( ) they didn't do a call [okay sure] uhm because he didn't actually [yeah okay] you know it wasn't a respiratory arrest [yeah] as such [sure] and he responded really quickly to the [yeah ((soft))] hydrocortisone and he responded very quickly [yeah] to that

In summary, clinical information is shared between participants in all of the encounters by Sandra providing a narrative about the clinical history and management so far, punctuated by questions (some specific, some more general) from the doctor participants. With the exception of the encounter involving Fara and Sandra, this component of the handover is achieved in a "clinical information" frame. By contrast, Fara invokes frames that involve explicit discussion of her clinical responsibilities, as well as the roles of different staff members in the hospital context.

14.4.3 The Family Context

At various points in the interaction, Sandra offers information to the doctor-participants about Aaron's family situation. This information includes the fact that he has been staying with his grandparents as his parents are currently on holiday in another state, which explains why it is his grandfather who is waiting at the hospital. She also gives the grandfather's name, and (in some of the interactions) even mentions the parents' given names. Interaction that focuses on these elements can be seen as part of a "family context" frame. In some instances, it is the nurse who initiates the shift into this frame, while in other instances the doctor participants initiate the frame shift.

In contextualizing the handover discussion in the initial turns, the nurse and five of the six doctor participants chose to refer to the patient by referring to him by name. Both parties then continued to use the name "Aaron" throughout the conversation. The establishment of the patient's name was achieved in various ways. Rebecca, Anne and Ali use his name in their opening statements. In the interaction with Bron, it is Sandra who uses the name first, and Bron reciprocates in the following turn. In all of these interactions, Aaron's name is brought into the conversation without an actual shift of frame. However, in the case of Nina, a brief frame shift occurs (Extract 7) when Nina does not recall the patient's name, but deliberately moves to establish what it is at the beginning of the encounter.

Extract 7

```
11 Nina  Uh I just got a handover from one of my (0.2) colleagues [yeah] about a
         patient? [yes] Six-year old boy? [yes] now what was his name again? =
12 S     =Aaron
13 Nina  =I have forgotten
14 S     Aaron's the name
15 Nina  Aaron that's right. Okay so I just wanted to follow up on (1.0) what's
         been happening with him...
```

When it comes to the use of names, Fara's approach, once again, is different. Unlike the other participants, she continues to talk of "the patient" throughout, rather than referring to him by name. In handing over to Fara, Sandra does refer to him as Aaron throughout, although at certain points in the encounter she appears to mirror Fara's use of "the patient", particularly when discussing his current condition and providing assurances that he is medically stable following the allergic reaction.

The use of names in one sense may seem a trivial point of difference. However, it is noteworthy that five of the six participants establish the name of the patient near the beginning of the encounter and use it throughout. The fact that Fara does not use the name of the patient at all during the interaction could be attributed to a personal communication style (some people are less inclined than others to use names) or a cultural difference in the use of names to refer to patients in a professional context such as this. Another possible explanation is that Fara prioritizes her interactional and information processing resources to focus on the essential medical details. While it is a convenient and personalizing way to refer to him, the name "Aaron" is not an essential medical detail. Fara's unfamiliarity with the system, as evidenced by her shifts into the "roles and responsibilities" frame, adds to the cognitive burden for her in keeping track of information offered as part of the handover.

In each of the encounters, Sandra explains to the doctor why it is the grandfather who is present, and not the parents. In some encounters, this information is elicited by a question from the doctor. In the interaction with Anne, for instance, Sandra mentions (in her initial recapitulation of Aaron's history) the fact that it was his grandfather who came to the hospital with him. Anne does not follow this up immediately, but has evidently made a note of it, as she returns (several turns later) to the topic to clarify the situation (Extract 8). Anne's utterance at turn 35 initiates a shift into the "family context" frame, which is picked up by Sandra.

Extract 8

```
35 Anne  Grandfather in the car with him when he was, or or driving, or what was
          happening?
36 S      No they were actually outside the grandfather's house [okay yup] So
          they've got (apparently) like a cul-de-sac [yup], a quiet street [yup]
          and he has been riding his bike up there with the other kiddies [sure].
          His grandfather is in the house changing a light bulb [ah:: okay], got
          a knock on the door from the neighbour saying [yup] "Aaron's been hit
          by a car" [ah:: I see] Cause who hit him was the neighbour [yup yup]
          quite distressed herself [okay alright] uhm
37 Anne  And the neighbour's not here at the moment [no] and the grandfather's
          the only family here? Where is the –
38 S      He's the only family here, yes.
39 Anne  No mum and dad? Where are they?
40 S      Mum and dad are on holidays in Cairns [ah:::] yes.
41 Anne  And have they been notified?
42 S      No! the grandfather, Jim is his name = ( )
43 Anne  =ah, Jim, okay yup
```

Similarly, Rebecca asks Sandra to clarify why it is Aaron's grandfather who has accompanied him to the hospital.

Extract 9

```
47 Rebecca  I just need a bit of background why is there a
            grandparent there?
```

Bron does not ask explicitly about the reasons why his grandfather is there, but Sandra offers the information. Interestingly, Bron (in Extract 10) takes this information as a clue that something may be amiss in the relationship between the grandfather and Aaron's parents. While this was not Sandra's intended meaning, the exchange below does provide evidence that Bron was ready to engage with the "family context" frame that Sandra had initiated.

Extract 10

```
58 Bron Yeah so please [yeah] uh pass on the message [absolutely] and I will
         talk to the uh relative of Aaron [yes]. His grandfather =
59 S     =so if you could
60 Bron  =(you said)?
61 S     see the grandfather before you see Aaron [yeah] because his grandfather
         is quite anxious
62 Bron  Yes no problem I talk to him. Thank you! Please also ((starts moving
         towards the door and out of the frame)) ( ) to your colleague
63 S     Yeah you might also want to know that uhm his mum, Aaron's parents,
         uh the reason he's staying with his grandfather is because they're on
         holidays in Cairns [okay] and the parents don't yet know anything about
         Aaron [aha aha] so it's just the grandfather wanted to get all the
         information before he uh:m spoke to Emma =
64 Bron  =ah okay
65 S     =Aaron's mum
66 Bron  So basically okay so only the grandfather is the closest relative
67 S     Yeah [yeah] closest relative at the time
68 Bron  Okay okay well I pass on to the
69 S     =so he's feeling
70 Bron  =grandfather
71 S     a bit guilty
72 Bron  And I find out a little bit more about the relation with the parents
         [yeah] so that we you know uh=
73 S     Oh I think
74 Bron  = ( )
75 S     I think it's pretty good [okay] it seems that the grandpa, Emma is uh
         his daughter, Jim is, Jim Lancaster is the grandfather [okay], Emma is
         his daughter they seem to have, as far as I can ascertain, good rela-
         tionship. It's just that he didn't express that Emma is quite you know
         reactionary person so [yeah, of course] he wanted to get all the medical
         facts [yeah ( )] But he wanted all the information [yeah] first before
         he spoke to her [yeah]. So yeah he's feeling a bit guilty and stuff so
         you know he prob, he'll be happy to see=
```

In the interaction with Nina (Extract 11), Sandra initiates a shift into the "family context" frame, which Nina follows up by asking first about the grandfather's emotional state, and later about the grandfather's name (in preparation for talking to him).

Extract 11

```
32 S     Aaron's okay [okay] uhm he seems quite calm and you know he's a bit
         (0.2) concerned about up there [yeah]. His pain seems to be under con-
         trol [uh-hm] we splinted his leg [mmh] so he's a pretty tough little
         fella ((smiles)) [okay, very good]. So he seems to be okay my only con-
         cern is with the grandfather [okay] cause he's been waiting for so long
         [mm-hm] that uhm he doesn't know anything [okay, alright] u:hm
33 Nina  Is he quite angry and upset? Have you=
34 S     =Uhm oh he's not
35 Nina  = (seen him or)
36 S     so much angry it's, he's feeling really guilty you know [ah okay]
         because [alright] Aaron's mum and dad are on holidays [uh-hm] and he's
         been looking after Aaron [(1.0) okay] so he's feeling quite guilty that
         this actually happened [alright] you know [okay] while he was in his
         care and uhm he's quite distressed [okay] as you can imagine
37 Nina  Yeah, that's fair enough okay
38 S     He hasn't actually rung the parents the because he wanted to get the
         full story [the full story yeah] before he did that [okay]=
39 Nina  =that's fine
40 S     =as far as I understand
41 Nina  And what's his=
42 S     =unless he's rung
43 Nina  =name?
44 S     them all up anyway
45 Nina  Yeah, and what's his name?
46 S     The grandfather?
47 Nina  Yeah do y'know?
48 S     Jim. [( )] Jim Lancaster
49 Nina  Okay very good. So I'll have a chat with (1.0) Jim=
```

In the handover interaction with Fara, we see that Sandra attempts on two separate occasions to initiate a shift into the "family context" frame, explaining why
Aaron's grandfather, and not his parents, are present (see Extracts 4 and 5). On both
occasions, however, Fara does not follow Sandra into the family context frame, but
shifts (as discussed above) into the "roles and responsibilities" frame. It thus appears
that Sandra's attempts to leave the "medical information" frame to provide information about the family context cause Fara to express concerns about her role and the
medical stability of Aaron. The turns at which Sandra initiates shifts into a "family
context" frame, which are resisted by Fara, are provided in Extracts 12 and 13.

Extract 12

```
14 S      I can show you his observations charts [okay that's fine] He's
          totally fine [okay ((soft)) ] uhm but the grandfather is quite dis-
          tressed [uh-hm] because he hasn't seen Aaron and you know he is he's
          feeling guilty because Aaron has been staying with him [mm-hm] for
          a holiday [oh yeah]
15 Fara   But uh no one explained them? You didn't explain to the (grandfather)?
```

Extract 13

```
137 S     Okay. So can you, I show you where the grandfather is [yeah yeah] and
          you can see the grandfather [yeah]. You might need to know also the
          reason that he is with his grandfather, his parents are on holidays
          in Queensland
138 Fara  Okay, but at the time when I'm talking with the parent is there any-
          one to take of the, what's the, the patient?
```

In Extract 13 (line 138) it is apparent that Fara is still referring to "talking with the parent", which suggests that she has not fully processed the fact that it is the grandfather whom she is about to see. At the end of the interaction (Extract 14), we see again that Fara needs to hear the information about the grandfather's role and the parents' whereabouts a third time.

Extract 14

```
154  Fara      Who knows about this condition? = the par-
155  S         = uh
156  Fara      Uh from uh the family?
157  S         Who knows about the fracture you mean?
158  Fara      Yeah.
159  S         The accident?
160  Fara      Yeah yeah.
161  S         Just the grandfather [just grandfather] only the =grandfather
162  Fara      =the parent doesn't know =
163  S         =Parents are on holidays
164  Fara      =don't know
165  S         And the grandfather wanted to get all the [oh okay] information
                before he phoned [yeah] the his parents, yeah.
166  Fara      Thank you =
```

14.5   Discussion and Conclusions

An analysis of interactive framing in these handover encounters leads to several key observations. First, the way in which the "handover recipients" framed the encounter from the start provided some clues as to their beliefs about "what they were doing" in the scenario that they had been presented with. Second, we saw the way that participants' past experiences (in Australia, for Anne, Nina and Rebecca, and in other parts of the world for Fara, Ali and Bron) led them to particular expectations, embodied in knowledge schemas. These knowledge schemas related to the typical features of a handover interaction in a given cultural context, but also to issues of medicine and surgery, hospital systems, and the typical roles and responsibilities in such systems. They also related to more general social knowledge, such as the common use of first names to talk about patients in a particular linguistic and cultural context. Finally, where such knowledge schemas were mismatched, this triggered shifts in frames in which participants negotiated the space between their respective experiences and expectations as they worked to accomplish the goals of the encounter.

From a framing perspective, the encounter involving Fara was distinctive in two principal respects. First, it contained frames relating to staff roles and clinical responsibilities that were not evident in any of the other encounters. Second, Fara's reluctance to engage with the "family context" frame was conspicuous. This was, in all probability, not a conscious resistance, but a mechanism for managing the cognitive burden associated with the handover and ensuring that "life and death" medical issues were fully canvassed. In the opening lines of her interaction with the grandfather (not discussed here), Fara expresses her sorrow at hearing about the accident and tries to reassure the grandfather that Aaron is in good hands.

On one level, the repeated shifts into a "roles and responsibilities" frame, as well as Fara's seeming unwillingness to engage with the "family context" frame, creates the impression of a handover event that did not run smoothly. However, Fara is coming to the encounter from a very different medical system, as well as a different cultural and linguistic background. While her apparent reluctance to rely on assurances about the condition of a patient's condition might be seen as a lack of trust in other members of the healthcare team, another perspective is that she is taking great care to leave nothing to chance. When one is dealing with an unfamiliar healthcare system, this is likely to be a wise approach. After all, with real experience in this new system, Fara's expectations (and thus knowledge schemas) will continue to evolve to take account of the observed realities of the system and the way that it works. In the meantime, she has little choice but to shift frames to negotiate the unfamiliar territory. An essential element here would be the language and discourse choices that Fara (as an international medical graduate) makes in such negotiations, as it would be important for her to build sound relationships and rapport with colleagues in any hospital system in which she was working. These issues, and how they can be addressed in training programmes, fall outside the scope of this chapter.

14.5.1 Practical Implications

How, then, can the concept of framing in interactions contribute to improving handover communication? The examples here have focused on ways in which differences in culture and medical practice experience in different healthcare systems can lead to different expectations, which in turn impact on professional communication. Cultural differences aside, however, the literature indicates that mismatched expectations are often expressed by parties involved in clinical handovers. In their study of handovers from ambulance crews to emergency department nursing and medical staff, Jenkin, Abelson-Mitchell and Cooper (2007) discuss the perspectives of the various parties. One of their findings was that ambulance personnel expressed some frustration when they perceived that emergency department (ED) staff were "not listening" or not taking due notice of the information being given to them. For their part, ED staff expressed dissatisfaction with some of the ambulance handover practices in the resuscitation room, which they saw as including non-essential or irrelevant details (ibid.). Furthermore, ED staff indicated the need for repetition of the handover for various reasons, with one participant commenting: "I like to hear the handover twice – once to get the base essentials to allow a complete primary survey, then again once things have calmed down, to get all of the details..." (ibid.: 144).

While on the surface it would seem likely that both parties in the study by Jenkin and colleagues (2007) shared the same idea of "what they were doing" when the handover was occurring, the fact that the communication was not always seen as satisfactory suggests that in fact participants may have been framing the events differently. Further investigation could determine whether this was the case. One possibility, suggested by the quote above, is that ED staff may mentally adopt an "urgent medical information" frame initially, meaning that they screen out details that do not fit this frame (thereby conveying the impression that they are not listening at times). Ambulance personnel, for their part, may be adopting a "thorough history" frame, knowing that they will soon need to leave the hospital and must ensure that all information is conveyed before they do so. Some information that is rightly part of the "thorough history" frame may not be relevant in the "urgent medical information" frame. Only by agreeing on the broad sequence of information sharing (i.e., explicit framing of the interaction at the outset) can such mismatches be overcome. This requires, as a first step, an understanding of the perspectives of both parties, as well as the constraints under which they operate.

The mismatched expectations in the setting investigated by Jenkin and colleagues (2007) share some important parallels with the role-played handover encounters that have been discussed in this chapter. Fara's contributions to the interaction suggest that she is primarily concerned with the medical stability and safety of the patient. Sandra, however, provides Fara with both a medical and a social history, as she is preparing Fara to speak with the waiting grandfather. As discussed earlier, Fara resists shifts into the "family context" frame, and does not appear to absorb non-medical information that is offered during the course of the interaction. For instance, her repeated references to "the parent" even after Sandra has explained that it is Aaron's grandfather who has accompanied him, could well give the impression that Fara was not listening. It seems more likely, however, that she was subconsciously screening out information that distracted from what she perceived as her primary responsibility for the patient's wellbeing. Interestingly the ED staff members quoted by Jenkin and colleagues (2007) appeared to be engaging in similar mental processes when dealing with acutely ill or injured patients arriving by ambulance. For Fara, the picture was complicated by linguistic and cultural differences between herself and her interlocutor, as well as the fact that her professional experience had been in a different medical system altogether. The other participants in the current study, by contrast, were more ready to accept the nurse's assurances that the patient was stable, and seemed to assume that the patient would be appropriately observed. From their contributions to the handover, it is clear that these participants regarded the details of the family context as relevant to their expectations of the encounter. Consistent with this picture, no overt framing ambiguities or tensions were observed in these handover interactions. When the nurse shifted into the "family context" frame, these participants "followed" her into this frame. Similarly, when the doctor participants initiated the "family context" frame,

Sandra followed. With the exception of Fara, the international medical graduates in this study had some local work, study or social experience; further research could explore the degree to which this might explain their different approaches to the handover scenario.

It is clear that when participants do not share the same expectations about what information needs to be conveyed and in what sequence, framing tensions are likely to ensue. Although these can be frustrating for participants, they are in fact useful signals that a mismatch is occurring, and needs to be addressed – explicitly, if necessary. As noted above, it is important that this is accompanied by an attitude of mutual respect, and one that seeks to understand the needs of the other professional involved in the encounter, as well as the constraints under which this person is operating.

How might this play out in practice? In the role-play scenario described here, Sandra quite properly "stuck to the script" in order to allow each of the doctor participants to move, within a few minutes, to a second role-play in the next room where the "grandfather" was waiting. In a real-life handover, Sandra could respond in a way that picked up on the apparent framing tensions that were occurring in her handover interaction with Fara, by saying (for instance):

"I can assure you that Aaron really is stable and that he's being closely monitored, but I can see you're really concerned to confirm this yourself before you talk to the grandfather. So how about you do that, and I'll make a short note in the file about why his grandfather is here with him and where his parents are. You can review that quickly before you talk to the grandfather. Would that work?"

Of course, not all health professionals would be willing to "tailor" their handover practices in this way, and in some handover contexts there may be constraints that work against such flexibility. However, persisting in following a "fixed" information-sharing agenda when the other party is needing or expecting something else may lead to essential information being lost, to the detriment of patient care and safety. Healthcare practitioners thus need to be sensitive to the kinds of framing tensions discussed here, and take steps to align their expectations in order for handover communication to be genuinely effective.

14.5.2 Future Research Directions

In order to enable comparisons between the approaches of individual participants, the present study has used a standardized role-play design to examine issues of framing in inter-professional clinical handovers. The next step will be to apply similar analytical approaches to authentic handover interactions. Analysis of these interactions could be supplemented with interviews with the professionals involved, in order to explore individual, cultural and professional underpinnings of the individuals' approaches to clinical handovers. Interviews could be expanded to include stimulated recall activities, where participants review the video-recorded interactions together and reflect aloud on their approaches to the interaction at critical junctures. In this way, the expectations that underlie the way that individual professionals frame the handover process could be made explicit and addressed. An understanding of the role of interactive framing in handover encounters can be the first step in working towards negotiated solutions that will ultimately facilitate the transfer of clinical information and enhance the quality of patient care.

Acknowledgements

This project was funded by the Partnership Seeding Scheme at Macquarie University, Sydney, Australia.

Transcription Conventions

`[yeah sure]`	square brackets indicate a short interjection by the other speaker
`=`	an equal sign indicates that another speaker continues without pause from the previous speaker
`=because`	
`=trust me`	indicates the that the two utterances overlapped
`(0.6)`	indicates a pause of a certain duration (in tenths of a second)
`((softly))`	double parentheses indicate a nonverbal cue or transcriber's comment
`::`	colons indicate prolongation of the immediately prior sound, and multiple colons indicate a more prolonged sound
`,`	a comma indicates that the intonation suggests that the speaker will continue
`.`	a period indicates a stopping fall in intonation
`li-`	a dash indicates an incomplete word
`( )`	empty parentheses indicate an inaudible utterance
`(you said)`	parentheses indicate the transcriber's uncertainty about the exact utterance

References

Bataller, Rebeca, and Rachel Shively. 2011. Role Plays and Naturalistic Data in Pragmatics Research: Service Encounters during Study Abroad. *Journal of Linguistics and Language Teaching*, 2(1): 15–50.

Bateson, Gregory. 1955. A Theory of Play and Fantasy. In *Psychiatric Research Reports, II*, December. American Psychiatric Association.

Beck, Christina S., and Sandra L. Ragan. 1992. Negotiating Interpersonal and Medical Talk: Frame Shifts in the Gynaecologic Exam. *Journal of Language and Social Psychology*, 11(1–2): 47–61.

Candlin, Sally, and Peter Roger. 2013. *Communication and Professional Relationships in Healthcare Practice.* Sheffield: Equinox.

Cleland, Jennifer A., Sarah Ross, S.C. Miller and Rona Patey. 2009. "There Is a Chain of Chinese Whispers...": Empirical Data Support the Call to Formally Teach Handover to Prequalification Doctors. *Quality and Safety in Health Care* (18): 267–71.

Coupland, Justine, Jeffrey D. Robinson and Nikolas Coupland. 1994. Frame Negotiation in Doctor-Elderly Patient Consultations. *Discourse and Society* 5(1): 89–124.

Coupland, Nikolas, and Adam Jaworski. 1997. Relevance, Accommodation and Conversation: Modeling the Social Dimension of Communication. *Multilingua* 16(2–3): 233–58.

Dahm, Maria R. 2011. Patient Centred Care: Are International Medical Graduates "Expert Novices"? *Australian Family Physician* 40(11): 895–900.

Goffman, Erving. 1974. *Frame Analysis.* Cambridge, MA: Harvard University Press.

Gumperz, John J. 1982. *Discourse Strategies.* Cambridge: Cambridge University Press.

Haig, Kathleen, Staci Sutton and John Whittington. 2006. SBAR: A Shared Mental Model for Improving Communication between Clinicians. *Journal on Quality and Patient Safety* 32(3): 167–75.

Hymes, Dell. 1974. Ways of Speaking. In *Explorations in the Ethnography of Speaking*, edited by Richard Bauman and Joel Sherzer, 433–52. Cambridge: Cambridge University Press.

Iedema, Rick, Eamon T. Merrick, Dorrilyn Rajbhandari, Alan Gardo, Anne Stirling and Robert Herkes. 2009. Viewing the Taken-for-Granted from a Different Aspect: A Video-Based Method in Pursuit of Patient Safety. *International Journal of Multiple Research Approaches* 3(3): 290–301.

Jenkin, Annie, Nadine Abelson-Mitchell and Simon Cooper. 2007. Patient Handover: Time for a Change? *Accident and Emergency Nursing* 15(3): 141–7.

Jorm, Christine M., Sarah White and Tamsin Kaneen. 2009. Clinical Handover: Critical Communications. *Medical Journal of Australia* 190(11): 108–9.

Manser, Tanja, and Simon Foster. 2011. Effective Handover Communication: An Overview of Research and Improvement Efforts. *Best Practice & Research Clinical Anaesthesiology* 25(2): 181–91.

Mazzocco, Karen, Diana B. Petitti, Kenneth T. Fong, Doug Bonacum, John Brookey, Suzanne Graham, Robert E. Lasky, J. Bryan Sexton and Eric J. Thomas. 2009. Surgical Team Behaviors and Patient Outcomes. *The American Journal of Surgery* 197(5): 678–85.

Randell, Rebecca, Stephanie Wilson and Peter Woodward. 2011. The Importance of the Verbal Shift Handover Report: A Multi-Site Case Study. *International Journal of Medical Informatics* 80(11): 803–12.

Ribeiro, Branca Telles. 1993. Framing in Psychotic Discourse. In *Framing in Discourse*, edited by Deborah Tannen, 77–113. New York: Oxford University Press.

Roger, Peter, and Chris Code. forthcoming. Diverging Professional Orientations to Content and Form in Interpreter-mediated Aphasia Assessments. In *Interpreter-Mediated Healthcare Consultations*, edited by Srikant Sarangi. Sheffield: Equinox.

Symons, Nicholas R.A., Helen W.L. Wong, Tanja Manser, Nick Sevdalis, Charles A. Vincent and Krishna Moorthy. 2012. An Observational Study of Teamwork Skills in Shift Handover. *International Journal of Surgery* 10(7): 355–9.

Tannen, Deborah, and Cynthia Wallat. 1993. Interactive Frames and Knowledge Schemas in Interaction: Examples from a Medical Examination/Interview. In *Framing in Discourse*, edited by Deborah Tannen, 57–76. New York: Oxford University Press.
Thomassen, Gøril. 2009. The Role of Role-play: Managing Activity Ambiguities in Simulated Doctor Consultation in Medical Education. *Communication and Medicine* 6(1): 83–93.

Peter Roger is a Senior Lecturer in Linguistics at Macquarie University, Sydney. After completing his MBBS and working for several years in clinical medicine, he went on to obtain a PhD in communication sciences and disorders. He has research interests in healthcare communication as well as in the area of linguistic diversity and the assessment and management of language disorders. He is co-author (with Sally Candlin) of *Communication and Professional Relationships in Healthcare Practice* (2013, Equinox).

Maria R. Dahm completed an Early Career Research Fellowship in Linguistics at Macquarie University, Sydney, and is currently working with the Australian Institute of Health Innovation at Macquarie where she combines her passion for patient-centred health research with her expertise in qualitative and mixed methods research. Her PhD (completed in 2012) examined the impact of medical terminology on English-medium consultations involving non-native speakers. Her research interests include communication and culture in intercultural health and other workplace contexts, health informatics and English for Specific Purposes.

John A. Cartmill is a senior consultant surgeon at Nepean Public and Macquarie University Private Hospitals and a founding Professor in the Faculty of Medicine and Health Sciences at Macquarie University, Sydney. Professor Cartmill has played a leading role in developing the emerging area of postgraduate surgical education in Australia. A fortunate introduction to David Butt and Alison Moore has led to a fascination with the power of linguistics to unlock many of the (hitherto) intangibles of the specialty he enjoys so much.

Lynda Yates, PhD, is a Professor of Linguistics at Macquarie University, Sydney. Her professional experience teaching adult TESOL and consulting to industry has fuelled an interest in research that can feed into the practical concerns of adult language learners and their teachers, and in particular the pronunciation and pragmatic needs of immigrants and transnational professionals. She has a strong commitment to the translation of research findings into professional practice.

15 Open Disclosure in Surgical Practice

Stewart Dunn

15.1 Introduction

Open disclosure is not new and most clinicians have been practising it in some form throughout their careers. But it is not easy and, like all areas of clinical practice, it is being gradually refined as we acquire more knowledge about the impact of an adverse event on patients, their families and health professionals. In this chapter I will focus on responses of clinical staff in the early phases of open disclosure prior to the implementation of administrative and legislative guidelines.

Here are three examples of open disclosure, modified from actual cases.

Erin is a 45-year-old woman who is extremely anxious about her first chemotherapy for metastatic bowel cancer. The nurse mistakenly gives the chemotherapy without the charted antiemetic. As a consequence Erin vomits copiously in front of all the other patients and is exceptionally distressed. The nurse, deeply embarrassed about her mistake, tells Erin that her anxiety was the major factor contributing to her vomiting. Erin does not attend the next two chemotherapy appointments.

Anne presents with her three-year-old daughter suffering convulsions. The registrar, who is new to paediatric ED, mistakenly gives an adult dose of anticonvulsant. The child arrests and the resuscitation is unsuccessful. The hospital, acting on legal advice, forbids attending staff to communicate with the parents. Ten months later, at the inquest, Anne recognizes one of the nurses, to whom she has been denied access. They both burst into tears and console each other.

Riana is receiving radiation therapy for breast cancer. Riana is seriously burned through the chest wall and lung and is left with a fistula that needs ongoing management. After 12 months of investigation the radiotherapy department admits the mistake to Riana. Her surgeon writes up the case.

These three cases are true, with only the names and minor details altered. They capture the essential ingredients of what patients need when things go wrong and people are damaged (Vincent, Phillips and Young 1994). Open disclosure is a return to connection and responsibility. It is not a maintenance of connection because medical error is inevitably experienced as a breach of trust and a break in the relationship between patient and practitioner. Open disclosure is part of the process that seeks to rebuild.

Like a tripod, there are three key elements that give open disclosure its stability and promote rebuilding. They are based on the premise that all parties involved in the adverse event are suffering.

Research shows that medical and nursing staff experience anguish and remorse when things go wrong (Serembus, Wolf and Youngblood 2001). People go into healthcare to do good and to ease suffering. The thought that you have contributed to suffering, or made it worse, is horrendous. From 2007–9, during workshops around Australia with senior clinical and administrative staff (Iedema et al. 2009), we heard real-life stories confirming the anguish that medical error precipitates in staff: self-doubt, disappointment, self-blame, shame, fear, impotence, depression, loss of clinical confidence and, occasionally, suicide (Gladstone 1995; Newman 1996).

Research with patients who sue following medical error shows that they experience anger, bitterness, a sense of betrayal and humiliation (Vincent, Phillips and Young 1994). They want honesty, a clear explanation of how and why the injury happened; they want appropriate compensation for actual losses, pain and suffering; they want staff and the organization to account for their actions; and they want an appreciation of their trauma and assurances that lessons have been learned (Newman 1996).

The tragedy of adverse events is mired with the human reactions that ensue: clinicians recoil in horror whilst patients reach out for reconnection (sometimes in despair or confusion, sometimes anguish, sometimes anger).

Yet that human response is variable and teachable. In actor-based workshops with first-year medical students, we explored the students' reaction to their discovery of a missed chest x-ray in a lung cancer patient (which meant the diagnosis should have been made 15 months earlier). Some students began by declaring that they were not in the hospital 15 months ago and could not be held accountable, literally holding the offending notes at arms' length; they then offered to find a senior person to help. Other students took ownership of the notes and shared their confusion over the apparent discrepancy with the patient, before also offering to find a senior person. The impact on the actor/patient was profoundly different: abandoned versus included. That initial impact set the scene for the patient's subsequent responses to open disclosure.

There is a world of difference between an offer of help from outside the patient's experience and an offer of help that comes from within that space.

15.1.1 Explanation

Erin needed an honest explanation of what had happened in order to move on. The nurse needed to salve her own anguish and embarrassment. But in shifting responsibility away from herself she caused Erin to blame herself and default on subsequent treatments.

The **explanation** gives patients certainty and maintains connection with the reality they have experienced. Without it they are left with further anxiety, loss of control and a sense of abandonment. It is hard for clinicians, when personal compassion is injured by error to maintain a focus on the best interests of the patient.

An honest **explanation** of error is the first leg of the open disclosure tripod.

15.1.2 Apology

Anne suffered 10 months of believing the people who were with her daughter when she died were uncaring monsters. When she finally met one of them, it was instead a person who was as traumatized as she was by the child's death and who had suffered throughout those 10 months. The nurse's suffering was not an admission of guilt; it was a gift – an empathic expression of shared suffering.

An **apology**, however it is expressed, is a reaching out to the harmed person – a willingness and a courage to acknowledge their suffering and to maintain the connection that began with the first clinical contact.

An **apology** is the second leg of the open disclosure tripod.

15.1.3 Reassurance

Rianna's surgeon published the case and also followed through with her fistula management over many months. They remained closely bound by the experience. Rianna, for her part, was overjoyed that her case had been published, written into the culture of medical practice. She believed that publication of her case meant it would never be visited on another patient.

The **reassurance** arising from continued connection with clinical staff and the clear evidence that the system had learned from her experience were critical to Rianna's recovery.

Reassurance is the third leg of the open disclosure tripod.

EAR (Explanation, Apology, Reassurance) is a summary of the literature on what patients need from us when there has been an adverse event. And we have two EARs: one for the patient and their family, and one for the staff involved. Because everyone is harmed by medical error. Staff need a clear **explanation** of how they got into a situation where the event could occur; they also need an **apology** because the system has failed to protect them; and **reassurance** that we will change the system. This is why open disclosure is as much the responsibility of administration as it is of clinicians.

15.2 Why Is It So Difficult to Implement Open Disclosure?

Despite a clear knowledge of these principles, practising open disclosure is incredibly difficult. Some people seem to be innately gifted in this sort of communication while the majority of us are good at some aspects and less so at others. A small cluster of recent studies is assembling a profile of people who demonstrate mastery of this sort of communication. Students who excel appear to be instantly recognizable to actor/patients, other students and staff. Austin and colleagues (2007), in a study of empathy levels in 273 medical students, found that students who score high on emotional intelligence, and those who are good at reading the emotions of others, are perceived by their peers to be more effective in these groups. Gender, too, plays a role: a study of 512 final-year medical students suggested that female students are better at communicating successfully under the stress of examination conditions (Wiskin, Allan and Skelton 2004).

Differences in the ways we learn and solve problems are also robust determinants of how we approach medical communication. These differences have been demonstrated among clinical teachers and among surgical trainees, and an understanding of one's own learning style allows people to develop different strategies beyond what they instinctively do well. The original Honey and Mumford classification (1992) identified four learning styles: *Reflector* (analytical focus on feelings and intuition), *Theorist* (analytical focus on facts and theories), *Pragmatist* (action-oriented focus on protocols and evidence-based practice) and *Activist* (action-oriented focus on feelings and intuitions).

Perhaps not surprisingly, the predominant learning styles among surgical trainees were *Pragmatist* (60 per cent) and *Activist* (26 per cent), leaving only 10 per cent *Theorist* and 4 per cent *Reflector* styles. The majority of surgical trainees rely principally on hands-on experience to learn and to solve problems (Drew et al. 1999). This is clearly beneficial in surgical trainees: cut along the dotted line, follow best practice, and stick to the protocol...but also be willing to act quickly on limited evidence when action is essential.

So what is the relevance of learning styles to open disclosure? Quite simply, learning styles determine what we do well when we communicate with patients and, indeed, with each other.

During workshops with thousands of experienced clinicians and senior managers we found there are some who manage the first key task of open disclosure well, i.e., explaining clearly to patient and family exactly what happened. They are instinctively researchers with a clear focus on theory and structure to explain clinical findings and to develop a deeper understanding of events. Their approach to problem-solving is inherently logical and linear and they will rise to the task of deciphering and delivering an **explanation** of an adverse event to patients and families. Theirs is a *Theorist* approach. However, their preference to advance logic and eschew emotion means they are less comfortable with, or maybe even unaware of, the benefits of apologizing for suffering.

Another group are adept at investigating the adverse event and taking steps, by tweaking systems, to minimize the chances it will happen again. These are the people who invent incident reviews, Incident Information Management Systems (IIMSs) and Root Cause Analyses (RCAs). They are *Pragmatists*. They operate in a world of documented actions and coordinated systems. Extrapolating from Drew and colleagues' (1999) study, we would expect the large majority of surgical trainees to excel in providing concrete **reassurance**. Like Theorists, however, Pragmatists are less attentive to the emotional context and likely to have no impulse to apologize.

An **apology**, on the other hand, is likely to be the first response for a *Reflector* or *Activist*, who are both primed instinctively to experience personally, and express regret for, the patient/family's loss and suffering and to find exactly the right words to reassure the patient of their sympathy and understanding.

There is a critical point here. Open disclosure calls on different approaches to solving the problems raised by an adverse event. Most of us seem to be hard-wired to deal spontaneously with some of the issues while being less conscious and skilful in others. Few people are adept across everything and research suggests that all three elements are required to begin the process of healing.

There is an additional element to understanding the impact of learning styles on open disclosure. This is apparent if one examines what happens when the learning styles of doctor and patient are mismatched. A sample of 464 doctors differed significantly from UK adult population norms on most of the dimensions of personality measured, including learning style (Clack et al. 2004). While 40 per cent of the UK population preferred the *Reflector* mode they would have only a 1 in 6 chance of seeing a doctor with the same preference. The 31 per cent of doctors with preferences for the *Theorist* mode would have only a 1 in 11 chance of a match with the patient. As Clack and colleagues put it:

> If the two individuals involved in the interaction differ to this extent, they are likely to be talking on different wavelengths, resulting in potential misunderstandings unless there is some adjustment or "flexing" of style. (2004: 184)

The authors suggest that a lack of accommodation of doctors' interaction styles to these differences may partly explain complaints about poor communication, and patients' lack of understanding and poor adherence. Presumably experienced clinicians learn how to do this, to shift from one style to another as appropriate, through trial and error over many years.

A simple solution to the high risk of leaving out one leg of the open disclosure tripod is to always practice open disclosure as a team, utilizing all the skills of different learning styles. That is, of course, unless you are one of those rare individuals who has acquired the full spectrum of skills through years of experience.

15.3 So What Is Open Disclosure?

The *Australian Open Disclosure Framework* defines open disclosure as:

> ...an open discussion with a patient (or family/carers) about an incident(s) that resulted in harm to that patient while they were receiving health care. The elements of open disclosure are an apology or expression of regret (including the word "sorry"), a factual explanation of what happened, an opportunity for the patient to relate their experience, and an explanation of the steps being taken to manage the event and prevent recurrence.
>
> Open disclosure is a discussion and an exchange of information that may take place over several meetings. (Australian Commission on Safety and Quality in Health Care 2013: 4)

It sounds straightforward, and eminently desirable, and yet it proves incredibly difficult to implement consistently. Gallagher and Levinson posed the dilemma thus:

> Improving the disclosure process could enhance patients' satisfaction and their trust in physicians' integrity. Furthermore, as error disclosure becomes better integrated with patient safety activities, such disclosure could promote higher quality of care. Yet, physicians may feel that the medical malpractice climate poses an insurmountable barrier to disclosing errors more fully to patients. (2005: 1819)

The 2011–12 review of the 2003 *Australian Open Disclosure Standard* emphasized that patients appreciate an honest open dialogue rather than a formal transfer of information. In the ideal world open disclosure would improve doctor-patient relationships, underlining humanity, building resilience and strengthening trust. But surgeons (and other health professionals) are concerned about medico-legal consequences of disclosure, about how to prepare for it, and the conflict between open, timely communication and the need to seek early advice from their insurers.

Gallagher and Levinson conclude:

> there is no published evidence to suggest that more open disclosure of errors dramatically increases liability. Fortunately, the vast majority of patients who are injured by medical errors never sue. Thus, we believe that physicians can presume

that disclosure will lead to an overall reduction in the likelihood of a successful lawsuit. (2005: 1823)

One other main finding of the 2011–12 review of the 2003 *Australian Open Disclosure Standard* was that disclosure works better when it is approached as *learning from error* rather than a risk management strategy. The terminology of the *near miss* is unhelpful. It encourages an attitude of dismissive bravado when an adverse event is avoided and diminishes the opportunity for systemic learning. How much better to adopt the terminology and mindset of the *near hit* that encourages people to examine carefully how that incident almost occurred and what prevented it from happening.

15.4   The First Disclosure Interview is Breaking Bad News

Open disclosure is an iterative process. The information available will change with each meeting and with each conversation and it is critical that the discussion is limited to what is known at each stage. There is rarely justification for presumption or prognostication and there have been several examples of people making admissions of liability that subsequently proved to be incorrect, causing significant suffering for patients, families and professionals.

In most instances the first discussion about an adverse event is a case of breaking bad news. When an adverse event occurs, people want to know first and foremost: Is the patient safe? And what will be the outcome? In the emotional intensity of realizing that something has gone wrong, most people's initial reaction is fear for the safety of the patient. Questions about how the harm came about are often secondary for the patient and family at this stage.

In medical communication workshops using trained actors, we regularly observe very senior clinicians who handle a breaking bad news scenario with skill, compassion and transparency. But if we tweak the scenario so that the identical clinical outcome has even a whiff of medical error, the very same clinicians will interrupt and talk over the patient, close off certain avenues of discussion, and fail to address the critical need of the family for information about the patient's safety.

So it is helpful, and consistent with the recommendation in the review of the *Open Disclosure Standard*, to approach the first discussion following an adverse event, as breaking bad news: the patient is in a less desirable situation than they were expecting to be. There are several models for breaking bad news, e.g., the SPIKES (Baile et al. 2000) model: **S**et up the interview – assess the patient's **P**erception – obtain the patient's **I**nvitation – give **K**nowledge to the patient – address the patient's **E**motions with **E**mpathy – **S**trategy and **S**ummary.

What is missing from the SPIKES protocol is awareness of the emotion of the doctor, which, unacknowledged, can quickly sabotage continuing efforts at effective disclosure. In fact, it is this lack of awareness of the clinician's state of arousal that promotes blocking of responses from the patient/family members and a failure to address their needs. We know that physicians, even senior ones, react with strong physiological arousal to the task of breaking bad news (Brown et al. 2009; Shaw, Dunn and Heinrich 2012). People who are not strong on insight into their own emotional state can wreak havoc on attempts at constructive open disclosure.

Our own research suggests that ISBAR (**I**ntroduction – **S**ituation – **B**ackground – **A**ssessment – **R**ecommendation) is an effective summary of the steps involved in breaking bad news and builds on experience with a clinical handover protocol used widely in practice.[1]

Subsequent discussions with the patient and family, with clinical teams, senior staff and administration, will engage with issues of how the harm occurred and focus on continuing management of the patient. But it is the quality of these early interactions that critically sets the scene for the success of open disclosure.

In closing this chapter, and in accordance with Drew and colleagues' data (1999) suggesting that a majority of surgeons are likely to favour practical, bullet-point guides to evidence-based practice, here is a list of frequently asked questions on open disclosure, with answers.

15.5   FAQs on Open Disclosure

Why should I practise open disclosure?

- *It reduces the chances of getting sued or a formal complaint*
- *It will enhance your reputation*
- *It might save your patient from additional distress*
- *It is good medicine*

When should I practise open disclosure?

- *Anytime something goes wrong*
- *Perhaps not every time if the adverse event is truly trivial*
- *As negotiated with the patient during pre-operative consent*
- *Mindful that most often the patient might find out later*

Who should I disclose to?

- *The patient*
- *My boss*
- *The family*

---

1   A good summary of ISBAR, with a video example, is available at: http://nswhealth. moodle.com.au/DOH/DETECT/content/00_worry/when_to_worry_06.htm.

- *The team*
- *Administration*

What should I say to a patient or relative when something goes wrong?

- *What have you experienced?*
- *This is what happened*
- *I am sorry you have suffered*
- *This is what I have done to make it unlikely to happen again*

What should I not say or do to a patient or relative?

- *Avoid them*
- *Cover it up*
- *Use jargon*
- *Blame anyone*
- *Not say sorry (about the patient's suffering)*
- *Not follow up*

What should I say to my boss?

- *This is what happened*
- *How does this affect you?*
- *I am sorry this has happened*
- *This is what I have done to make it unlikely to happen again*

What should I say to hospital admin?

- *This is what happened*
- *How does this affect you?*
- *I am sorry this has happened*
- *This is what I have done to make it unlikely to happen again*

Who else should I involve in open disclosure?

- *Mentors or colleagues who have been there*
- *People who have open disclosure training*
- *Close family or friends*
- *Someone quite independent, e.g., a psychologist if necessary*

How can I remember to say the right things?

- *Remember EAR – Explanation, Apology, Reassurance*
- *Take someone with you who complements your areas of weakness*

Should I say "sorry"?

- *Every time*
- *Only if you mean it*
- *Mean it*

References

Austin, Elizabeth J., Phillip Evans, Belinda Magnus and Katie Hanlon. 2007. A Preliminary Study of Empathy, Emotional Intelligence and Examination Performance in MBChB Students. *Medical Education* 41(7): 684–9. doi: 10.1111/j.1365-2923.2007.02795.x

Australian Commission on Safety and Quality in Health Care. 2013. *Australian Open Disclosure Framework*. Sydney: ACSQHC.

Baile, Walter F., Robert Buckman, Renato Lenzi, Gary Glober, Estela A. Beale and Andrzej P. Kudelka. 2000. SPIKES – A Six-Step Protocol for Delivering Bad News: Application to the Patient with Cancer. *The Oncologist* 5(4): 302–11.

Brown, Rhonda, Stewart Dunn, Karen Byrnes, Richard Morris, Paul Heinrich and Joanne Shaw. 2009. Doctors' Stress Responses and Poor Communication Performance in Simulated Bad-News Consultations. *Academic Medicine* 84(11): 1595–602. doi: 10.1097/ACM.0b013e3181baf537

Clack, Gillian B., Judy Allen, Derek Cooper and John O. Head. 2004. Personality Differences between Doctors and Their Patients: Implications for the Teaching of Communication Skills. *Medical Education* 38(2): 177–86. doi: 10.1111/j.1365-2923.2004.01752.x

Drew, Phil J., N. Cule, Martin Gough, Kamal Heer, John R. Monson, Peter W. Lee, Michael J. Kerin and Graeme S. Duthie. 1999. Optimal Education Techniques for Basic Surgical Trainees: Lessons from Education Theory. *Journal of the Royal College of Surgeons of Edinburgh* 44(1): 55.

Gallagher, Thomas H., and Wendy Levinson. 2005. Disclosing Harmful Medical Errors to Patients: A Time for Professional Action. *Archives of Internal Medicine* 165(16): 1819–24.

Gladstone, Jill. 1995. Drug Administration Errors: A Study into the Factors Underlying the Occurrence and Reporting of Drug Errors in a District General Hospital. *Journal of Advanced Nursing* 22(4): 628–37. doi: 10.1046/j.1365-2648.1995.22040628.x

Honey, Peter, and Alan Mumford. 1992. *The Manual of Learning Styles*. 3rd ed. London.

Iedema, Rick, Christine Jorm, John Wakefield, Cherie Ryan and Stewart Dunn. 2009. Practising Open Disclosure: Clinical Incident Communication and Systems Improvement. *Sociology of Health & Illness* 31(2): 262–77. doi: 10.1111/j.1467-9566.2008.01131.x

Newman, Marc C. 1996. The Emotional Impact of Mistakes on Family Physicians. *Archives of Family Medicine* 5(2): 71–5. doi: 10.1001/archfami.5.2.71

Serembus, Joanne Farley, Zane Robinson Wolf and Nancy Youngblood. 2001. Consequences of Fatal Medication Errors for Health Care Providers: A Secondary Analysis Study. *MEDSURG Nursing* 10(4): 193–201.

Shaw, Joanne, Stewart Dunn and Paul Heinrich. 2012. Managing the Delivery of Bad News: An In-Depth Analysis of Doctors' Delivery Style. *Patient Education and Counseling* 87(2): 186–92. doi: 10.1016/j.pec.2011.08.005

Vincent, Charles, Angela Phillips and Magi Young. 1994. Why Do People Sue Doctors? A Study of Patients and Relatives Taking Legal Action. *The Lancet* 343(8913): 1609–13. doi: 10.1016/S0140-6736(94)93062-7

Wiskin, Connie M.D., Teresa F. Allan and John R. Skelton. 2004. Gender as a Variable in the Assessment of Final Year Degree-Level Communication Skills. *Medical Education* 38(2): 129–37. doi: 10.1111/j.1365-2923.2004.01746.x

Stewart Dunn, PhD, is Professor of Psychological Medicine in the Sydney Medical School, University of Sydney, and Associate Dean for Admissions. He is based at Royal North Shore Hospital (RNSH) where his clinical specialty is psycho-oncology. He has extensive teaching commitments in the University of Sydney Medical Program and he has received nine research travel awards and seven teaching awards. Stewart has published extensively on research into doctor-patient communication, and psychological predictors of morbidity and mortality in medical illness. His current interests include multidisciplinary teams, medical error and open disclosure, and physiological responses of doctors breaking bad news. He is Director of the Pam McLean Centre, which develops evidence-based simulations of difficult medical communication situations for health professionals, working with professional actors.

16 Clinical Communication Education for Surgeons

Suzanne M. Kurtz

16.1 Introduction

During the last 30 years, medical education and the profession it serves have taken on communication education and training as an important component of undergraduate and postgraduate curricula. In many countries substantive communication training has become a requirement for accreditation of both undergraduate and postgraduate programmes. Continuing education offerings on communication in medicine have also become widespread. These advances notwithstanding, strong communication training is still a relatively recent development, particularly at the postgraduate level where specialty surgical training is most intense.

Each chapter of this book has, in effect, presented compelling arguments for enhancing communication in surgical contexts and, to that end, for also raising the bar on communication education for surgeons. This final chapter explores: (a) the evidence-based scaffolding – the conceptual framework – that is necessary for the development of coherent, comprehensive communication education programmes for surgeons or, for that matter, any other doctor (sections 16.2 and 16.3) and (b) successful strategies for teaching and learning clinical communication effectively (section 16.4). Both the conceptual framework and the strategies are essential if we want to develop programmes at any level (from undergraduate to residency level and beyond) that significantly impact how surgeons actually communicate.

Because how we think about communication has such a significant impact on what we do, both in the practice of medicine and in our teaching and learning of clinical communication, the chapter begins by highlighting *four underlying assumptions* that replace commonly held misperceptions about communication and answer the question: Is it really necessary to teach communication to surgeons – can't they just get what they need later through experience? Continuing to build the conceptual framework, the chapter discusses several elements that help us decide what is worth teaching. These elements include three interdependent *types of communication skills*, *domains* that this field incorporates, *paradigms* that influence how we interact in healthcare, *first principles* of effective communication, the *goals* of communication in healthcare and the more *specific skills* that research has shown to make a difference. The final section of the chapter considers specific evidence-based approaches and strategies that comprise *"best practices" for teaching and learning clinical communication*, that is, teaching and learning that enhances not only surgeons' understanding of communication but also the clinical communication skills and capacities surgeons (choose to) apply in actual practice.[1]

16.2   Deciding Whether to Teach Communication in Surgery

The first part of the conceptual framework provides an important foundation by highlighting four evidence-based underlying assumptions (italicized below) that replace commonly held misperceptions about communication in medicine.

*Assumption 1: Communication is an essential **clinical** skill, not an optional add-on and not "simply" a social skill at which we are already adept.* Like the other components of clinical competence (medical technical knowledge, physical examination skills, surgical and other procedural and diagnostic skills, clinical reasoning), communication makes a substantial difference to outcomes of care. The preceding chapters of this book bear witness to the importance of communication in surgical contexts. So does a large and substantive body of research on healthcare communication developed over the past 45-plus years that has relevance across the specialties and for medical education at all levels. While a review of that literature is beyond the scope of this chapter, it is useful to summarize it here in terms of a variety of relevant findings. Research demonstrates consistently that there are problems with communication in healthcare and that specific improvements in communication have a significant positive impact on outcomes of care (see Silverman, Kurtz and Draper 2013 for an extensive review of this literature). Research shows that improving clinical communication in specific ways leads to:

(a) More effective consultations for patients, clients and clinicians:
  - Greater accuracy
  - Heightened efficiency

1　For a more in-depth description and analysis of the ideas and material in this chapter, including the theory and research evidence on which it is grounded, please see two companion books: Kurtz, Silverman and Draper (2005) and Silverman, Kurtz and Draper (2013). I wish to acknowledge my co-authors, Jonathan Silverman and Juliet Draper, and these texts as primary resources for this material. The books' co-authors have previously published various versions of this material in other articles and book chapters. Additional collaborators are noted in the text.

- Enhanced supportiveness and trust
- Relationships characterized by collaboration and partnership

(b) Better coordination of care (between healthcare professionals, with patients and their significant others, etc.)

(c) Improved outcomes of care:
- Greater patient satisfaction
- Better understanding and recall
- Greater adherence and follow-through
- Enhanced symptom relief
- Better physiological outcomes
- Enhanced patient safety, fewer clinician errors
- Greater clinician satisfaction
- Reduced costs, shorter hospital stays and fewer complications
- Fewer conflicts, complaints and malpractice claims

Clearly, improving communication is not just about "being nice" to patients, nor is it only about the so-called "soft", psychosocial side of medicine. That is not to say that relationships and other psychosocial elements are unimportant. The literature also shows that:

- The medical perspective and the patient's perspective are different and require different management; both are important
- Resolving relational, cultural and physical barriers improves outcomes
- Patients who are *active* partners have better outcomes

Establishing communication as an influential clinical skill, these findings and the interdependence between clinical communication, clinical reasoning and medical problem-solving answer the question of "why bother" with communication in medicine. With so much depending on it, clinical communication is clearly worth teaching, but can we teach it and, in any case, do we need to?

Assumption 2: Like other clinical skills, clinical communication is a series of learned skills rather than a personality trait. Although personality may have a bearing on attitudes toward communication, the communication skills themselves can be learned. As long as there is not an underlying psychiatric problem, anyone with appropriate assistance who wants to can learn to communicate more effectively. And like athletic skills honed to a professional level of competence, clinical communication skills atrophy if we stop paying attention to them.

For those who doubt that communication is a learned skill that can be taught, Aspegren's (1999) literature review may be a useful reference. The review quality graded 180 studies on teaching and learning communication skills and selected 81 that met the high or medium quality criteria, including 31 randomized trials, 38 open effect studies and 12 descriptive studies. The review found overwhelming support for the positive effect of communication skills training – only one study found no change in skills, likely due to the brevity of the training period. Learners at all levels of medical education improved their communication skills, from medical students to residents to junior and senior practising clinicians. And specialists were as likely to benefit from learning communication skills as primary care clinicians.

A brief illustration may be useful here. Halfway into a senior ophthalmologist's four-hour clinic that I was observing, a no-show patient allowed us 20 minutes to discuss issues the specialist raised concerning what, if anything, makes a difference when it comes to adherence. We quickly discussed selected research findings showing that: (a) patients' recall and understanding – both of which impact adherence – can improve by 30 per cent if they are asked to repeat important information, thus also giving clinicians immediate insight as to the clarity and completeness of their explanations as well as patient errors in recall or interpretation; (b) adherence improved when physicians asked about their patients' beliefs regarding cause and other concerns and related subsequent explanations and plans to each patient's perspective; and (c) adherence improved when physicians asked whether the patient would be able to follow through with plans made. For the rest of the afternoon, he changed his mode of communication to incorporate all three suggestions and later reported surprise at what a difference the changes made, what he was finding out from familiar clients that he had never discovered before and how useful it all was.

Assumption 3: Experience alone can be a poor teacher of clinical communication. Although it is an excellent reinforcer of habit, experience tends not to discern very carefully between good and bad habits. Testing the frequently espoused sentiment that "I can get this later on my own – all I need is a little more practice", a longitudinal study assessed how physicians' communication skills changed over their careers. Findings showed that without explicit intervention, most communication skills were fixed in place by the end of residency training (Maguire, Fairbairn and Fletcher 1986a). The same researchers (1986b) found that information-gathering skills which doctors had learned by the end of medical school remained strong five years out, but these same doctors were weakest in many explanation and planning skills which had essentially been left to be learned through experience – six communication skills related to improved compliance were not even attempted 63 to 90 per cent of the time.

Another problem with relying on experience alone is that we often perceive our own communication inaccurately. For example, two studies showed that doctors overestimate the time they give to explanation and planning by up to 900 per cent (Waitzkin 1985; Makoul, Arntson and Schofield 1995). In a study measuring the use of patient-centred skills by senior primary care residents, Campion and colleagues (2002) showed that these behaviours (e.g., checking for patient understanding, responding to patients' emotional cues) occurred in only 58 per cent of recorded interviews, even though residents self-selected their videos for assessment and knew patient-centred skills would be a focus of the evaluation. Other studies found that physicians interrupted 18 (Beckman and Frankel 1984), 23 (Marvel et al. 1999) and 12 (Rhoades et al. 2001) seconds after asking patients to tell their stories. Physicians were largely unaware of this behaviour. Marvel and colleagues (1999) also checked to see if physicians followed through on their intentions to go back later and let their patients finish – only 8 per cent had actually done so. Clinicians have suggested that patients will take too long to tell their stories if left to their own devices. Yet in the Beckman and Frankel study the actual time primary care patients took to do so in response to a good open-ended question was only up to 150 seconds, with most finishing in less than 60 seconds. In a fourth study done with tertiary care patients, 78 per cent finished telling their stories in less than two minutes, with a mean time of 92 seconds; clinicians listening to tapes of those few patients who took longer deemed those patients to be giving essential information for the duration (Langewitz et al. 2002).

A third reason experience can be an ineffective teacher is our tendency to confuse intentions or feelings with actions. For example, consider Morse, Edwardsen and Gordon's (2008) findings. In their analysis of 20 audio-recorded thoracic surgery and oncology consultations, they identified 384 opportunities for making empathy statements. Physicians responded empathically to 39 of them and otherwise provided little emotional support; 50 per cent of these responses occurred in the last third of the interview despite even distribution of opportunity throughout the consultation. No one would expect responses to every opportunity for empathy, but considering the impact of trusting relationships on accuracy and efficiency and the role empathy plays in developing such relationships, these missed opportunities seem particularly unfortunate. Clinicians are empathic human beings, but developing a capacity for empathy is not the same as using communication skills effectively to demonstrate that capacity.

Assumption 4: Effective communication is possible in the time reasonably allotted for regular consultations. This fourth assumption reflects the troublesome misperception that there is too little time to apply effective, evidence-based communication skills in the "real world" of medical practice. Research confirms that once skills are mastered, effective communication results in more efficient interactions. One relevant study compared physicians who engaged in patient-centred practice with those who did not (Stewart 1985). The latter took 7.8 minutes on average per consultation. Physicians who had mastered the patient-centred skills took less than one minute longer. However while they were learning the skills, physicians took nearly 11 minutes. If we really want to improve communication in medicine, we have to figure out how to set up the system so that clinicians – be they students or senior surgeons – have time in their interactions with patients and others to learn, master and maintain effective communication skills. Furthermore, true efficiency must take accuracy and quality of outcomes into account along with time required over time, not just time required for a single consultation. At some point consultations become too short to do the job well from a communication or medical perspective (for a more detailed look at the question of time, see Stewart et al. 1999).

Understanding and acknowledging these underlying assumptions are important first steps in effective communication education and training. As Lara Cooke – a neurologist and Associate Dean of Continuing Medical Education and Professional Development at the University of Calgary – has suggested, the research on communication in healthcare puts communication skills teachers in a better position to implement programmes with strong credibility that have an essential element needed to motivate adult learners and even reluctant participants; that element is relevance (Kurtz and Cooke 2011).

16.3   Deciding What to Teach

So, if communication is an essential clinical skill worth teaching with the same degree of rigour and intention as other clinical and procedural skills, then the next question is: What exactly are we trying to teach and learn? This second part of the conceptual framework can be approached from several angles.

16.3.1 Three Interdependent Types of Communication Skills

Whether enhancing our own clinical communication skills, assisting others or designing communication education programmes, it is helpful to distinguish between three interdependent types of clinical communication skills:

- *Content skills* – what you say
- *Process skills* – how you communicate, e.g., how you structure interactions, ask and respond to questions, relate to patients, use nonverbal skills, involve clients in decision-making
- *Perceptual skills* – what you are thinking and feeling, e.g., your clinical reasoning skills; the emotions you feel and what you do with them; your values, attitudes, biases, assumptions and intentions; awareness and self reflection; inner capacities, such as integrity, respect, compassion, flexibility and mindfulness

These somewhat overlapping skill sets are interdependent – a weakness or strength in one weakens or strengthens all three. Developing (i.e., teaching and learning) communication process and content skills without ongoing and commensurate development of the values, personal ethics and capacities that underlie those skills can lead to manipulation rather than effective interaction. On the other hand, developing our values, capacities and other perceptual skills without ongoing development of the process and content skills needed to *demonstrate* those values and capacities is inadequate – no one will know we hold them.

For another example of the relationship between these types of skills, consider the interdependence of clinical reasoning and clinical communication as they impact medical problem-solving:

- Clinical reasoning = the thought processes you engage in as you collect information and opinions from various sources (e.g., the patient and their family, physical examination, diagnostic tests, other healthcare professionals, the medical record etc.) and synthesize that information with your knowledge and experience to generate hypotheses, differentials, diagnoses and action/treatment plans – these perceptual skills occur at the intrapersonal level of communication (i.e., communication within the self).
- Clinical communication skills and capacities = what you employ to initiate interactions with those involved; develop the relationships with patients and their significant others, referring doctors and other medical colleagues, nurses, allied health professionals etc. that are necessary to engage in effective (i.e., accurate, efficient, supportive) interactions; gather information from others accurately and efficiently; structure your interactions so all participants can engage in them at optimal levels; give explanations and participate in planning and decision-making; close interactions; and follow-up appropriately with those involved – communication content and process skills play major roles here, along with perceptual skills related to feelings, attitudes, values, biases, intentions and capacities.
- Medical problem-solving = what you get when you have well-developed clinical reasoning and clinical communication skills and capacities, and are adept at integrating all of them.

Said another way, the evidence-based process and content skills that are important in clinical communication have the potential to influence clinical reasoning significantly. Conversely, clinical reasoning has a considerable influence on the particular process and content skills used during interactions. Well-designed clinical communication programmes pay attention to the development – and interdependence – of all three types of skills.

16.3.2 Domains of Communication in Healthcare

Outlined in Figure 16.1, the domains that define the contexts in which communication in healthcare occurs represent another useful starting point for deciding what to teach (Kurtz, Silverman and Draper 1998).

1. Clinician-Patient interaction
- o Communicating with patients – accuracy, efficiency, relational competence; process and content skills on Calgary-Cambridge Guides
- o Communicating with family members, significant others
- o Special needs patients (elderly, young, challenged, low literacy)
- o Specific contexts, types of practice
- o Enhancing patients' ability to communicate with clinicians, with "the system"

2. Communication issues
- o Culture
- o Ethics
- o Gender
- o Dealing with feelings
- o Confrontation and conflicted situations
- o Breaking bad news, death and dying
- o Malpractice
- o One Health

3. Communicating with other professionals (relational competence, coordination of care)
- o Medical colleagues
- o Team members (formal and informal teams – nurses, allied professionals, technicians, family members etc.)
- o Administrators
- o Written communication (letters, medical records)
- o Researchers (directly and through lit)
- o Oral presentations, lectures, discussion leadership
- o Colleagues in other disciplines

4. Communication with(in) self
- o Clinical reasoning
- o Development of personal capacities (e.g., compassion, integrity, authenticity, flexibility, mindfulness)
- o Attitudes (awareness, expression of)
- o Feelings (awareness, use/expression of)
- o Reflection & self-assessment skills
- o Dealing with stress and tension
- o Handling mistakes
- o Handling failures
- o Biases and assumptions

5. Communicating at a distance
- o Telephone
- o Telemedicine
- o Computer assisted consults
- o Internet networks, databases, websites

6. Prevention and health promotion (communicating with the public)
- o Pamphlets, posters
- o Radio, TV, newspaper campaigns
- o Public speaking, discussion leadership
- o Talking to the press
- o Advertising

7. Communicating with "the system" (government, community, hospital etc.)
- o Influencing health policy
- o Talking with government, community and agency representatives
- o Influencing and coping with change

Adapted from Kurtz, Silverman and Draper (2005: 298–9).

Figure 16.1: Domains of communication in healthcare

The main sections of this book suggest additional contexts specific to surgery that fit into these domains: namely, the consultation, the operating theatre and the aftermath beyond the theatre. Again specific to surgery, the chapters within each section identify a variety of issues in surgical practice as well as a variety of process, content and perceptual skills related to those issues that teachers and learners can take up in each context.

It makes sense for communication programmes in surgery to focus first on communication with patients both pre- and post-op and to take into account the potential added complexity of needing to confer with the patient's family or significant others and with referring doctors as well as other physicians who are caring for the patient in multiple services/units. Communication during the consultation is the most obvious domain and the one we know most about since a large majority of the research on communication in healthcare has been about physician-patient interaction.

Most medical schools focus on students' history-taking and relationship-building skills and on how they structure interactions, with this training often occurring most systematically during the early years of medical school and on a more limited basis (if at all) during clerkship or clinical rotations. The focus on explanation and planning is begun but is rarely extensive, presumably because of time pressures, lack of opportunity and undergraduate medical students' limited knowledge and experience. Even when communication skills and capacities are well taught and learned at the undergraduate or any other level, trainees (at all levels) frequently have difficulties taking skills gained in one context and applying them to a different context requiring the same skills. Intentional application, ongoing development and deepening of communication skills in these different and often more complex contexts is necessary.

Based on these issues and on the research evidence showing that experience alone is not the best teacher and that when communication skills are not attended to they tend to atrophy or decline, residency programmes are a particularly important venue for continuing formal communication training. It is at this level and beyond that clinical communication skills need to be reinforced, honed and expanded as learners encounter increasingly difficult medical problems and issues; have opportunities to care for patients and work with patients' significant others over time; interact frequently with other healthcare professionals face-to-face and via electronic means, with medical colleagues both within and outside the operating theatre, and with referring and referral surgeons and physicians; begin to understand how to work with and influence healthcare organizations and systems, etc.

16.3.3 Shifting Paradigms

Historically three shifting paradigms have influenced how we communicate in healthcare and what we teach. The first is *doctor-centred care*, wherein the clinician holds most of the control and tells essentially passive patients what to do. This corresponds to what Barbour (2000) calls the "shot-put" approach which views effective communication as content, delivery and persuasion – you prepare your message carefully, heave it out there, and your job is done. Telling is central. Feedback and interaction are nowhere in the picture. Part of the difficulty we have with clinical communication may be due to the fact that, from the time of the ancient Greeks almost to the end of the 20th century, communication training in the professions emphasized or considered only the shot-put approach.

Eventually healthcare moved to *patient-centred care* (see Stewart et al. 2003, 2013 for more detailed explanations and research substantiating this approach). This paradigm requires that clinicians understand their patients' *perspectives* as well as their problems. Strongly substantiated through research in many contexts and cultures, patient-centred care places emphasis on eliciting and responding to the patient's ideas and beliefs regarding cause of illness and efficacy of treatments offered, concerns and other feelings, and expectations, as well as the effects of patients' problems on their lives and the lives of their significant others.

Building on patient-centred care, a third paradigm shift is in progress. Focusing on the wellbeing of both patients and clinicians, *relationship-centred care* (Beach et al. 2006; Suchman et al. 2002; Tresolini and Pew-Fetzer Task Force 1994) sees relationship as central to all healthcare and healing, including the clinician's relationship with patients, clients, self, colleagues and communities.[2] This paradigm emphasizes that "...the privileges of the healer are founded on meaningful relationships in healthcare, not just technically appropriate transactions" (Beach et al. 2006). Patient- and relationship-centred care correspond to what Barbour (2000) aptly calls the "Frisbee" approach to communication in which confirming/ acknowledging the other and developing mutually understood common ground are seen as essential foundations for trust and accuracy. The well-conceived, well-delivered message is still important, but emphasis shifts to feedback, inter-action and collaborative relationship.

A large study Gittell and colleagues conducted (Gittell 2003; Gittell et al. 2000) illustrates some of the benefits of relationship-centred care in surgical settings. She and her colleagues compared the efficiency and outcomes of nine hospitals (located in Boston, New York and Dallas) with respect to joint replacement surgery. Matched for size and surgery volume, some of these hospitals invested heavily in hiring and subsequent training for "relational competence", that is, the ability to interact with others to accomplish common goals. Others looked instead for the most highly qualified individuals – the tendency in this group of hospitals to neglect relational competence was most pronounced in physician hiring. This study found significant differences between hospitals in the strength of relational coordination among their care providers that significantly improved the patient care process. To illustrate, Gittell (2003: 48) reported that a 100 per cent increase in relational coordination enabled a 31 per cent reduction in the length of hospital stay, a 22 per cent increase

---

2   See also Suchman, Sluyter and Williamson (2011) for useful descriptions of relationship-centred skills and processes along with a series of in-depth case studies explaining how these relationship skills and processes have been used to promote significant changes in healthcare in a variety of contexts.

in the quality of service patients perceived, a 7 per cent increase in post-operative freedom from pain and a 5 per cent increase in post-operative mobility.

As Gittell and colleagues (2000) concluded, those in positions that require high levels of functional expertise also tend to need high levels of relational competence to integrate their work with others. A hospital administrator in their study put it this way: "We've moved from patients experiencing individuals as caregivers to patients experiencing systems as caregivers... It's not just individual brilliance that matters anymore. It's a coordinated effort." Since that earlier study, considerable research has verified the powerful influence of relational competence and relational coordination.[3] Relationship-building skills and relational competence are important to the patient-doctor consultation per se and also to relationships with patients' significant others and between healthcare professionals. In each of these contexts, relational competence and relational coordination are necessary to realize the potential contributions of individual experts.

Importantly, doctor-centred, patient-centred and relationship-centred care are not competing paradigms. Each is more or less appropriate depending on the context and needs/preferences of individual patients or others with whom surgeons are communicating at any given time. Surgeons and other clinicians need a full repertoire of relationships (i.e., paradigms) that they can employ skilfully and flexibly as appropriate (Lussier and Richard 2008).

16.3.4 First Principles of Effective Communication (and Teaching)

Another way to decide what communication skills to focus on is to work from "first principles" that characterize effective communication (Dance 1967; Dance and Larson 1972; Kurtz 1989). Interestingly, these same principles characterize effective teaching. Effective communication (or teaching):

- *Ensures interaction not just transmission* – only giving information or telling someone what to do is insufficient; accuracy, efficiency and relationship require two-way conversation, feedback, question and response from both patient and clinician, both you and your colleague, etc.
- *Reduces unnecessary uncertainty* – uncertainty distracts attention and interferes with accuracy, efficiency and relationship; for example, we can reduce uncertainty about the patient's problems and anticipated outcomes, the patient's expectations for a visit, the clinician's expectations, the structure of the interview, how the team works etc.

---

3 See http://rchcweb.com/Portals/0/Summary%20of%20Relational%20Coordination%20 Research.pdf, a website that summarizes some of this research and defines relational coordination more explicitly. For more detailed explanations see Gittell (2011).

- *Requires planning, thinking in terms of outcomes* – effectiveness can only be determined in the context of the particular needs and outcomes the clinician and the patient or are working toward and consideration of the patient's needs at any given moment. If I am angry and want to vent that anger then I communicate in one way, but if I want to get at the misunderstanding that caused the anger, then to be effective I must communicate in an entirely different way.
- *Demonstrates dynamism* – this principle includes engaging with the patient, being present in the moment and demonstrating flexibility; clinicians need to develop a repertoire of skills that allow different approaches with different individuals or with the same individual as circumstances change.
- *Follows a helical rather than a linear model* – saying something once is not enough; repetition and feedback are essential. Each reiteration moves us up the spiral to a higher level of understanding. Similarly, the helix is an excellent learning/teaching model. Developing communication skills and maintaining competence requires reiteration as skills are deepened and applied in different contexts.

These principles are a useful self-assessment tool. And as with first principles of surgery, when in doubt about what communication skills would be most useful or effective, go back to first principles.

16.3.5 Goals of Communication in Healthcare

Thinking in terms of outcomes provides a fifth way to conceptualize what to teach. In keeping with the evidence base and first principles, the goals of communication in medicine include:

- Ensuring increased accuracy, efficiency and supportiveness
- Promoting collaboration and partnership (relationship-centred care)
- Enhancing patient *and* clinician satisfaction
- Improving outcomes of care

Like the other elements of the conceptual framework, these broad goals of communication training remain the same across all levels of medical education. At more senior levels deeper mastery of skills and development of attitudes or capacities is expected, contexts and problems become more complex as learners advance, but the goals of training remain constant. The ultimate goal of communication training is, of course, not merely to improve knowledge and understanding about communication but to improve communication skills *in practice* to a *professional* level of competence. Professional competence implies heightened awareness, greater ability to reflect accurately and articulate with precision, heightened intentionality in choosing what to do and more consistent performance across all situations. Moreover, professional communication competence in medicine is evidence-based.

16.3.6 Specific Communication Skills

The three types of skills, domains, paradigms, first principles and goals (described in sections 16.3.1 to 16.3.5 above) all contribute to decisions regarding what to teach surgeons and other healthcare professionals about communication. But still, just what are the specific communication skills that enable everything else in practice? Ask any group of clinicians, learners or patients and they quickly come up with a convoluted list of clinical communication skills they deem important. Although it may seem counter-intuitive, surgeons and other specialists come up with remarkably similar lists as do learners at all points on the medical education continuum. How do we combine their long lists with research findings and translate it all into a comprehensive, yet manageable and memorable delineation and definition of skills that can be put into practice in the real world?

One answer to this question is the *Calgary-Cambridge Guides* (C-C Guides), a proven instrument for teaching and learning clinical communication skills that has been evolving since the early 1980s.[4] Over the years, the C-C Guides have gone through several iterations, drawing on the work of many individuals and their earlier communication models: Rob Sanson-Fisher in Australia, Peter Maguire in England, Don Cassata and Paula Stillman in the United States, Cathy Heaton and myself in Canada, and Jonathan Silverman in England. An American geneticist, Vincent Riccardi, and I published an earlier version (1983). Many clinicians from across all specialties, students and residents, faculty and other medical educators who teach communication, and a variety of patients from many cultures have added their feedback and ideas. Nonetheless, the primary resource behind this instrument continues to be the research evidence.

First published in two companion books in 1998 (Kurtz, Silverman and Draper 1998; Silverman, Kurtz and Draper 1998), the "Calgary-Cambridge Guides – Communication Process Skills" instrument has changed only slightly since then. This despite the explosion of research on clinical communication between 1998 and now, and the guides' authors' concerted efforts to identify evidence-based changes in the skills or new skills to add as they updated the literature in the second (Kurtz, Silverman and Draper 2005; Silverman, Kurtz and Draper 2005) and third (Silverman, Kurtz and Draper 2013) editions. Since 2003, the C-C Guides have included both a process and a content guide (Kurtz et al. 2003). The content guide outlines a patient- and relationship-centred approach to structuring the content of the medical history, explanation and planning and the medical record (see Kurtz et

---

4   To view the complete Calgary-Cambridge Guides (human medicine and veterinary versions) see www.vetmed.wsu.edu/ClinicalCommunication. The only difference in the veterinary version of the process guide is the use of veterinarian instead of physician and client instead of patient (where appropriate). Some headings in the content guide are altered to fit the veterinary context.

al. 2003; Kurtz, Silverman and Draper 2005; Silverman, Kurtz and Draper 2005, 2013, for more detailed explanations and substantiation of the C-C Guides).

As of 2013, the C-C communication process skills guide summarizes approximately 800 references in terms of 58 highly evidence-based communication process skills that make a difference in healthcare, plus another 15 process and content skills related to common focuses in explanation and planning. To make the evidence-based list of skills in the C-C Process Guide more memorable and coherent, it is organized in a way that corresponds directly to how we structure consultations in real life (see Figure 16.2).

We admit without apology that the list of skills is long – effective communication in medicine is complex and the research on it extensive. There is, of course, no need to use or assess every skill in the guides at every consultation. Which clinical communication skills are needed depends on the specific outcomes clinician and patient are trying to achieve at any given moment in the consultation. The good news is that the skills are highly adaptable. Useful in the gamut of healthcare contexts from clinic to home visit to surgery or intensive care unit, the skills are applicable whether clinicians are giving bad news or finding out that someone has nothing more than a common cold. Context changes and with it the content of what you say as well as the level of intensity, intention and awareness that you need to employ. But the repertoire of communication process skills you need remains the same. A sports analogy is helpful: Playing good basketball requires a full repertoire of well-developed skills and you do have to stay focused – but that doesn't always require the intensity of a full court press.

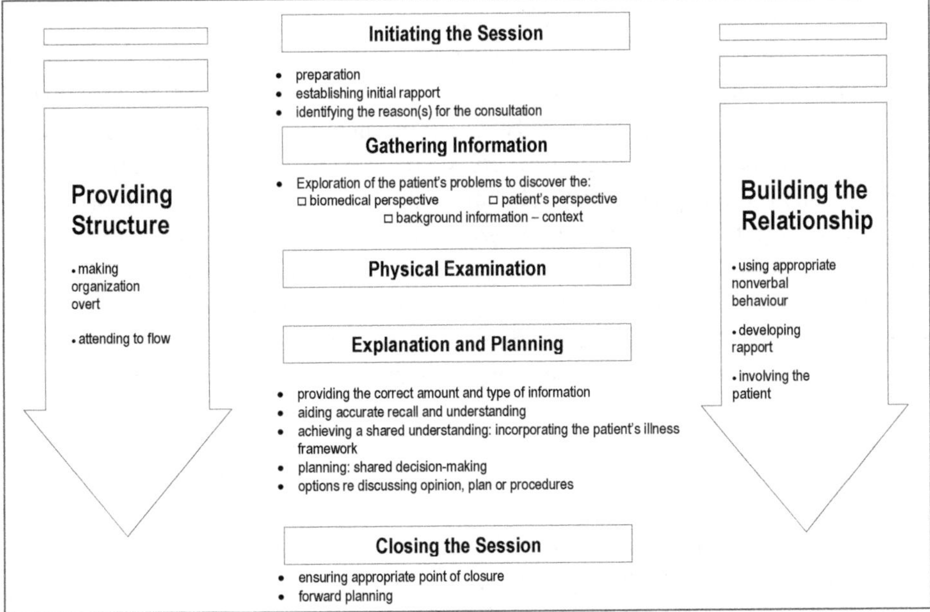

Figure 16.2: Expanded framework for medical consultations in the Calgary-Cambridge Guides

To illustrate, a senior surgeon at a major tertiary care teaching hospital asked me for a laminated copy of the C-C Process Guide. He explained that whenever a consultation seemed not to be working well, he made an excuse to leave the room and quickly scanned the guide until he pinpointed the specific skill(s) that he was forgetting to use effectively. Re-entering the consultation room, he would apply the pinpointed skill(s) with care and attention, whereupon he usually found that the problem(s) with the consultation would be resolved. We responded to the surgeon's request by making a pocket-card version of the guide for him that we have since used widely with learners at all levels.

The C-C Guides offer several advantages. They provide an overview of the state of the art – or perhaps it is more accurate to say the state of the evidence – for enhancing communication skills in healthcare. Translated into several languages as diverse as French and Arabic and used in countries around the world, the C-C Guides have remarkably wide cross-cultural applicability. In addition to providing an accessible and comprehensive summary of the literature, the guides give a definitive, evidence-based answer to the question of what skills to focus on in order to raise the bar on clinical communication. Offering guidance with considerable latitude for personal style, they serve as a memory aid for keeping the skills in mind and provide the basis for systematic skill development and for comprehensive (as opposed to hit-and-miss) development, feedback and assessment of skills. Useful as research instruments as well as teaching tools, they provide a common language for labelling communication behaviour. A foundation for self-directed learning and communication programmes at all levels of training from undergraduate medical education through residency and continuing medical education, the guides have been used across virtually all the specialties.

There is one additional reason to invest the time required to master the skills on the guides, namely, that all of the skills – with the obvious exception of physical examination – are applicable not only to communication with patients, but also to interaction between teachers and learners, with colleagues or within teams. In other words, this is the comprehensive delineation of skills that make a difference wherever accuracy, efficiency, supportiveness and collaboration are needed. Taken individually the skills appear to be disarmingly straightforward. Keeping the repertoire of skills in mind, using them consistently and appropriately while doing everything else clinicians need to do, integrating them effectively with the other clinical skills in both difficult and routine circumstances – that becomes more complex.

16.4 Deciding How to Teach and Learn Clinical Communication

This section on strategies and approaches for teaching and learning clinical communication effectively is already well begun – the first strategy is to develop a conceptual framework, like the one described in the second and third sections of this chapter. The framework provides essential rationales for teaching and learning clinical communication and is a significant aid in making decisions about what is worth teaching and learning, whether in surgery or other medical contexts. Understanding and using the conceptual framework is a foundational first step toward the development of a comprehensive, coherent and systematic communication education programme that extends over time and across a variety of contexts. What else is needed? The rest of this chapter outlines a variety of evidence-based teaching and learning methods, and strategies for teaching and learning clinical communication effectively.

As implied earlier in the chapter, surgeons learn communication skills just like everyone else does and can benefit from what others have found successful – i.e., there's no point in starting from scratch; the principles and other elements of the conceptual framework and the strategies that make for good communication teaching and learning in surgery are the same as those that are useful in other specialties. The setting and some of the content of what surgeons communicate may change but not the communication teaching and learning process.

16.4.1 Skills vs Attitudes and Capacities vs Issues

The debate is ongoing about how best to bridge the gap between doctors' real-life communication behaviours during consultations or in other contexts, and the behaviours that research has shown to make a positive difference in the outcomes of care. Three views on how to structure communication training and education have emerged. The *skills perspective* structures learning around the three types of communication skills: what surgeons and other doctors say (content skills), how they say it (process skills), and what they are thinking and feeling (perceptual skills, including capacities such as compassion, integrity, flexibility, mindfulness). Skills-based programmes give primary attention to the development of process skills since they are the least emphasized in most curricula at all levels of education, and secondary but significant attention to content and perceptual skills since they are the focus of other parts of the curricula. The *attitude or mindfulness perspective* focuses teaching on preparation of the inner ground, that is, on enhancing attitudes, capacities, intentions, assumptions and psychological factors that influence how doctors communicate. Here the rationale is that these underlying factors block effective communication and attending to these factors will improve communication. The *issues perspective* suggests that we structure learning around communication issues such as delivering bad news, death and dying, obtaining informed consent, communicating treatment risks and benefits, and reducing error as well as issues related to gender or culture and to communication with children, geriatric patients, neurologically compromised patients etc.

What we choose here is important, because content and teaching methods can vary considerably for each of the views. All of the views have validity, but the skills approach is at the top of the educational hierarchy. It is true that, as explained earlier in the chapter, without preparation and development of the "inner ground" of attitudes, intentions and capacities, the masterful use of skills becomes manipulation. So focusing on the "inner ground" is important. On the other hand, the best of intentions and the most well-developed capacities are essentially useless if we do not have well-developed skills to demonstrate or apply those capacities in practice. Issues, too, have their place in communication teaching and assessment. The dilemma in using issues as the primary focus is inefficiency. This perspective can promote the mistaken notion that each issue requires a different set of skills, when in fact the same communication process skills (for example, as delineated in the C-C Guides) are useful in responding to each of these issues. The context changes from issue to issue, the content of the communication changes, the skills may need to be applied with greater intentionality or intensity or mastery, but the process skills themselves remain the same.

This chapter primarily reflects the Calgary-Cambridge approach that chooses to use the skills perspective to structure teaching and learning. The skills-based approach emphasizes development of evidence-based communication process, content and perceptual skills and their application in a variety of real-life contexts. Using appropriate methods to teach clinical communication skills in the contexts of patient care and simulation exercises with carefully trained simulated and standardized patients, the Calgary-Cambridge approach works from this primary focus on skills to enhance crucial values, attitudes and capacities without generating undue defensiveness and to explore issues as they arise.[5] In other words, the skills perspective allows us to focus attention on the primary outcome of enhancing communication skills in practice to a professional level of competence.

Reporting on a workshop in which a large international group of clinicians and medical educators participated, Cary and Kurtz (2013) provide a detailed example of a skills-based approach that integrates the teaching of communication skills, clinical reasoning, attitudes and issues. Using a well-chosen, simulated, longitudinal, surgical case (i.e., a case that unfolds across several months, but through simulation can be presented in a matter of hours) in a problem-based learning exercise that can be adapted for use with specialty residents, faculty or practising physicians and surgeons, the article demonstrates how to teach:

---

5 For a useful way to conceptualize and identify the universal values that are relevant and necessary in all healthcare interactions across international and disciplinary boundaries, see the International Charter for Human Values at: http://charterforhealthcarevalues.org and Rider et al. (2014).

- the interconnectedness of content, process and perceptual skills
- the influence of these three types of skills on clinical reasoning
- follow-up with patients and their significant others over time
- ways to integrate the teaching of communication with clinical reasoning and with a variety of issues, including cognitive errors, clinicians' response to such errors, clinical uncertainty and delivering bad news.

16.4.2 Six Elements Necessary to Change Behaviour and Master Any Clinical Skill

We know that knowledge about the clinical communication skills learners are trying to enhance and the research behind those skills is useful and important. Yet, as with other clinical skills, knowledge does not translate directly into either competence (can you do it?) or performance (do you [choose to] do it in practice?). Nor does simply watching the experts. I can read a lot of books on tennis and watch a lot of excellent tennis and still improve my skills very little.

Six elements are necessary to change behaviour and master any skill set (see detailed explanations and review of research evidence regarding these elements in Kurtz, Silverman and Draper 2005: chs 2 to 7):

(1) Systematic delineation and definition of the evidence-based skills to be learned
(2) Observation and assessment of learners performing the skills (live and/or on video, but for communication skills preferably with some video or at least audio-recording of the interaction)
(3) Well-intentioned, detailed, descriptive feedback (guided reflection, coaching)
(4) Practice and rehearsal of skills
(5) Planned reiteration (a helical, reiterative teaching/learning model rather than a linear, once and done model; usually this includes applying the skills in increasingly complex situations or contexts)
(6) Interactive small group or one-on-one experiential teaching/learning format.

Finding or making the time and opportunity to bring all six elements into play is a primary challenge for anyone who wants to enhance clinical communication skills in surgery, be they individual surgeons who want to improve their own clinical communication skills or the skills of their practice group; clinical faculty or programme directors involved in clerkship (rotation), residency or continuing education programmes; or hospital or other organizational administrators. How these challenges are met depends on what is available or can be made possible in each of those contexts.

Placing the delineation of the communication skills at the top of the list is not accidental. All the other components are dependent on that first nitty-gritty element. Developed in a variety of countries, several models exist that delineate the skills in various ways, for example, the Three-Function Model (USA), Maastricht's Maas Global (The Netherlands), the Segue Model (USA), Patient-Centered Care (Canada), the Model of the Macy Initiative in Health Communication (USA), CanMEDS (Canada), and the Calgary-Cambridge Guides already introduced in some detail above (Canada, England and USA). Most effective communication programmes are based upon and heavily use models such as these. Without a well-constructed, evidence-based model – i.e., instrument that delineates and organizes the skills and makes them memorable – communication training can all too often deteriorate into a bag of tricks that is neither effective nor evidence-based.

Of course, once the task of identifying the skills is accomplished, the five other elements of effective communication training still need to be brought into play. As already noted all six elements apply to teaching and learning any clinical skill. In surgery residency programmes and continuing medical education, communication skills and capacities can be taught in many of the same contexts and using many of the same methods that are used to teach, learn and hone any other clinical skills. Lectures/demonstrations can be helpful to raise awareness and enhance knowledge, but one-on-one or facilitated small groups, experiential teaching and learning formats accompanied by guided self reflection as well as peer and expert feedback are essential for developing skills, learning how to use them appropriately in routine as well as (increasingly) complex healthcare situations, deepening and refining communication skills over time etc. Such formats include workshops, rounds, clinics, the bedside, the operating theatre – i.e., anywhere learners' clinical communication performance can be observed and discussed in a timely manner (and generally away from patients).

Simulation is as useful a tool for enhancing clinical communication as it is in teaching and learning the medical technical aspects of surgery. While role-playing is a possibility, simulation exercises can be even more efficacious when they employ well-trained simulated patients (SPs) portraying carefully selected real cases (with enough details changed to protect real patients' anonymity). Well-facilitated communication simulations offer safety for learners and patients alike and the advantages of being able to try out a variety of alternative communication skills or approaches, make mistakes, call timeouts for assistance, start over at any point or do "rewinds" of particular parts of an interaction – and all without any adverse consequences. While surgical programmes may wish to develop their own simulated cases and SPs, many undergraduate medical schools already have well-established SP programmes and sizeable case banks that include surgical and other relevant cases. Medical school programmes also often have SP trainers who can work with surgeons to develop specific simulations involving patient cases or other scenarios. Video or audio recording of interactions with real and/or simulated patients and their significant others for later review and feedback is especially helpful.

16.4.3 Differences between Teaching and Learning Clinical Communication and Other Clinical Skills

While teaching and learning communication skills has much in common with what it takes to teach/learn other clinical skills, it is also substantively different. Communication is more complex than simpler procedural skills, so many more variables influence it. Although it is not a personality trait, communication is closely bound to self-concept. No one is invested in how they palpate a liver before they learn how to do it, but most of us are heavily invested in how we communicate – we tend to think of it as part of our personal style or who we are. There is no achievement ceiling. Even when we apply communication skills masterfully today, an unfamiliar situation, a hit to our confidence or a variety of distractions can substantially reduce our effectiveness tomorrow. What we did to communicate successfully with a given patient on one occasion may not work with another or even with the same patient in different circumstances. Considerable flexibility is required. From a communication standpoint, we can always improve on what we are doing. Finally, while faculty are generally acknowledged and perceive themselves to be experts in the other clinical skills that they teach, many of those charged with teaching clinical communication have had little formal training in this area.

These differences influence in important ways how we teach and learn clinical communication. This is particularly true for how we choose to engage in feedback, regardless of whether we are reflecting on our own performance or another clinician's communication skills. As discussed earlier in this chapter, structuring observation, feedback discussions and self-reflection around an evidence-based instrument such as the Calgary-Cambridge Guides is advisable.

Because so many preceptors and other faculty who are in a position to facilitate communication teaching and learning have had considerable experience but limited formal communication education themselves, they often benefit from workshops focusing, for example, on:

- the conceptual framework above
- the evidence base and the evidence-based clinical communication skills that are worth teaching (including the many similarities and occasional differences reported between the efficacious use of a particular skill in surgical as compared with other medical contexts)
- evidence-based model(s) that make the delineation of skills memorable
- teaching methods that are most efficacious, such as how to make effective use of skills guides and simulated patients, how to work optimally one-on-one or with rounding and other small learning groups to teach clinical communication, how to engage learners in feedback sessions about their communication skills using a particular model and specific feedback techniques, and how to demonstrate/model clinical communication skills and capacities to advantage.

16.4.4 Agenda-Led Outcome-Based Analysis – The Feedback Process

Because of some of the differences related to teaching and learning clinical communication skills, the feedback process itself needs to be engaged in with care. The purposes of feedback include enhancing what learners already do well, looking at alternatives and "next steps" learners can take to expand their repertoire of skills and become even more effective, learning to apply familiar skills in more complex circumstances, and breaking habits that serve neither clinician nor patient well.

To be more specific, Agenda-Led Outcome-Based Analysis (ALOBA) is a protocol Kurtz, Silverman and Draper (2005) have developed for engaging in the feedback process and facilitating experiential, learner-centred, problem-based sessions while using the C-C Guides. ALOBA maximizes participation of individuals as well as small learning groups, reduces defensiveness and enhances learning. The protocol is not cast in stone; it is intended as a flexible guide, a framework that facilitators can adapt to their learners' changing needs and purposes. As you will see, the ALOBA protocol resembles the tasks on the C-C Guides. Furthermore, the specific skills required to facilitate a feedback session effectively using ALOBA are very similar to the skills listed in the C-C Guides but are here applied to the individual learner in a group of learners.

ALOBA begins with participants exchanging greetings and, in the initial meeting, getting to know each other briefly and agreeing on rules of conduct (confidentiality, participation, attendance, experimentation etc.). Next the facilitator prepares the learner(s) for observation of an interaction that will be the basis for feedback discussion with the individual(s) being observed as well as a gift of "raw" material for the learning of all participants if others are present. Before the interaction begins, the facilitator asks for the agenda of the learner who is about to engage in a simulation, interact with a patient and/or other(s), or share their video. For example, the facilitator might ask: What do you want me/us to watch for? What do you want feedback on? The facilitator and other participants, if present, then observe the interaction, making concrete and specific notes as they observe using the Guides. The learner or the coach may call "time-outs" during the interaction to get ideas if a problem arises or the learner wants to try something over, but time-outs are generally kept to a minimum. Once the observation is complete the facilitator, in true learner-centred fashion, again requests information about the learner's perspectives and insights before allowing others to weigh in with their ideas on the interaction: How do you think that went? What are your feelings about the interaction? Anything else you'd like us to look at now regarding the interaction?

Spotting skills and engaging in a feedback discussion regarding selected skills is the next step. After the observers (and the patient, if present) respond to the learner's agenda, others may add in their agendas, as well, or point out things the learner may not have thought to ask about. By offering well-intentioned, descriptive feedback that is as concrete and specific as possible, the observers are essentially holding up a mirror to reflect what they saw or heard. The facilitator and all group members are responsible for ensuring that the feedback is well-intentioned and balanced between reinforcing what worked and discussing problem areas and next steps to make the interaction even better. Participants offer and, in selected cases, try out alternative approaches to specific parts of the interaction with the simulated patient or, when simulators are not present, with the facilitator playing the role of the patient or other. These "rewinds" are often more effective than just talking about alternative approaches or what you would do differently.

The outcome-based part of ALOBA comes into play when trying to determine what communication skills and approaches would be most effective. Instead of trying to evaluate what is good or bad or attempting to reach consensus about the "best" approach, ALOBA urges consideration of the outcomes the learner was trying to accomplish at a given moment in the interaction as well as the outcomes the patient (or their significant other) was trying to work on. The facilitator or a group member might ask: What were you trying to accomplish just then? And what was the patient needing or working on? So was what you were doing getting at both sets of outcomes? What else would be an effective way to get at those outcomes? With communication skills, effectiveness can only be determined in the context of the outcomes the various players in an interaction are after.

16.4.5 Two Essential Contexts for Teaching and Learning Clinical Communication

There are two essential contexts for clinical communication teaching and learning:

- The formal curriculum in which lectures, demonstrations, modules, workshops and rounds offer explicit focus on clinical communication teaching and learning
- The informal curriculum, including "in-the-moment" teaching that occurs in clinic, hospital and other "real world" contexts; intentional and unintentional modelling that surgeons and other clinicians do as they interact with patients, colleagues and others, including what surgeons and other clinicians choose to focus on and discuss with learners and each other during rounds and in clinic settings; and the "hidden" curriculum of how learners are treated and see their colleagues and mentors treating others.

Like the formal curriculum, modelling can have a profound effect on attitudes, values and beliefs as well as communication skills and capacities (e.g., compassion, integrity, respect etc.). This effect, of course, can be either positive or negative, depending on what we (choose to) do as well as the explicit commentary and questions we offer to focus attention on what we are doing. Optimal learning occurs when the formal curriculum consisting of experiential learning opportunities structured around a model that delineates evidence-based communication skills combines forces with the informal curriculum in which we engage during daily practice.

16.4.6 Ideas for Implementing Clinical Communication Teaching and Learning

Several examples drawn from both formal and informal curricula illustrate a variety of creative ways in which surgeons, other physicians and veterinarians, medical students, residents, clinical communication specialists and medical educators have implemented communication teaching and learning in practice and educational contexts.[6] Ideally these would be part of a coherent communication curriculum rather than stand-alone events. The intent here is for this sampling of ideas, grouped into four categories, to stimulate thinking and serve as a springboard as you consider how you might enhance or implement clinical communication teaching and learning in your own settings.

<u>Rounds</u>

- A senior surgeon explicitly and routinely discussed communication skills she or members of her rounding group were using or considering using with patients and significant others just as they discussed history taking, physical examination and other procedural skills, clinical reasoning, treatment options etc. The surgeon invited a communication specialist to participate in these rounds, especially when she first started to do them.
- A medical director scheduled periodic communication rounds in which surgical and other residents or their mentors presented and discussed recently encountered clinical communication problems and issues they had encountered with patients. These communication rounds followed the familiar format used in grand rounds or morbidity and mortality rounds, but appropriate medical/surgical specialists along with a health communication specialist and/or a psychologist were present to facilitate or add their perspective.
- A family medicine doctor initiated monthly "communication rounds" for cross-specialty training, including issues regarding communication between referring and referral clinicians.

---

6 The author had the privilege of observing first-hand or participating in the listed examples and gratefully acknowledges the numerous individuals who initiated or implemented these ideas over a period of many years in their practices and medical training programmes at: the Universities of Calgary, Edmonton, Dalhousie and Cambridge; the Canadian Orthopaedic Resident Forum; Washington State University's College of Veterinary Medicine.

- During surgical rounds a senior surgeon asked for two additional pieces of information after each learner's presentation of their patient – doing so demonstrated and reinforced the value of gathering information about and reporting the patient's perspective and made presentations more useful to the senior surgeon as s/he followed up on the patient's care:
  - *What questions will this patient want me to answer?*
  - *What concerns does this patient have that I need to address?*
- During patient care rounds, an endocrinologist focused attention on what he wanted junior doctors to emulate. He:
  - asked questions about communication just as he did about PE or medical problem solving or medical technical knowledge
  - reflected out loud on what he was doing regarding his communication with the patient
  - thought out loud and invited learners and sometimes the patient to think with him
  - talked about his own errors or mistakes regarding communication and how he handled them (usually this was done away from the bedside).

Clinic or bedside teaching

- A senior orthopaedic surgeon invited a communication specialist to observe him during several pre- and post-operative clinics where residents and medical students were in attendance, and immediately afterwards invited feedback and discussion on the communication skills he had used with patients and their families as well as those skills he had used while teaching the residents and students. Observation notes and feedback discussion were based on the C-C Guides. This approach opened the way for observation, feedback and discussion of clinical communication the residents or students used with patients and their families during subsequent clinics.
- During bedside teaching, an internal medicine staff doctor explicitly distinguished between teaching about problem-solving and patient care.
- Instead of just discussing alternative ways to talk with or respond to a patient, a senior doctor demonstrated alternative approaches in mini-simulations either away from or with the real patient; the senior doctor asked learners to do the same.
- As an extension of their own communication training, surgery residents and residents in other specialties intentionally modelled effective communication skills and relational competencies with medical students, and then asked questions and talked about what they were modelling.

Assessments

- The director of an anaesthesiology residency programme developed a version of the C-C Guides for pre-op interaction with patients and included it in the daily faculty evaluation protocol for residents – she saw positive changes in the communication of both faculty and residents as a result.
- Serving as a bridge between residency and full-fledged practice for the past 13 years, the Canadian Orthopaedic Resident Forum (CORF) is attended most years by over 95 per cent of fifth-year orthopaedic surgery residents in Canada. For most of the four-day forum, the residents engage in expert-facilitated small group learning sessions focused around the orthopaedic surgery sub-specialties. In each small group session, expert faculty present actual cases relevant to their sub-specialty and case-based simulated orals similar to those that have been encountered in Canadian orthopaedic surgery board examinations. Expert orthopaedic surgery faculty from across Canada joined together with communication specialists to facilitate feedback on the way individual residents handle cases and simulated orals – that feedback focuses not only on the surgical and medical issues that arise but also on residents' communication skills and capacities, on how residents present themselves and their comments, how they come across during each small group session. The communication specialists have also offered individual tutorials on request regarding any communication issue an individual resident wants to explore.
- A medical school postgraduate dean worked with a communication specialist to implement an Objective Structured Clinical Examination (OSCE) type assessment of communication skills that all incoming residents and students were required to take. Feedback on this assessment was provided to each individual. A similar assessment was repeated after several months, again with feedback. This assessment established baseline data and opened the way for clinical communication training and a focus on communication skills and issues in teaching hospital and clinic settings.

Workshops and other teaching contexts

- The director of an orthopaedic surgery residency programme invited a communication specialist (with whom he had often worked) and his residents to observe him for several pre- and post-operative clinics and during patient care rounds and then to do a "roast" focused on how they perceived his communication with his patients (including the good, the bad and the ugly, of course offered as constructively as possible). In subsequent clinics and rounds he discussed what he had learned from the "roast", both about his communication with patients and how to phrase feedback constructively. He used this experience to open the way for including constructive discussion about clinical communication as a routine part of surgical rounds and clinics (including what worked well and less well), how to engage in feedback effectively etc.

- A neurologist scheduled a series of noon communication sessions for residents to work through communication issues or difficulties they had experienced in the past week or anticipated experiencing in the near future with patients and their families or with mentors, colleagues or other co-workers; facilitators for these sessions included a faculty physician/surgeon, a communication specialist and an experienced simulated patient. To set up these sessions residents first participated in a one- to two-hour orientation to develop "rules of engagement" to ensure safety (e.g., confidentiality) and to introduce and discuss foundational communication concepts and principles, the C-C Guides, approaches for giving feedback on communication skills (ALOBA) etc. Initially residents were asked to submit brief (half-page) descriptions of the issues or difficult situations they wanted to work through – participants would then chose one or two of the submitted scenarios they most wanted to work on. Playing whatever role was called for, the SP helped to simulate the scenario based on the written description, with needed details added in-the-moment. The submitting resident could choose to participate in the simulation as him/herself and try out alternative ways to deal with the situation or ask someone else to take their place to see how they would handle the issue(s). After hearing self-reflection from the resident(s) who participated in the simulation, all other participants engaged in feedback and discussion, including during frequent timeouts and rewinds. After a few sessions residents began bringing very recent dilemmas to the group verbally as well as in written format.

- Residency programme administrators asked a surgeon and communication specialists to provide a 2.5-day session on clinical communication during the five-day orientation programme for incoming veterinary surgery and medicine residents in which the new house officers worked through a carefully selected variety of simulations based on real cases – these included acute and longitudinal cases complete with complications (where, for example, four months could be condensed into a two- to four-hour simulation), cases that involved issues regarding referring clinicians and other colleagues, telephone communication, interactions with students like those the residents would soon be teaching, etc. Well-trained simulators portrayed clients/colleagues/students/staff with whom the residents would soon be working.

- This orientation was followed by a semester-long elective on communication skills and professional development where the communication and teaching skills introduced during the orientation programme were pursued and where residents routinely discussed communication dilemmas they encountered and solutions to those dilemmas as well as communication successes.

- A residency director invited a representative from an agency that insured physicians and surgeons and a communication specialist to join forces for a weekend workshop with ob/gyn residents, including surgical specialists. The workshop reviewed data on complaints and litigation involving communication issues (comprising approximately 80 per cent of all such complaints, with about half of those involving a communication issue along with a medical technical error or adverse event and half involving only communication issues), described a variety of such cases, and engaged participants in exercises to enhance their understanding and effective application of relevant clinical communication skills.
- A large surgical practice invited their referring doctors to join them for a workshop facilitated by a communication specialist that focused on each group's perception of what communication practices worked and what posed challenges or issues regarding interaction between referring and referral clinicians.
- A senior surgeon organized a session on dealing with errors and adverse outcomes for the surgical faculty and residents that was facilitated by a lawyer who represented physicians and surgeons when complaints were brought, senior hospital administrators, a communication specialist and senior faculty. It included two well-written case scenarios that the participants role-played (complete with time-outs and rewinds) involving patients and their significant others, surgeons and other physicians, nurses and other relevant staff.
- A hospital administrator organized a panel and discussion in which hospital surgeons, physicians and nurses came together to work on resolving coordination of care and other communication issues they were experiencing.
- During a lecture, a nephrologist who was also Associate Dean of Medical Education invited junior doctors to conduct a review of a recent video recording he had made with one of his patients and requested that participants focus on his communication skills with the patient.
- A general practice doctor joined forces with a surgical oncologist and a simulated patient to organize and facilitate lunchtime "improv" simulations based on residents' current communication dilemmas.

16.5 Conclusion

The goal of this chapter has been to enhance communication in surgical contexts by raising the bar on communication education for surgeons. To that end, the chapter has offered a conceptual framework for systematically developing coherent, evidence-based clinical communication programmes as well as a variety of strategies for teaching and learning clinical communication effectively in surgery and the wider healthcare context. Taken together, the scaffolding in the conceptual framework and the specific strategies suggested for teaching clinical communication to surgeons and other healthcare professionals, and for learning, provide responses to three essential questions:

(1) Should we teach clinical communication to surgeons and surgical residents?
(2) If so, what should we teach them regarding clinical communication in surgical contexts?
(3) What strategies and approaches to teaching and learning have proven to be successful?

The rest of this book has provided numerous complementary ideas and strategies for enhancing surgeons' communication. Certainly no one individual will put all of these ideas into practice. But consider what might happen to communication in surgical practice if each reader of this book chose to implement consistently over time just a few of the ideas we have presented in these pages!

References

Aspegren, Knut. 1999. BEME Guide No. 2: Teaching and Learning Communication Skills in Medicine – A Review with Quality Grading of Articles. *Medical Teacher* 21(6): 563–70.

Barbour, Alton. 2000. Making Contact or Making Sense: Functional and Dysfunctional Ways of Relating. Humanities Institute Lecture 1999–2000 Series, Denver, CO.

Beach, Mary Catherine, Debra L. Roter, Nae-Yuh Wang, Patrick S. Duggan and Lisa Cooper. 2006. Are Physicians' Attitudes of Respect Accurately Perceived by Patients and Associated with More Positive Communication Behaviors? *Patient Education and Counseling* 62(3): 347–54. doi: 10.1016/j.pec.2006.06.004

Beckman, Howard B., and Richard M. Frankel. 1984. The Effect of Physician Behavior on the Collection of Data. *Annals of Internal Medicine* 101(5): 692–6.

Campion, Peter, John Foulkes, Roger Neighbour and Peter Tate. 2002. Patient Centredness in the MRCGP Video Examination: Analysis of Large Cohort. *BMJ: British Medical Journal* 325(7366): 691–2.

Cary, Julie, and Suzanne Kurtz. 2013. Integrating Clinical Communication with Clinical Reasoning and the Broader Medical Curriculum. *Patient Education and Counseling* 92(3): 361–5. doi: 10.1016/j.pec.2013.07.007

Dance, Frank E.X. 1967. Toward a Theory of Human Communication. In *Human Communication Theory: Original Essays*, edited by Frank E.X. Dance. New York: Holt, Rinehart and Winston.

Dance, Frank E.X., and Carl E. Larson. 1972. *Speech Communication: Concepts and Behaviour*. New York: Holt, Rinehart and Winston.

Gittell, Jody Hoffer. 2003. *The Southwest Airlines Way: Using the Power of Relationships to Achieve High Performance*. New York: McGraw-Hill.

Gittell, Jody Hoffer. 2011. New Directions for Relational Coordination Theory. In *The Oxford Handbook of Positive Organizational Scholarship*, edited by Kim S. Cameron and Gretchen M. Spreitzer. Oxford: Oxford University Press.

Gittell, Jody Hoffer, Kathleen M. Fairfield, Benjamin Bierbaum, William Head, Robert Jackson, Michael Kelly, Richard Laskin, Stephen Lipson, John Siliski, Thomas Thornhill and Joseph Zuckerman. 2000. Impact of Relational Coordination on Quality of Care, Postoperative Pain and Functioning, and Length of Stay: A Nine-Hospital Study of Surgical Patients. *Medical Care* 38(8): 807–19.

Kurtz, Suzanne M. 1989. Curriculum Structuring to Enhance Communication Skills Development. In *Communicating with Medical Patients*, edited by Moira Stewart and Debra Roter. Newbury Park: Sage.

Kurtz, Suzanne and Lara Cooke. 2011. Learner-Centered Communication Training. In *Handbook of Communication in Oncology and Palliative Care*, edited by David W. Kissane, Barry Bultz, Phyllis Butow and Ilora G. Finlay, 583–96. Oxford: Oxford University Press.

Kurtz, Suzanne, Jonathan Silverman, John Benson and Juliet Draper. 2003. Marrying Content and Process in Clinical Method Teaching: Enhancing the Calgary-Cambridge Guides. *Academic Medicine* 78(8): 802–9. doi: 10.1097/00001888-200308000-00011

Kurtz, Suzanne, Jonathan Silverman and Juliet Draper. 1998. *Teaching and Learning Communication Skills*. Oxford and San Francisco: Radcliffe Medical Press.

Kurtz, Suzanne, Jonathan Silverman and Juliet Draper. 2005. *Teaching and Learning Communication Skills*. 2nd ed. Oxford and San Francisco: Radcliffe Medical Press.

Langewitz, Wolf, Martin Denz, Anne Keller, Alexander Kiss, Sigmund Rüttimann and Brigitta Wössmer. 2002. Spontaneous Talking Time at Start of Consultation in Outpatient Clinic: Cohort Study. *BMJ: British Medical Journal* 325(7366): 682–3.

Lussier, Marie-Thérèse, and Claude Richard. 2008. Because One Shoe Doesn't Fit All: A Repertoire of Doctor-Patient Relationships. *Canadian Family Physician (Médecin de famille canadien)* 54(8): 1089.

Maguire, Peter, Susan Fairbairn and Charles Fletcher. 1986a. Consultation Skills of Young Doctors – I: Benefits of Feedback Training in Interviewing as Students Persist. *British Medical Journal (Clinical Research Edition)* 292(6535): 1573–6.

Maguire, Peter, Susan Fairbairn and Charles Fletcher. 1986b. Consultation Skills of Young Doctors – II: Most Young Doctors Are Bad at Giving Information. *British Medical Journal (Clinical Research Edition)* 292(6535): 1576–8.

Makoul, Gregory, Paul Arntson and Theo Schofield. 1995. Health Promotion in Primary Care: Physician-Patient Communication and Decision Making about Prescription Medications. *Social Science & Medicine* 41(9): 1241–54. doi: 10.1016/0277-9536(95)00061-b

Marvel, M. Kim, Ronald M. Epstein, Kristine Flowers and Howard B. Beckman. 1999. Soliciting the Patient's Agenda: Have We Improved? *JAMA* 281(3): 283–7.

Morse, Diane S., Elizabeth A. Edwardsen and Howard S. Gordon. 2008. Missed Opportunities for Interval Empathy in Lung Cancer Communication. *Archives of Internal Medicine* 168(17): 1853–8.

Rhoades, Donna R., Kay F. McFarland, W. Holmes Finch and Andrew O. Johnson. 2001. Speaking and Interruptions during Primary Care Office Visits. *Family Medicine* 33(7): 528.

Riccardi, Vincent M., and Suzanne M. Kurtz. 1983. *Communication and Counseling in Health Care*. Springfield, Ill.: Charles C. Thomas Publisher.

Rider, Elizabeth A., Suzanne Kurtz, Diana Slade, H. Esterbrook Longmaid III, Ming-Jung Ho, Jack Kwok-hung Pun, Suzanne Eggins and William T. Branch. 2014. The

International Charter for Human Values in Healthcare: An Interprofessional Global Collaboration to Enhance Values and Communication in Healthcare. *Patient Education and Counseling* 96: 273–80.

Silverman, Jonathan, Suzanne M. Kurtz and Juliet Draper. 1998. *Skills for Communicating with Patients*. Oxford: Radcliffe Publishing.

Silverman, Jonathan, Suzanne M. Kurtz and Juliet Draper. 2005. *Skills for Communicating with Patients*. 2nd ed. Oxford: Radcliffe Publishing.

Silverman, Jonathan, Suzanne M. Kurtz and Juliet Draper. 2013. *Skills for Communicating with Patients*. 3rd ed. Oxford: Radcliffe Publishing.

Stewart, Moira. 1985. Comparison of Two Methods of Analysing Doctor Patient Communication. North American Primary Care Research Group Conference, Seattle, April 14–17.

Stewart, Moira, Judith B. Brown, Heather Boon, Joanne Galajda, Leslie Meredith and M. Sangstar. 1999. Evidence on Patient-Doctor Communication. *Cancer Prevention Control* 3(1): 25–30.

Stewart, Moira, Judith Belle Brown, W. Wayne Weston, Ian R. McWhinney, Carol L. McWilliam and Thomas R. Freeman. 2003. *Patient-Centered Medicine: Transforming the Clinical Method*. 2nd ed. Oxford: Radcliffe Medical Press.

Stewart, Moira, Judith Belle Brown, W. Wayne Weston, Ian R. McWhinney, Carol L. McWilliam and Thomas R. Freeman. 2013. *Patient-Centered Medicine: Transforming the Clinical Method*. 3rd ed. London and New York: Radcliffe Medical Press.

Suchman, Anthony L., Edward Deci, Susan McDaniel and Howard B. Beckman. 2002. Relationship Centred Administration. In *The Biopsychosocial Approach: Past, Present, Future*, edited by Richard Frankel, Timothy Quill and Susan McDaniel. Rochester NY: Univerity of Rochester Press.

Suchman, Anthony L., David J. Sluyter and Penelope R. Williamson. 2011. *Leading Change in Healthcare: Transforming Organizations Using Complexity, Positive Psychology and Relationship-Centered Care*. Oxford: Radcliffe Publishing.

Tresolini, Carol P., and Pew-Fetzer Task Force. 1994. *Health Professions Education and Relationship-Centered Care*. San Francisco: Pew Health Professions Commission.

Waitzkin, Howard. 1985. Information Giving in Medical Care. *Journal of Health and Social Behavior* 26: 81–101.

Suzanne M. Kurtz, PhD, has been Clinical Professor and founding Director of the Clinical Communication Program, College of Veterinary Medicine, Washington State University, Pullman, since 2006, and is Professor Emeritus, University of Calgary. Prior to this she was joint-appointed to the Faculties of Education and Medicine (1976–2005), where she directed Calgary's medical communication programme and co-developed the Calgary-Cambridge Guides and approach to teaching clinical communication. Having served as advisor to numerous healthcare organizations, she consults internationally at all levels of medical and veterinary education and across the specialties in both professions regarding effective communication in healthcare. A founding member of the International Research Centre for Communication in Healthcare, she serves on its Management Council.

Index

CPSIA information can be obtained
at www.ICGtesting.com
Printed in the USA
BVHW042344030319
541507BV00008B/67/P

9 781781 790502